AF768893

EVA

the

DEAN VAUGHN
LEARNING SYSTEM

applied to

BASIC HUMAN ANATOMY

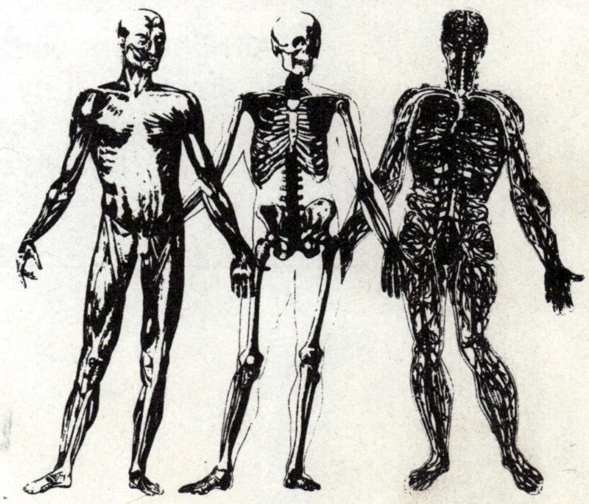

LEARNING GUIDE

DCM/INSTRUCTIONAL SYSTEMS

WESTWOOD, MASS. 02090

ISBN 0-914901-09-5

TABLE OF CONTENTS

SKELETAL SYSTEM SUPPLEMENT

INTRODUCTION

THE DEAN VAUGHN LEARNING SYSTEM

This unique learning system was developed by Dean Vaughn, whose applied memory techniques are used in thousands of academic and business institutions with unprecedented success. His revolutionary learning systems have been acclaimed by many educators as the most significant breakthrough in the history of formal education.

As a student of BASIC HUMAN ANATOMY, you are fortunate to have the opportunity to use these organized, effective memory techniques to learn and remember the subject. This is the only course ever developed that teaches **how to learn** and **how to remember** BASIC HUMAN ANATOMY.

Millions of others have had to learn anatomy without the benefit of a memory system. The inefficient conventional method of learning by repetition discourages, rather than encourages, the learning process. Through the use of these effective memory techniques you will learn incredibly faster and you will be able to remember what you learn — with ease and self confidence.

DESIRE

The most important factor in assuring your success in this course is **your desire to learn**! If you do not want to learn, this program will be no more effective than any other method of learning. If you do **want** to learn BASIC HUMAN ANATOMY, there is no known method that can approach the effectiveness of this proven memory system.

PURPOSE OF COURSE

The purpose of this course is to teach you BASIC HUMAN ANATOMY. You will learn the names and locations of the principal parts of the body systems, including the structure of the eye and the ear (sensory organs).

IMPORTANCE OF AUDIO-VISUAL PRESENTATION

All of the lessons include an audio-visual presentation. The importance of this audio-visual instruction cannot be overemphasized. Please **do not** take any notes during the audio-visual presentation. Instead, concentrate completely on the memory techniques. Since the memory system is based on words (objects) that sound like the body part to be remembered, it is absolutely necessary that you **pronounce aloud** all the words the narrator asks you to pronounce. It is also imperative that you **visualize** the words as you pronounce them.

IMPORTANCE OF LEARNING GUIDE

This is a multipurpose workbook, carefully designed to serve numerous functions as follows:

PRE-TEST: The pre-test is designed, not just to determine how much you know about anatomy before you begin the course, but, rather, as an honest measuring device for you to compare how much you learn with how much you knew before the course began. That is why the pre-test and final test are identical in content.

REVIEW: This section appears after each lesson. It is a review of what you should know upon completion of the lesson. You should spend sufficient time reviewing this section to satisfy yourself that you honestly know everything being reviewed. This will enable you to complete the worksheet section with ease and with accuracy.

WORKSHEET: This section is identical in content to the review section. You will have no difficulty completing this section if you have properly completed the review section. If you can complete all of the worksheet sections of the workbook, you will have no difficulty completing the final test with ease and self-confidence.

FINAL TEST: The final test has no surprises. It is identical in content to all of the worksheets combined. If you complete the review and worksheets after each lesson, you will have no difficulty scoring 100% on the final test!

After completing the course use your Learning Guide as a valuable reference and for occasional review to confirm your retention of BASIC HUMAN ANATOMY.

<u>100% AWARD</u>

This award is earned by every individual who achieves 100% on the final test. It is truly an award for excellence and demonstrates an individual's desire to achieve. It is an award which is displayed with great pride.

HOW TO ACHIEVE 100% ON YOUR FINAL EXAM

1. **Concentrate** and carefully **observe** the audio-visual presentation of each lesson.
2. **Pronounce** aloud and **visualize** the anatomical terms, names and audionyms along with the narrator when he asks you to do so.
3. **Review** each lesson in your workbook before completing the worksheet for that lesson so that you know the audionym and its location or meaning..
4. **Complete** the worksheet section of each lesson before continuing to the next lesson.
5. After completion of the last lesson, review the questions and illustrations of the final test. Make certain that you know the meaning or name and location of every term or body part indicated.

Suggestion: Have a fellow student test you on your knowledge of all the lessons before taking your final test.

The use of the Dean Vaughn Learning System is only a means to an end. Soon it will be unnecessary for you to use the audionym or the illogical association. Instead, you will immediately **KNOW** the actual meaning.

It is most important that you always use the audionym and the illogical association until the actual meaning is permanent in your mind. Do not try to rush the process. The actual meaning will soon come to mind naturally, but only if you first use the system.

PRE TEST

______________ ____

Date Name

POSSIBLE SCORE: 500

NUMBER CORRECT: ______

PERCENT CORRECT: ______%

IMPORTANT:

Please do not feel uncomfortable with the results of your pre test. You are not expected to know all of the answers before the course begins. The pre test is used only to establish a basis for measuring your accomplishment upon completion of the program.

PRE TEST
COMPLETE THE BLANKS

ANATOMICAL TERMS AND LOCATIONS

WORD	MEANING
CRANIAL	Skull
CEPHAL	Head
CAUDAL	Tail
SUPERIOR	above
INFERIOR	below
x EPI	upon
HYPO	under
PROXIMAL	nearest
DISTAL	Far
VENTRAL	Front
ANTERIOR	Front
DORSAL	back
POSTERIOR	back
LATERAL	Side
GASTR	Stomache
RENAL	Kidney
CHONDR	Cartlidge
PULMONARY	Lung
x VISCERA	Ventral Organs

PRE TEST
PRINT THE CORRECT LETTER WITHIN THE PARENTHESES

ANATOMICAL TERMS AND LOCATIONS

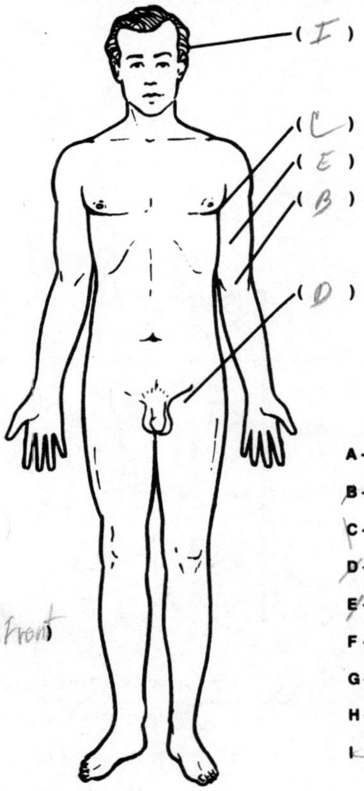

A - POPLITEAL
B - CUBITAL
C - AXILLARY
D - INGUINAL
E - BRACHIAL
F - POSTERIOR
G - ANTERIOR
H - LATERAL
I - CEPHAL

VIEW (front)

ANATOMICAL TERMS AND LOCATIONS

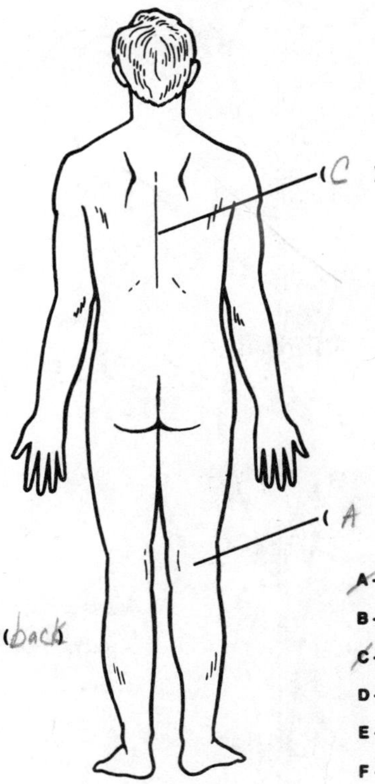

A - POPLITEAL
B - CUBITAL
C - DORSAL
D - VENTRAL
E - POSTERIOR
F - ANTERIOR

VIEW (back)

ANATOMICAL POSITION

1. (E)
2. (H)
3. (B)
4. (G)

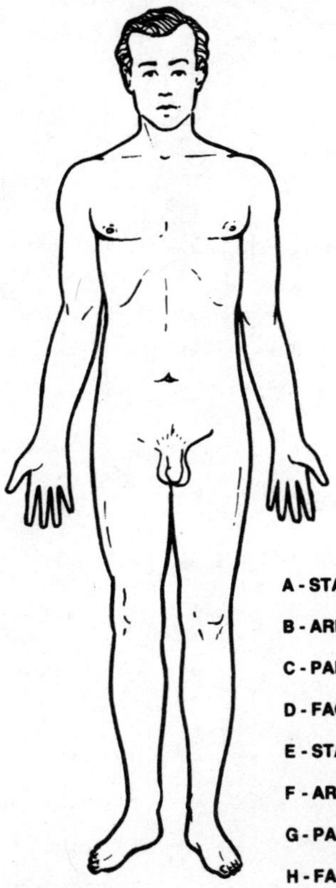

A - STANDING OBLIQUE
B - ARMS HANGING AT SIDES
C - PALMS AT SIDES
D - FACING LATERALLY
E - STANDING ERECT
F - ARMS AT REST
G - PALMS FORWARD
H - FACING FORWARD

BODY PLANES

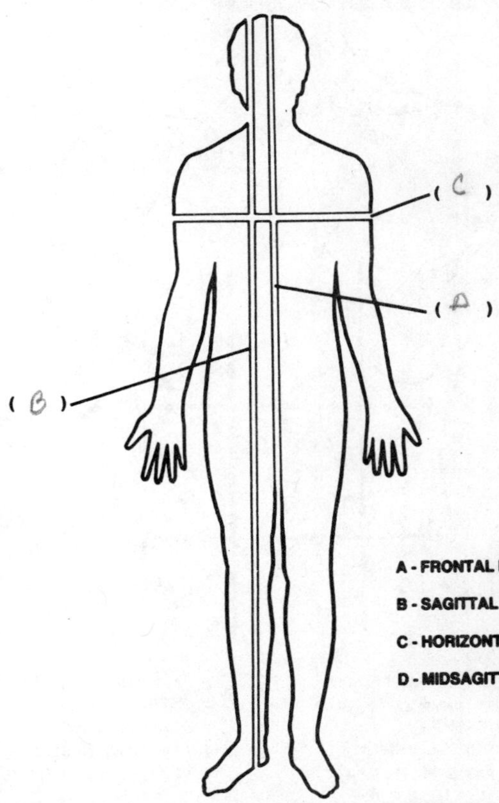

A - FRONTAL PLANE
B - SAGITTAL PLANE
C - HORIZONTAL PLANE
D - MIDSAGITTAL PLANE

PRE TEST
PRINT THE CORRECT LETTER WITHIN THE PARENTHESES

BODY PLANES

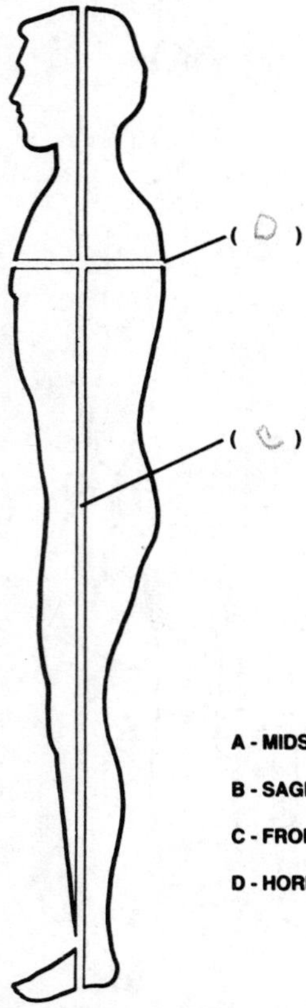

A - MIDSAGITTAL PLANE
B - SAGITTAL PLANE
C - FRONTAL PLANE
D - HORIZONTAL PLANE

ABDOMINOPELVIC QUADRANTS

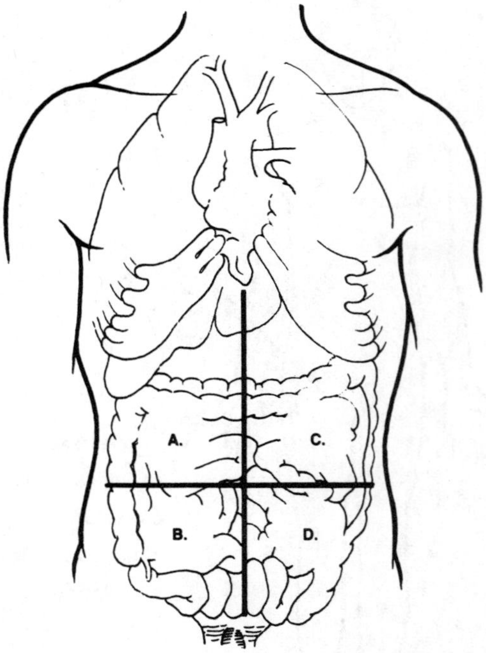

(B) RIGHT LOWER QUADRANT
(C) LEFT UPPER QUADRANT
(A) RIGHT UPPER QUADRANT
(D) LEFT LOWER QUADRANT

REGIONAL SUBDIVISIONS OF THE ABDOMINOPELVIC CAVITY

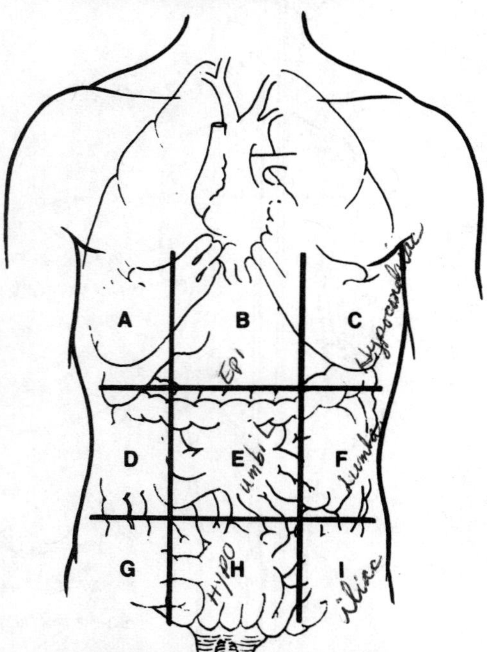

(F) LEFT LUMBAR REGION
(A) RIGHT HYPOCHONDRIAC REGION
(E) UMBILICAL REGION
(B) EPIGASTRIC REGION
(I) LEFT ILIAC REGION
(C) LEFT HYPOCHONDRIAC REGION
(G) RIGHT ILIAC REGION
(H) HYPOGASTRIC REGION
(D) RIGHT LUMBAR REGION

BODY CAVITIES

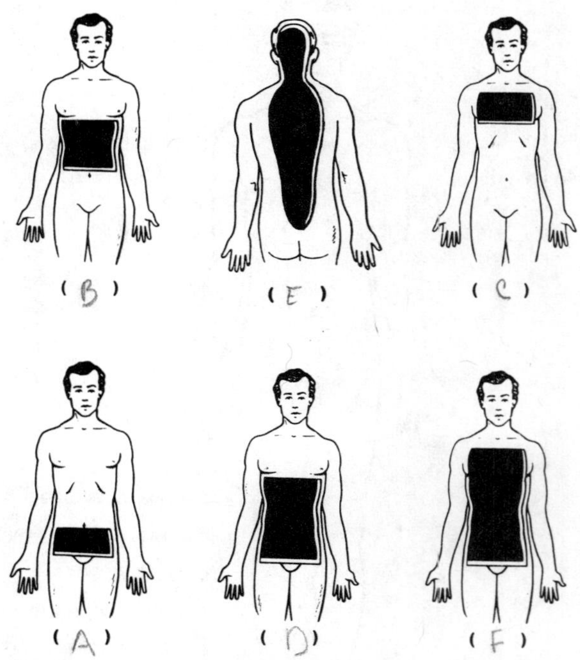

A - PELVIC CAVITY
B - ABDOMINAL CAVITY
C - THORACIC CAVITY
D - ABDOMINOPELVIC CAVITY
E - DORSAL CAVITY
F - VENTRAL CAVITY

PRE TEST
PRINT THE CORRECT LETTER WITHIN THE PARENTHESES

Skull

BONES OF THE CRANIUM

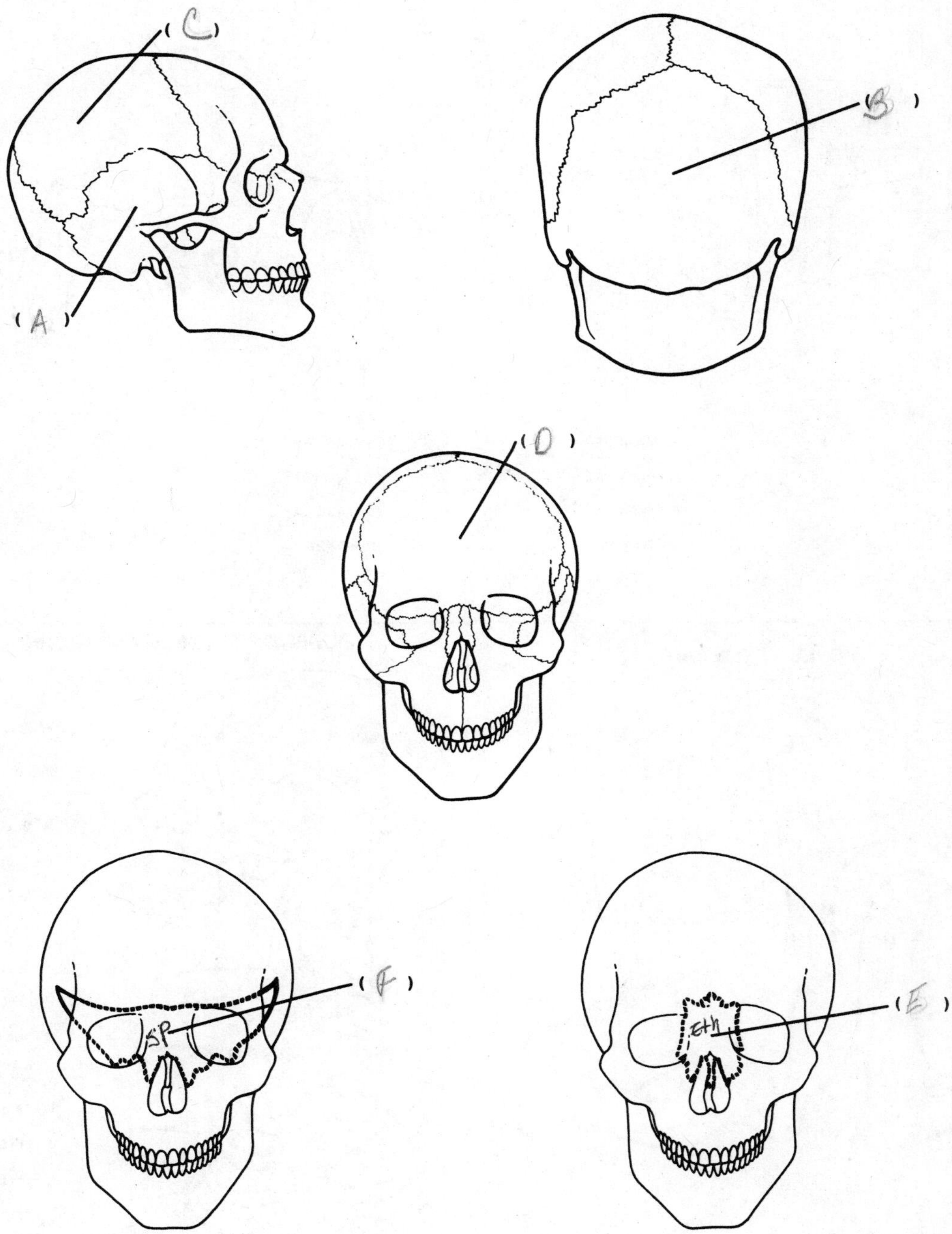

A - TEMPORAL
B - OCCIPITAL

C - PARIETAL
D - FRONTAL

E - ETHMOID
F - SPHENOID

PRE TEST
PRINT THE CORRECT LETTER WITHIN THE PARENTHESES

BONES OF THE FACE

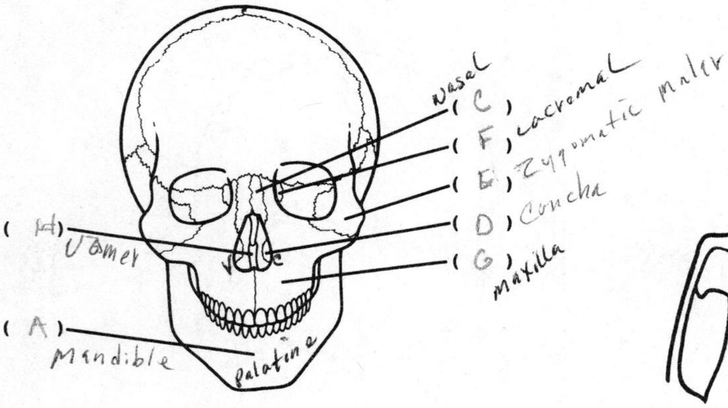

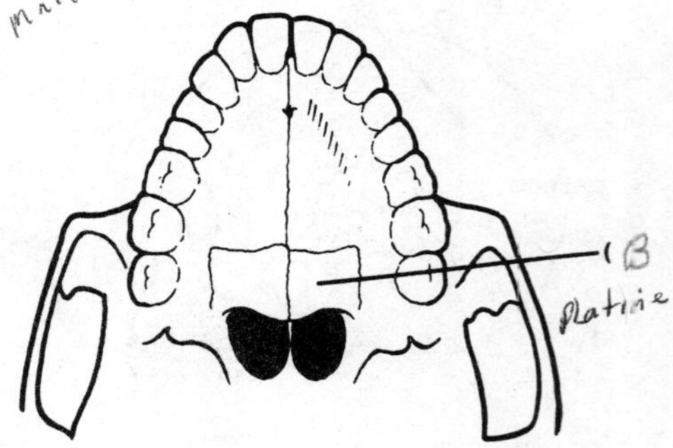

A - MANDIBLE
B - PALATINE
C - NASAL
D - CONCHA
E - ZYGOMATIC/MALAR
F - LACRIMAL
G - MAXILLA
H - VOMER

BONES OF THE EAR

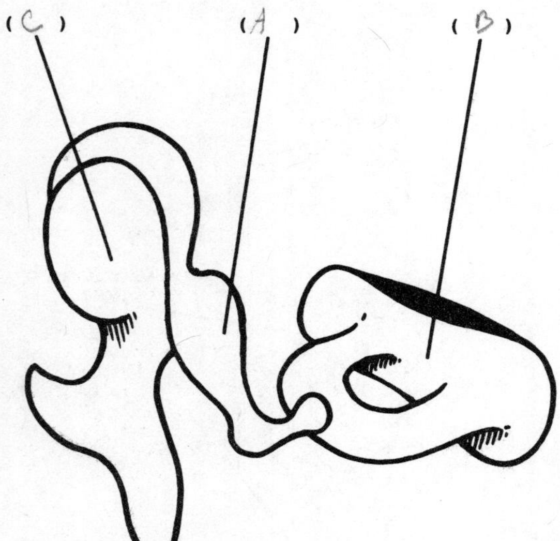

A - INCUS (ANVIL)
B - STAPES (STIRRUP)
C - MALLEUS (HAMMER)

BONES OF THE NECK AND TRUNK

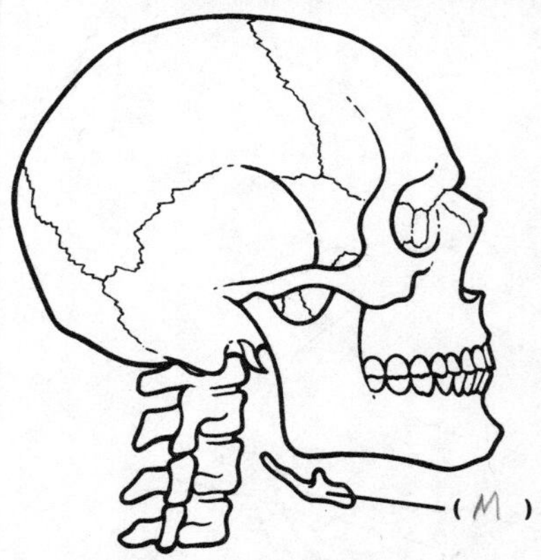

RIGHT LATERAL (SIDE) VIEW

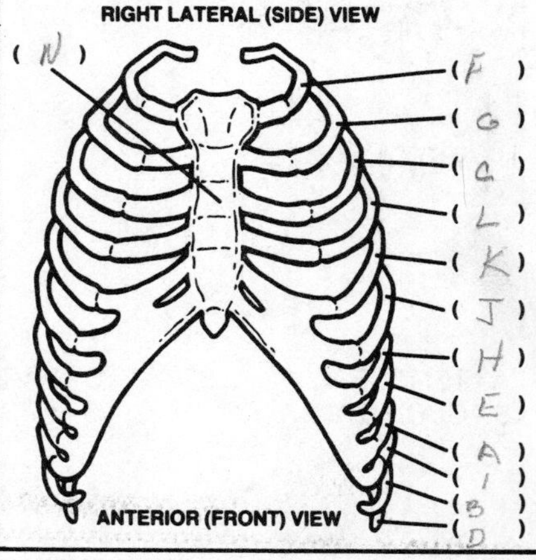

ANTERIOR (FRONT) VIEW

A - 9th LEFT RIB
B - 11th LEFT RIB
C - 3rd LEFT RIB
D - 12th LEFT RIB
E - 8th LEFT RIB
F - 1st LEFT RIB
G - 2nd LEFT RIB
H - 7th LEFT RIB
I - 10th LEFT RIB
J - 6th LEFT RIB
K - 5th LEFT RIB
L - 4th LEFT RIB
M - HYOID
N - STERNUM

PRE TEST

PRINT THE CORRECT LETTER WITHIN THE PARENTHESES

BONES OF THE TRUNK (THE SPINAL VERTEBRAE)

(D)— COCCYX
(C)— CERVICAL VERTEBRAE
(B)— SACRUM
(E)— LUMBAR VERTEBRAE
(A)— THORACIC VERTEBRAE

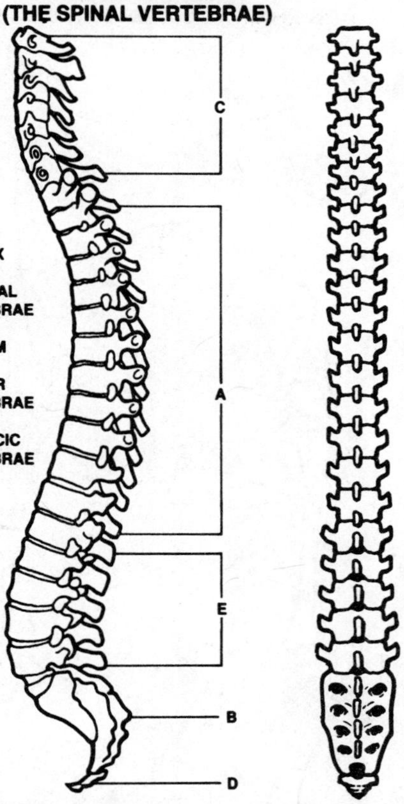

LATERAL (SIDE) VIEW | POSTERIOR (BACK) VIEW

BONES OF THE UPPER AND LOWER EXTREMITIES

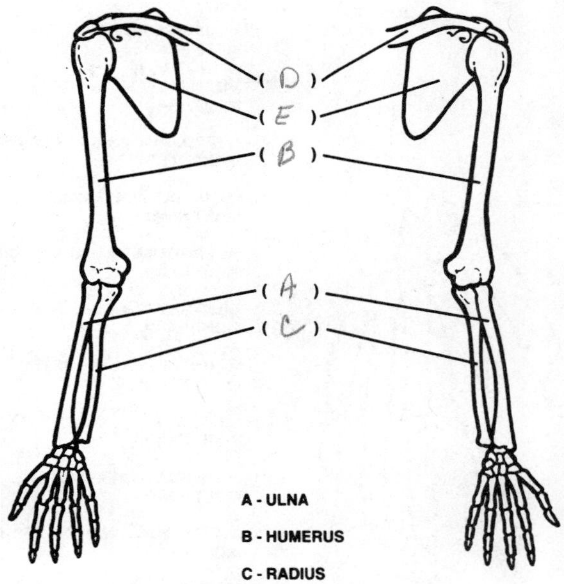

A - ULNA
B - HUMERUS
C - RADIUS
D - CLAVICLE
E - SCAPULA

ANTERIOR (FRONT) VIEW

BONES OF THE WRIST, HAND AND FINGERS

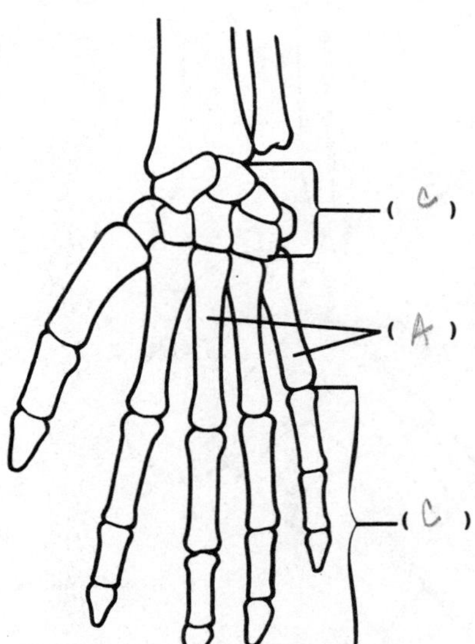

RIGHT HAND

A - METACARPALS
B - PHALANGES
C - CARPALS

BONES OF THE WRIST, HAND AND FINGERS

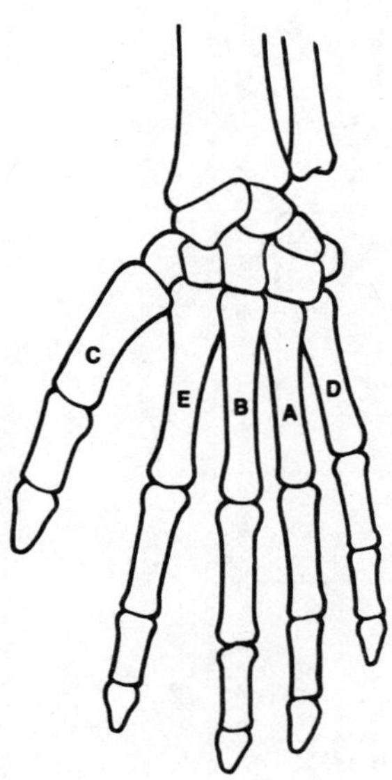

(A) - 4th METACARPAL OF THE RIGHT HAND
(B) - 3rd METACARPAL OF THE RIGHT HAND
(C) - 1st METACARPAL OF THE RIGHT HAND
(D) - 5th METACARPAL OF THE RIGHT HAND
(E) - 2nd METACARPAL OF THE RIGHT HAND

RIGHT HAND

PRE TEST
PRINT THE CORRECT LETTER WITHIN THE PARENTHESES

BONES OF THE WRIST, HAND AND FINGERS

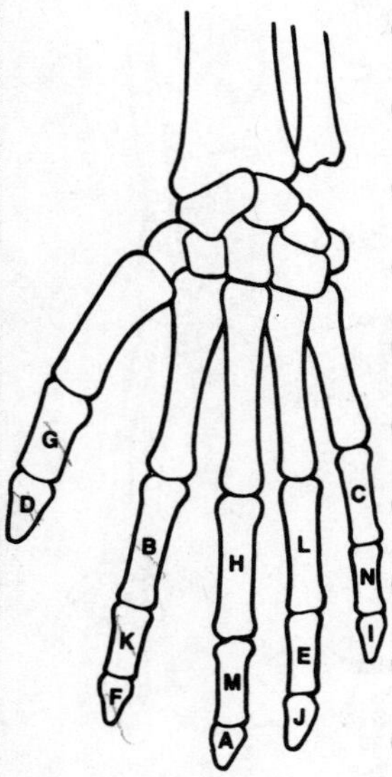

RIGHT HAND

(F) - 2nd DISTAL PHALANX OF THE RIGHT HAND
(A) - 3rd DISTAL PHALANX OF THE RIGHT HAND
(G) - 1st PROXIMAL PHALANX OF THE RIGHT HAND
(K) - 2nd MIDDLE PHALANX OF THE RIGHT HAND
(I) - 5th PROXIMAL PHALANX OF THE RIGHT HAND
(E) - 4th MIDDLE PHALANX OF THE RIGHT HAND
(C) - 5th DISTAL PHALANX OF THE RIGHT HAND
(D) - 1st DISTAL PHALANX OF THE RIGHT HAND
(M) - 3rd MIDDLE PHALANX OF THE RIGHT HAND
(B) - 2nd PROXIMAL PHALANX OF THE RIGHT HAND
(N) - 5th MIDDLE PHALANX OF THE RIGHT HAND
(H) - 3rd PROXIMAL PHALANX OF THE RIGHT HAND
(J) - 4th DISTAL PHALANX OF THE RIGHT HAND
(L) - 4th PROXIMAL PHALANX OF THE RIGHT HAND

BONES OF THE LOWER EXTREMITIES

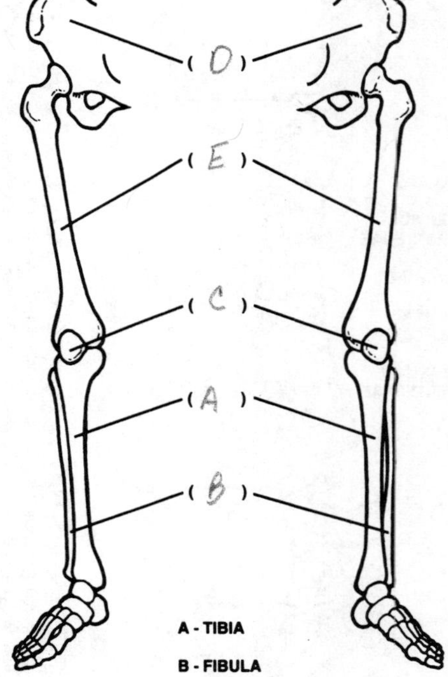

A - TIBIA
B - FIBULA
C - PATELLA
D - HIP
E - FEMUR

BONES OF THE ANKLE, FOOT AND TOES

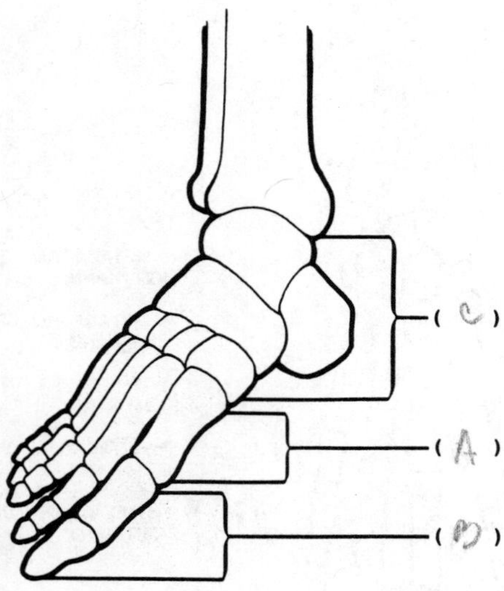

A - METATARSALS
B - PHALANGES
C - TARSALS

BONES OF THE ANKLE, FOOT AND TOES

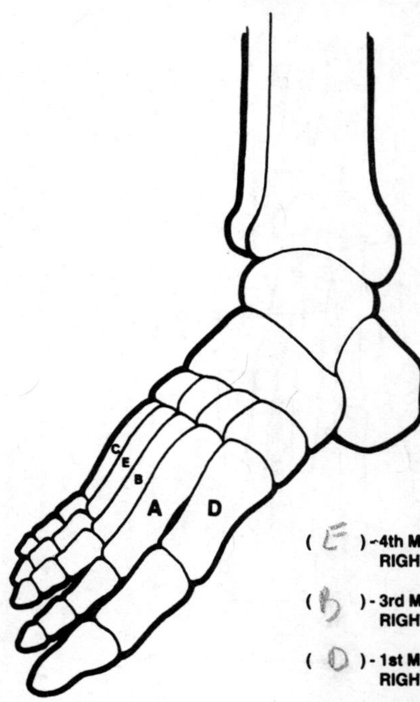

RIGHT FOOT

(E) - 4th METATARSAL OF THE RIGHT FOOT
(B) - 3rd METATARSAL OF THE RIGHT FOOT
(D) - 1st METATARSAL OF THE RIGHT FOOT
(C) - 5th METATARSAL OF THE RIGHT FOOT
(A) - 2nd METATARSAL OF THE RIGHT FOOT

PRE TEST
PRINT THE CORRECT LETTER WITHIN THE PARENTHESES

BONES OF THE ANKLE, FOOT AND TOES

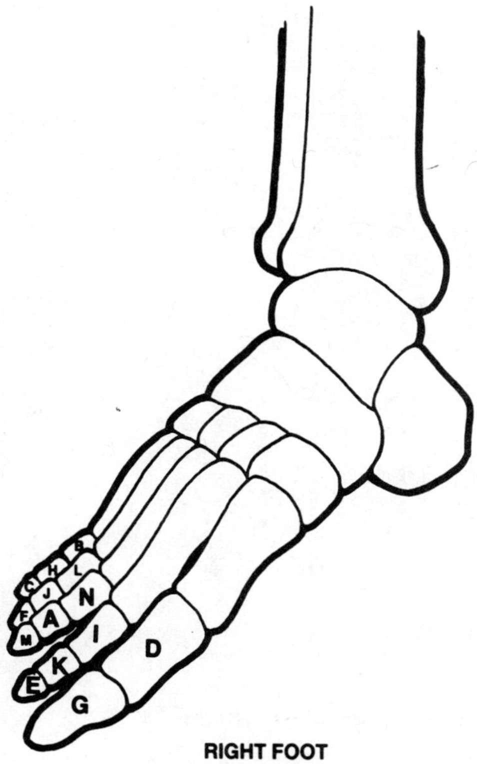

RIGHT FOOT

(K) - 2nd MIDDLE PHALANX OF THE RIGHT FOOT

(G) - 1st DISTAL PHALANX OF THE RIGHT FOOT

(A) - 3rd MIDDLE PHALANX OF THE RIGHT FOOT

(C) - 5th DISTAL PHALANX OF THE RIGHT FOOT

(J) - 4th MIDDLE PHALANX OF THE RIGHT FOOT

(D) - 1ST PROXIMAL PHALANX OF THE RIGHT FOOT

(E) - 2nd DISTAL PHALANX OF THE RIGHT FOOT

(I) - 2nd PROXIMAL PHALANX OF THE RIGHT FOOT

(N) - 3rd PROXIMAL PHALANX OF THE RIGHT FOOT

(H) - 5th MIDDLE PHALANX OF THE RIGHT FOOT

(M) - 3rd DISTAL PHALANX OF THE RIGHT FOOT

(L) - 4th PROXIMAL PHALANX OF THE RIGHT FOOT

(F) - 4th DISTAL PHALANX OF THE RIGHT FOOT

(B) - 5th PROXIMAL PHALANX OF THE RIGHT FOOT

MUSCLES NAMED BY LOCATION

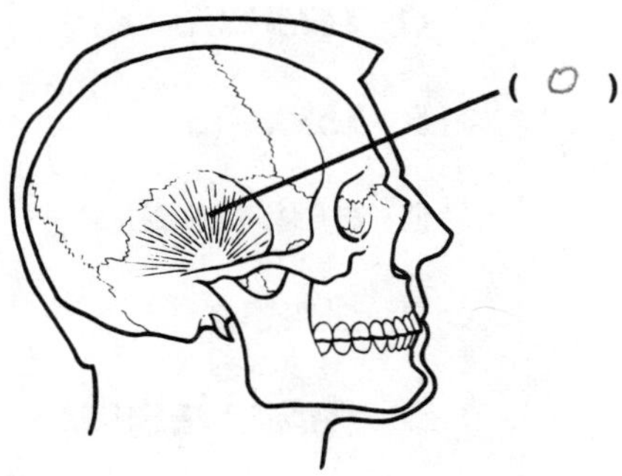

MUSCLES NAMED BY SIZE

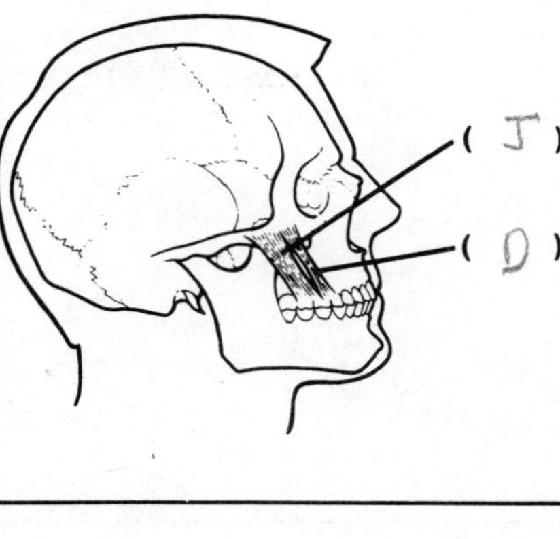

A - OBLIQUE MUSCLE
B - ROTATOR
C - EXTENSOR
D - ZYGOMATICUS MINOR
E - LEVATOR
F - DORSIFLEXOR
G - RECTUS MUSCLE
H - DEPRESSOR
I - ADDUCTOR
J - ZYGOMATICUS MAJOR
K - FLEXOR
L - SPHINCTER
M - TENSOR
N - EVERTOR
O - TEMPORALIS
P - INVERTOR
Q - PLANTAR FLEXOR
R - PRONATOR
S - SUPINATOR
T - ABDUCTOR
U - TRANSVERSE MUSCLE

MUSCLES NAMED BY DIRECTION

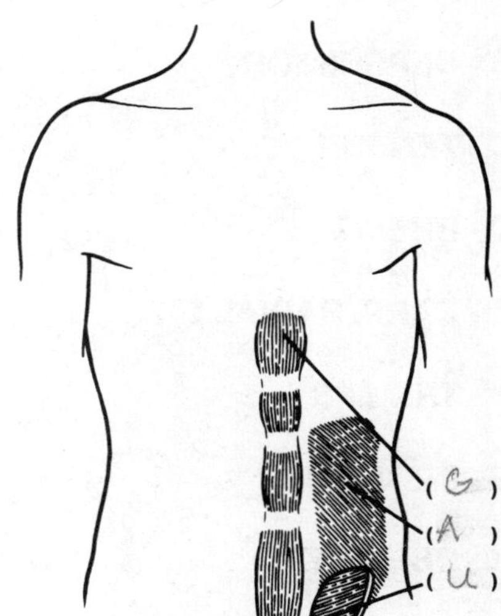

PRE TEST

PRINT THE CORRECT LETTER WITHIN THE PARENTHESES

MUSCLES NAMED BY NUMBER (OF ORIGINS)

From the list below, select **three** types of muscles named by their number of origins.

(BI=2) (TRI=3) (Quad=4)

MUSCLES NAMED BY SHAPE

From the list below, select **one** muscle named by its shape

( ) Trapezius, (Trapezoid)

MUSCLES NAMED BY ORIGIN AND INSERTION

From the list below, select **two** muscles named by their origin and insertion.

(S) (M)

A - OCCIPITALIS
B - DEPRESSOR
C - TENSOR
D - BREVIS
E - CARPI RADIALIS
F - TRICEPS
G - PRONATOR
H - OBLIQUE

I - ABDUCTOR
J - EVERTOR
K - LONGUS
L - RECTUS
M - TRAPEZIUS
N - INVERTOR
O - LEVATOR
P - TIBIALIS

Q - TEMPORALIS
R - MINIMUS
S - CARPI ULNARIS
T - BICEPS
U - TRANSVERSUS
V - MAXIMUS
W - ZYGOMATICUS
X - QUADRICEPS

PRE TEST
PRINT THE CORRECT LETTER WITHIN THE PARENTHESES

MUSCLES NAMED BY ACTION
(SKELETON USE TO ILLUSTRATE ACTION)

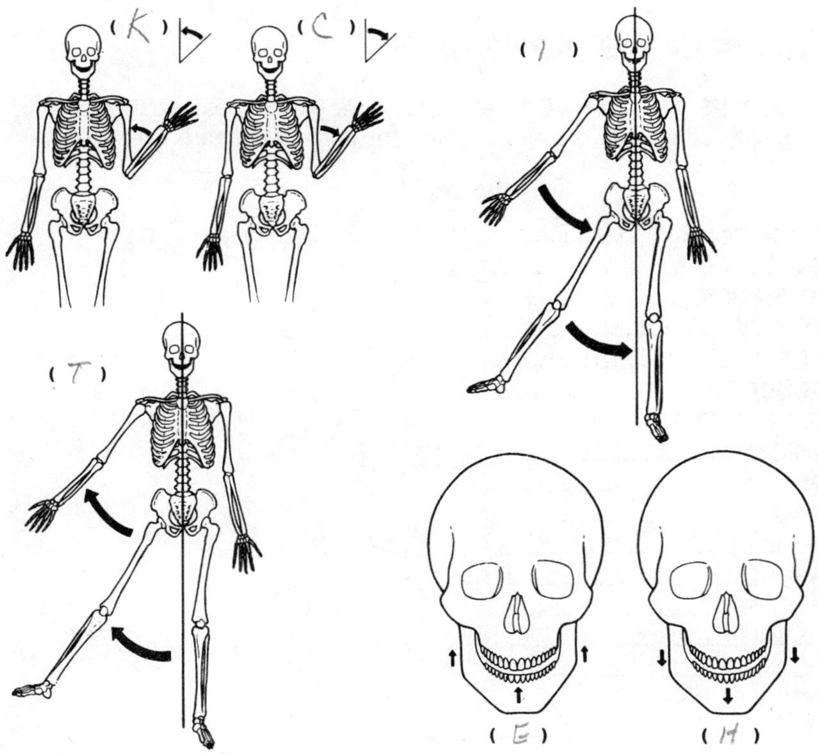

A - OBLIQUE MUSCLE
B - ROTATOR
C - EXTENSOR
D - ZYGOMATICUS MINOR
E - LEVATOR
F - DORSIFLEXOR
G - RECTUS MUSCLE
H - DEPRESSOR
I - ADDUCTOR
J - ZYGOMATICUS MAJOR
K - FLEXOR
L - SPHINCTER
M - TENSOR
N - EVERTOR
O - TEMPORALIS
P - INVERTOR
Q - PLANTAR FLEXOR
R - PRONATOR
S - SUPINATOR
T - ABDUCTOR
U - TRANSVERSE MUSCLE

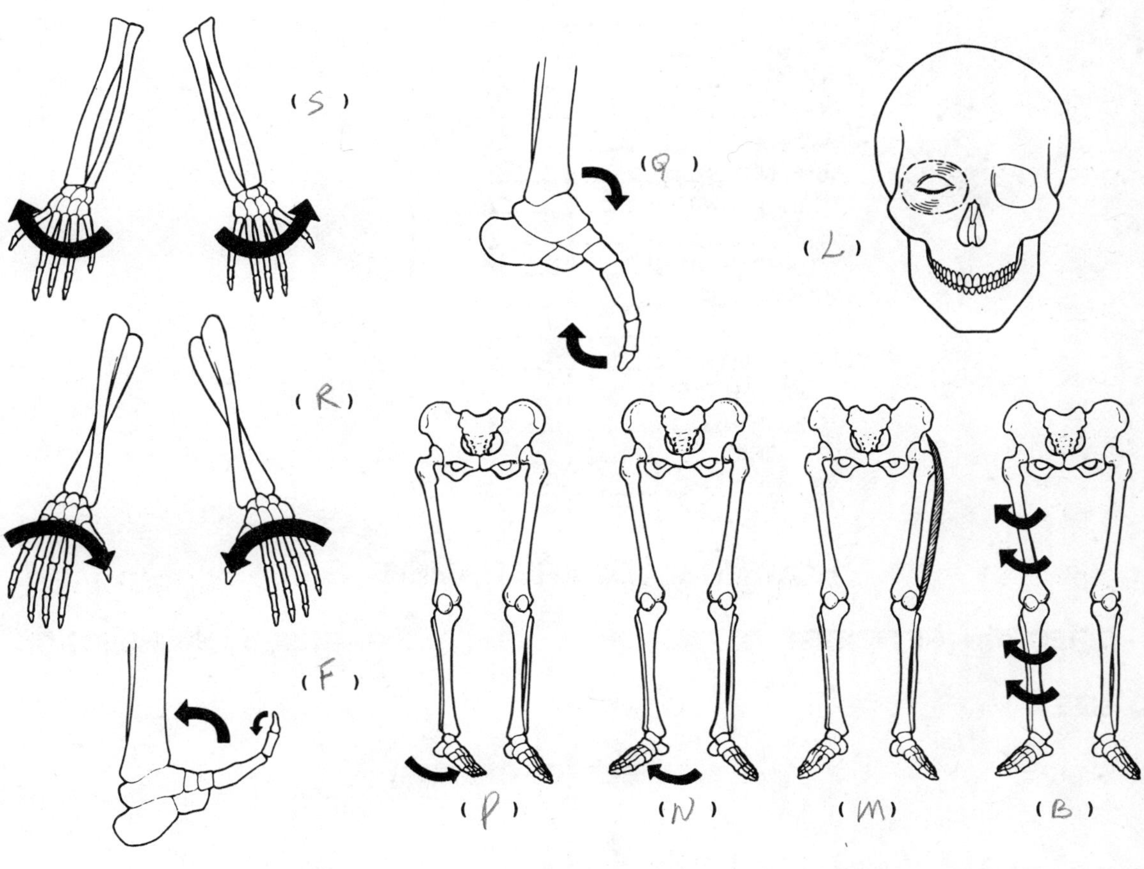

PRE TEST
PRINT THE CORRECT LETTER WITHIN THE PARENTHESES

HOW MUSCLES ARE NAMED

From the list marked "HOW MUSCLES ARE NAMED," select the letter which most closely describes how each of the following types of muscles are named. Mark the letter in the parentheses:

MUSCLE	NAMED BY:
OCCIPITALIS	(E)
DEPRESSOR	(D)
EXTENSOR	(D)
TENSOR	(D)
BREVIS	(B)
ADDUCTOR	(D)
CARPI RADIALIS	(G)
TRICEPS	(F)
PRONATOR	(D)
OBLIQUE	(A)
FLEXOR	(D)
ABDUCTOR	(D)
EVERTOR	(D)
LONGUS	(B)
RECTUS	(A)
DORSI FLEXOR	(D)
TRAPEZIUS	(C)
INVERTOR	(D)
LEVATOR	(D)
ROTATOR	(D)
TIBIALIS	(E)
TEMPORALIS	(E)
MINIMUS	(B)
SPHINCTER	(D)
CARPI ULNARIS	(G)
BICEPS	(F)
TRANSVERSUS	(A)
SUPINATOR	(D)
MAXIMUS	(B)
ZYGOMATICUS	(E)
PLANTAR FLEXOR	(D)
ABDOMINIS	(E)
FEMORIS	(E)
QUADRICEPS	(F)

HOW MUSCLES ARE NAMED

A - DIRECTION (OF FIBERS)

B - SIZE

C - SHAPE

D - ACTION

E - LOCATION

F - NUMBER (OF ORIGINS)

G - ORIGIN AND INSERTION

PRE TEST
PRINT THE CORRECT LETTER WITHIN THE PARENTHESES

THE INTEGUMENTARY SYSTEM

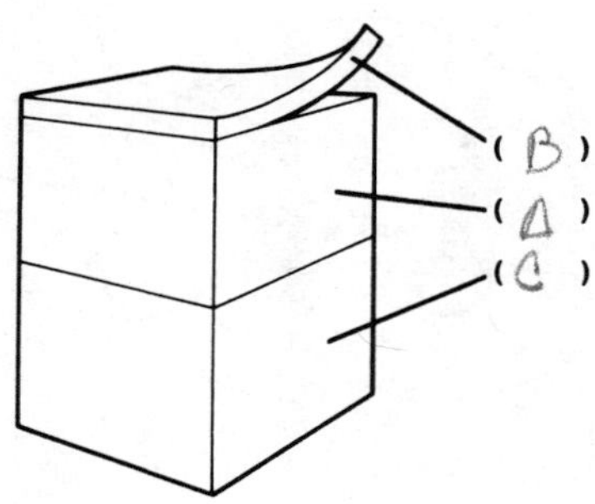

A - DERMIS

B - EPIDERMIS

C - SUBCUTANEOUS TISSUE

THE INTEGUMENTARY SYSTEM

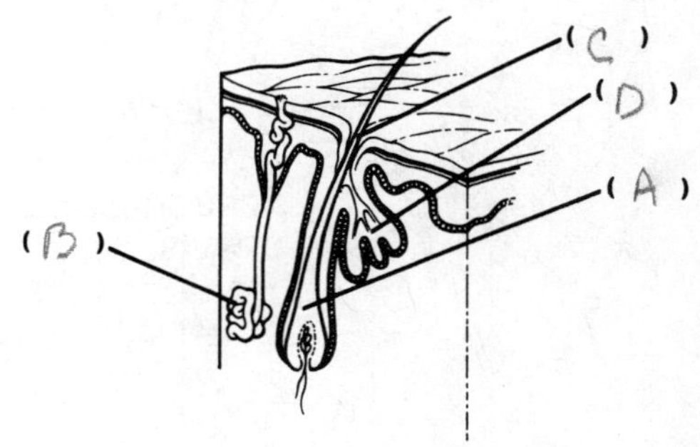

A - HAIR ROOT

B - SUDORIFEROUS (SWEAT) GLAND

C - HAIR SHAFT

D - SEBACEOUS (OIL) GLAND

THE INTEGUMENTARY SYSTEM

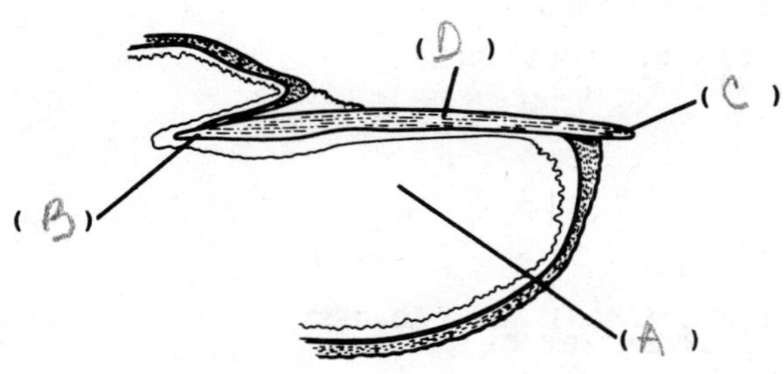

A - NAIL BED

B - NAIL ROOT

C - FREE EDGE

D - NAIL BODY

THE RESPIRATORY SYSTEM

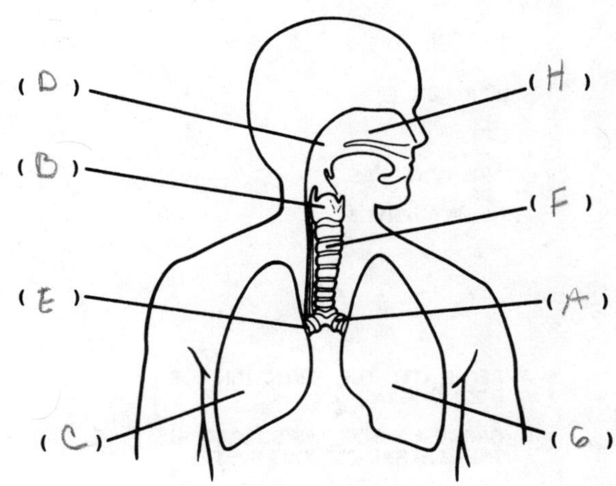

A - LEFT BRONCHUS

B - LARYNX

C - RIGHT LUNG

D - PHARYNX

E - RIGHT BRONCHUS

F - TRACHEA

G - LEFT LUNG

H - NASAL CAVITY

PRE TEST
PRINT THE CORRECT LETTER WITHIN THE PARENTHESES

PRINCIPAL PARTS OF THE BRAIN

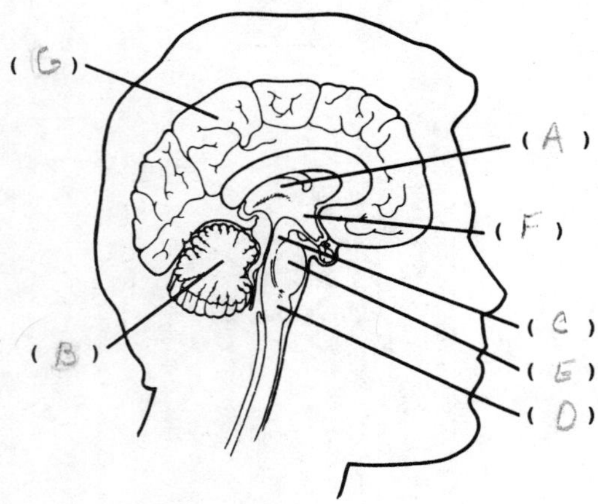

A - THALAMUS
B - CEREBELLUM
C - MIDBRAIN
D - MEDULLA
E - PONS
F - HYPOTHALAMUS
G - CEREBRUM

PRINCIPAL PARTS OF THE SPINAL CORD

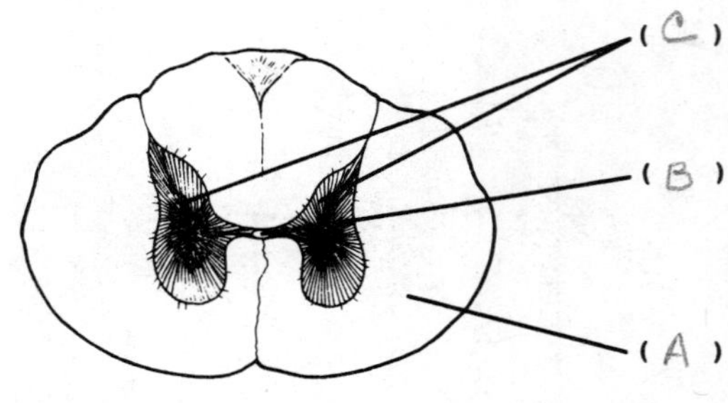

A - WHITE MATTER
B - CENTRAL CANAL
C - GRAY MATTER

THE PERIPHERAL NERVOUS SYSTEM

SCIATIC NERVE (E)
PLEXUS (G)
EFFERENT NERVES (D)
AFFERENT NERVES (B)

SYMPATHETIC NERVES (H) ( )
PARASYMPATHETIC NERVES (A) ( )
SOMATIC NERVOUS SYSTEM (VOLUNTARY) (F)

A - REGULATE THE FUNCTION OF BODY ORGANS
B - CARRY (SENSORY) MESSAGES TO THE CENTRAL NERVOUS SYSTEM
C - ORIGINATE IN CRANIOSACRAL REGION OF SPINAL CORD
D - CARRY (MOTOR) IMPULSES (MESSAGES) TO ALL PARTS OF THE BODY
E - THE LARGEST AND LONGEST NERVE IN THE BODY
F - SERVES THE SKELETAL MUSCLES
G - NETWORK OF SPINAL NERVES
H - ACT IN CASES OF EMERGENCY
I - ORIGINATE IN THORACOLUMBAR REGION OF SPINAL CORD

PRE TEST
PRINT THE CORRECT LETTER WITHIN THE PARENTHESES

CRANIAL NERVES

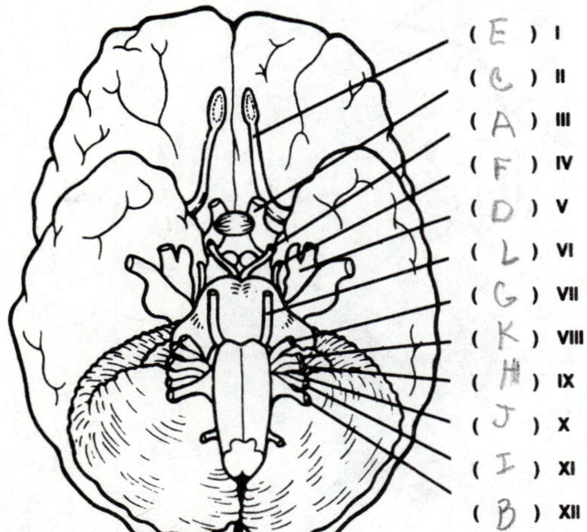

A - OCULOMOTOR
B - HYPOGLOSSAL
C - OPTIC
D - TRIGEMINAL
E - OLFACTORY
F - TROCHLEAR
G - FACIAL
H - GLOSSOPHARYNGEAL
I - ACCESSORY
J - VAGUS
K - VESTIBULOCOCHLEAR
L - ABDUCENS

SPINAL NERVES

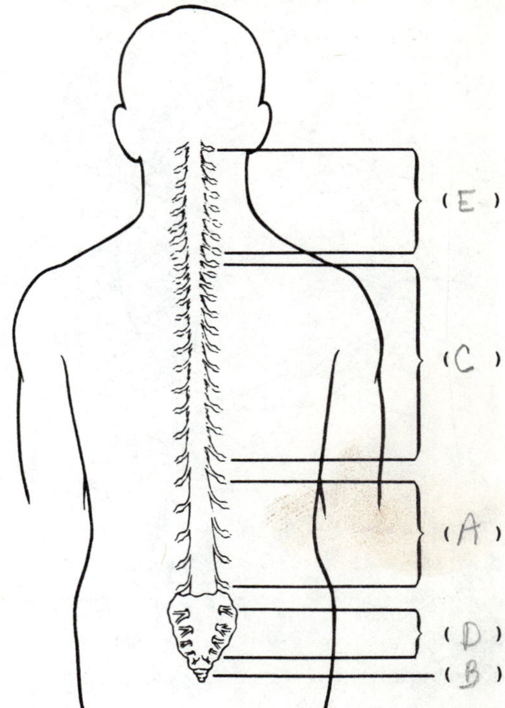

A - LUMBAR NERVES
B - COCCYGEAL NERVES
C - THORACIC NERVES
D - SACRAL NERVES
E - CERVICAL NERVES

POSTERIOR VIEW

PLEXUSES

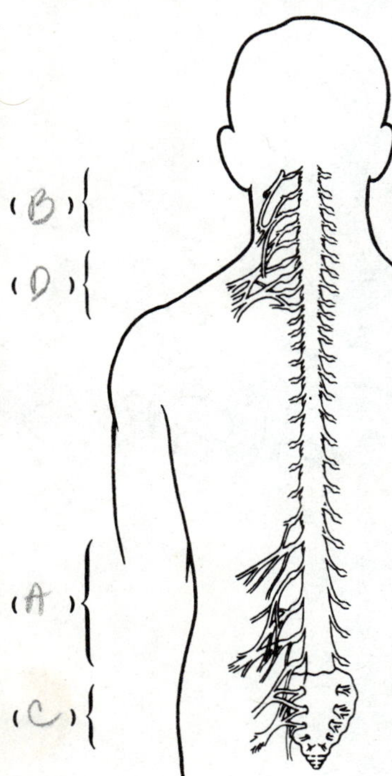

A - LUMBAR PLEXUS
B - CERVICAL PLEXUS
C - SACRAL PLEXUS
D - BRACHIAL PLEXUS

THE PERIPHERAL NERVOUS SYSTEM

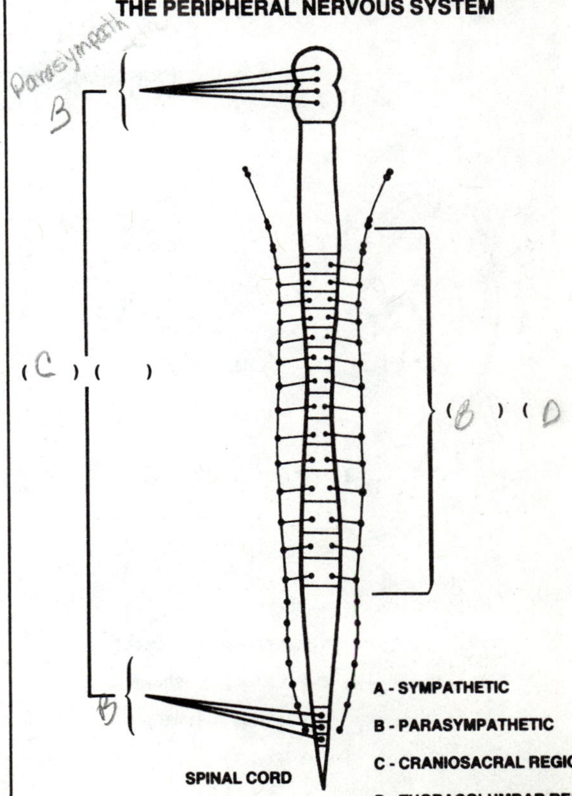

A - SYMPATHETIC
B - PARASYMPATHETIC
C - CRANIOSACRAL REGION
D - THORACOLUMBAR REGION

PRE TEST
PRINT THE CORRECT LETTER WITHIN THE PARENTHESES

PRINCIPAL PARTS OF THE EYE BALL

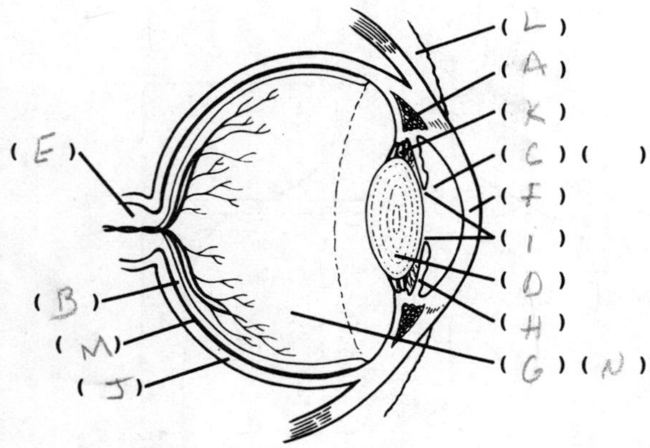

A - CILIARY BODY
B - RETINA
C - ANTERIOR CAVITY
D - LENS
E - OPTIC NERVE
F - CORNEA
G - POSTERIOR CAVITY
H - IRIS
I - PUPIL
J - SCLERA
K - SUSPENSORY LIGAMENT
L - CONJUNCTIVA
M - CHOROID
N - VITREOUS HUMOR
O - AQUEOUS HUMOR

PRINCIPAL ARTERIES OF NECK AND HEAD

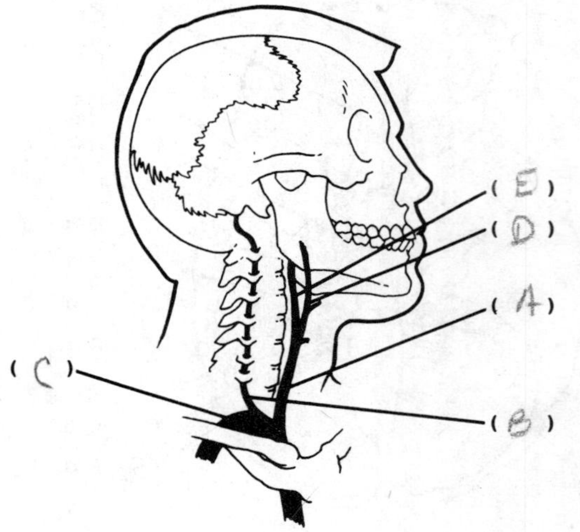

RIGHT LATERAL VIEW

A - RIGHT COMMON CAROTID
B - RIGHT VERTEBRAL
C - RIGHT SUBCLAVIAN
D - RIGHT EXTERNAL CAROTID
E - RIGHT INTERNAL CAROTID

PRINCIPAL PARTS OF THE EAR

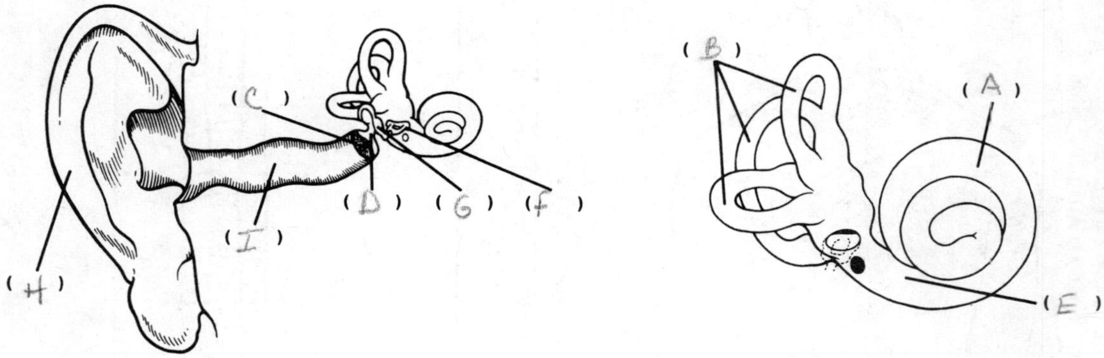

A - COCHLEA
B - SEMI-CIRCULAR CANALS
C - TYMPANIC MEMBRANE
D - MALLEUS (HAMMER)
E - VESTIBULE
F - STAPES (STIRRUP)
G - INCUS (ANVIL)
H - PINNA
I - AUDITORY CANAL

PRE TEST
PRINT THE CORRECT LETTER WITHIN THE PARENTHESES

PRINCIPAL ARTERIES OF THE RIGHT UPPER EXTREMITY

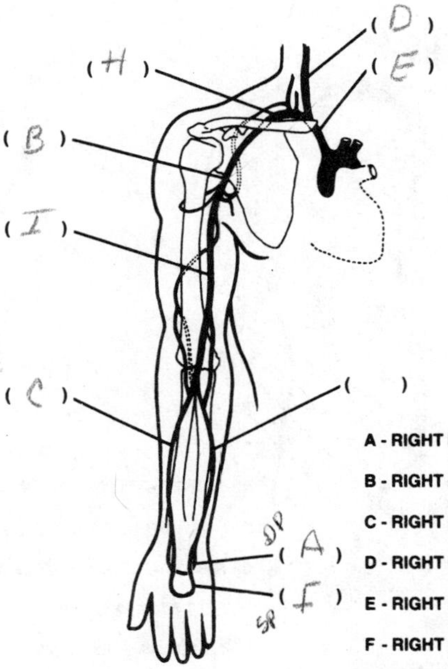

- A - RIGHT DEEP PALMAR
- B - RIGHT AXILLARY
- C - RIGHT RADIAL
- D - RIGHT COMMON CAROTID
- E - RIGHT BRACHIOCEPHALIC
- F - RIGHT SUPERFICIAL PALMAR
- G - RIGHT ULNAR
- H - RIGHT SUBCLAVIAN
- I - RIGHT BRACHIAL

ANTERIOR VIEW

PRINCIPAL DIVISIONS OF AORTA

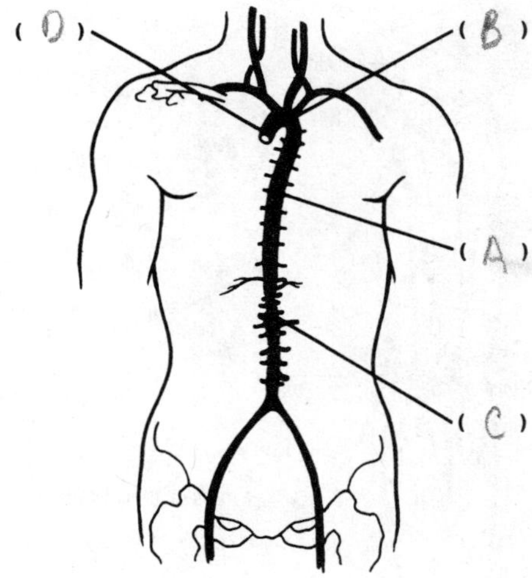

- A - THORACIC AORTA
- B - ARCH OF AORTA
- C - ABDOMINAL AORTA
- D - ASCENDING AORTA

PRINCIPAL ARTERIES OF PELVIS AND RIGHT LOWER EXTREMITY

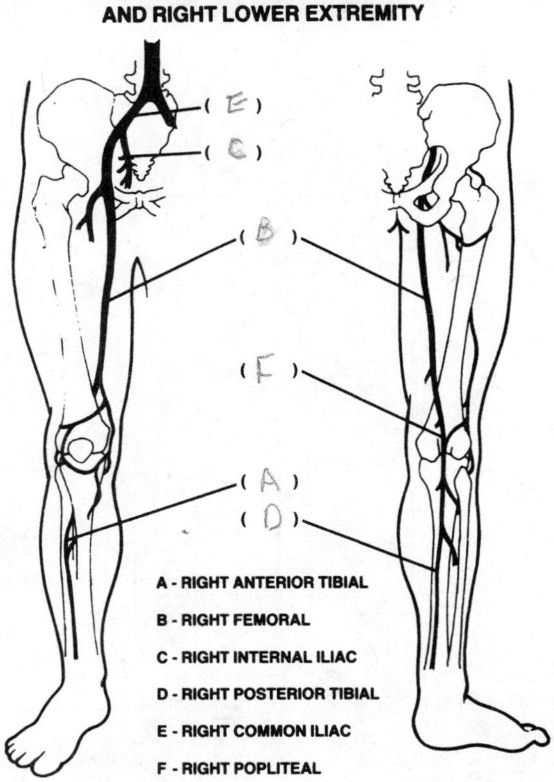

- A - RIGHT ANTERIOR TIBIAL
- B - RIGHT FEMORAL
- C - RIGHT INTERNAL ILIAC
- D - RIGHT POSTERIOR TIBIAL
- E - RIGHT COMMON ILIAC
- F - RIGHT POPLITEAL

ANTERIOR VIEW POSTERIOR VIEW

PRINCIPAL VEINS OF THE NECK AND HEAD

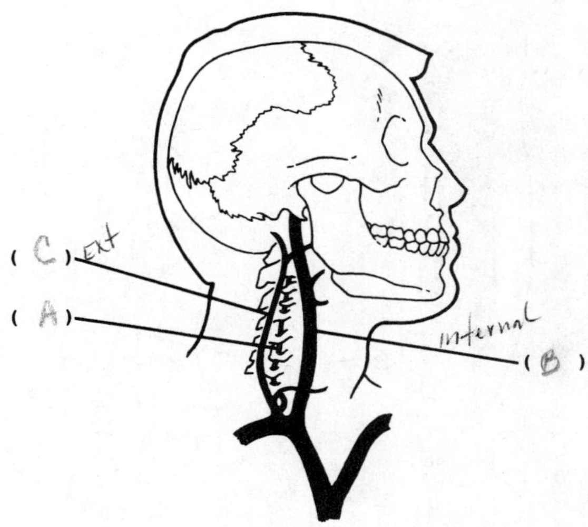

RIGHT LATERAL VIEW

- A - RIGHT VERTEBRAL
- B - RIGHT INTERNAL JUGULAR
- C - RIGHT EXTERNAL JUGULAR

PRE TEST
PRINT THE CORRECT LETTER WITHIN THE PARENTHESES

PRINCIPAL VEINS OF THE RIGHT UPPER EXTREMITY

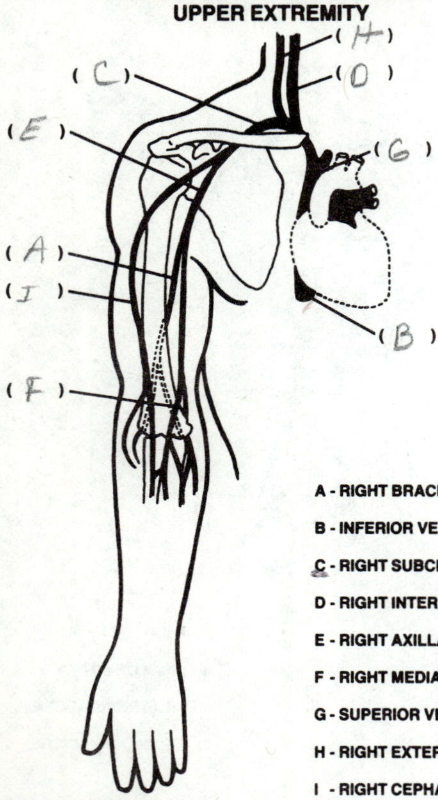

ANTERIOR VIEW

A - RIGHT BRACHIAL
B - INFERIOR VENA CAVA
C - RIGHT SUBCLAVIAN
D - RIGHT INTERNAL JUGULAR
E - RIGHT AXILLARY
F - RIGHT MEDIAN CUBITAL
G - SUPERIOR VENA CAVA
H - RIGHT EXTERNAL JUGULAR
I - RIGHT CEPHALIC

PRINCIPAL VEINS OF THE THORAX ABDOMEN AND PELVIS

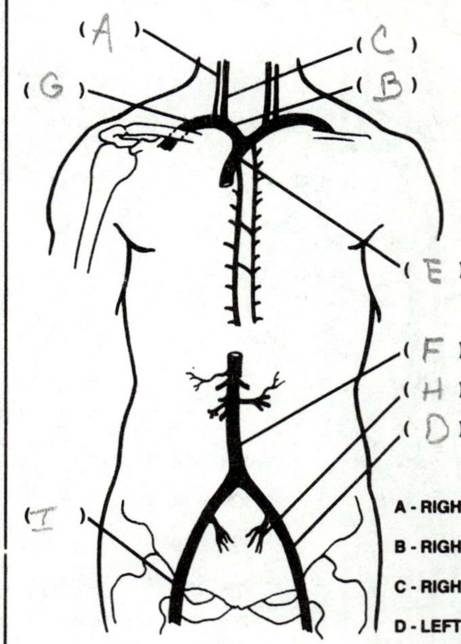

ANTERIOR VIEW

A - RIGHT EXTERNAL JUGULAR
B - RIGHT BRACHIOCEPHALIC
C - RIGHT INTERNAL JUGULAR
D - LEFT EXTERNAL ILIAC
E - SUPERIOR VENA CAVA
F - INFERIOR VENA CAVA
G - RIGHT SUBCLAVIAN
H - LEFT INTERNAL ILIAC
I - RIGHT FEMORAL

PRINCIPAL VEINS OF THE PELVIS AND RIGHT LOWER EXTREMITY

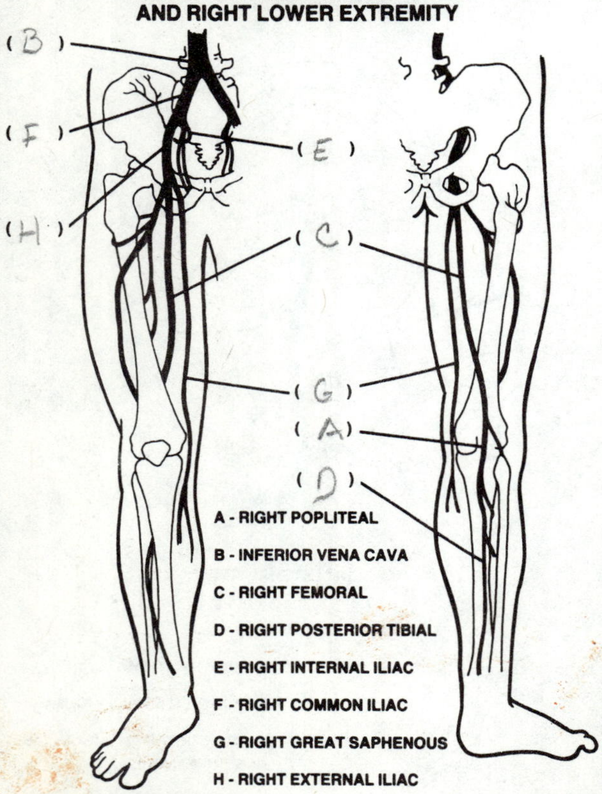

A - RIGHT POPLITEAL
B - INFERIOR VENA CAVA
C - RIGHT FEMORAL
D - RIGHT POSTERIOR TIBIAL
E - RIGHT INTERNAL ILIAC
F - RIGHT COMMON ILIAC
G - RIGHT GREAT SAPHENOUS
H - RIGHT EXTERNAL ILIAC

ANTERIOR VIEW

POSTERIOR VIEW

STRUCTURAL RELATIONSHIP OF VESSELS

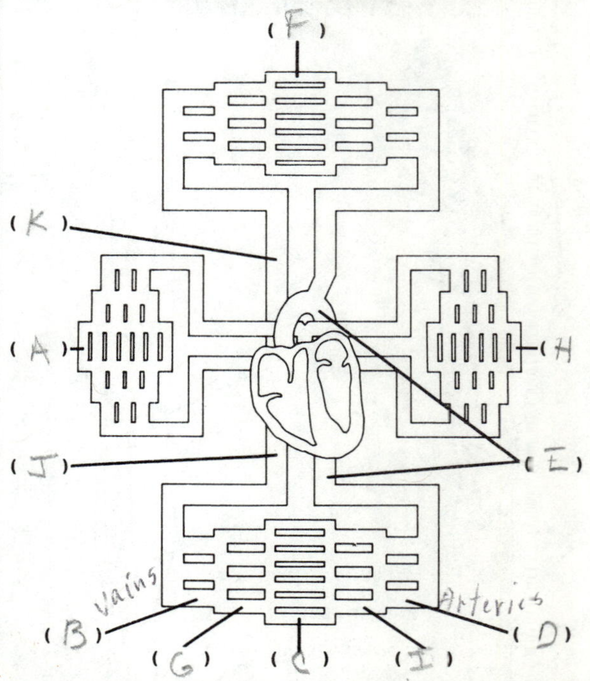

A - CAPILLARIES OF THE RIGHT LUNG
B - VEINS
C - CAPILLARIES OF LOWER EXTREMITIES
D - ARTERIES
E - AORTA
F - CAPILLARIES OF HEAD AND UPPER EXTREMITIES
G - VENULES
H - CAPILLARIES OF THE LEFT LUNG
I - ARTERIOLES
J - INFERIOR VENA CAVA
K - SUPERIOR VENA CAVA

PRE TEST
PRINT THE CORRECT LETTER WITHIN THE PARENTHESES

THE HEART

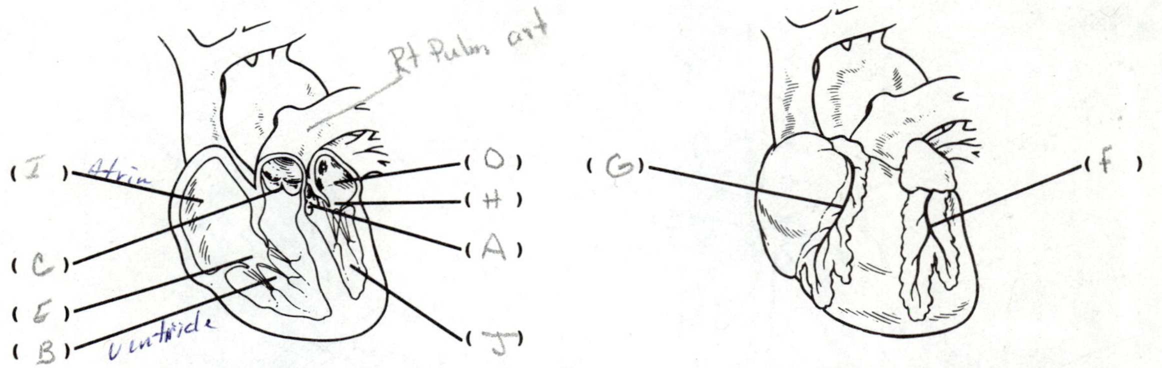

A - AORTIC SEMILUNAR VALVE
B - RIGHT VENTRICLE
C - PULMONARY SEMILUNAR VALVE
D - LEFT ATRIUM
E - TRICUSPID VALVE
F - LEFT CORONARY ARTERY
G - RIGHT CORONARY ARTERY
H - BICUSPID VALVE
I - RIGHT ATRIUM
J - LEFT VENTRICLE

PRINT THE CORRECT LETTER WITHIN THE PARENTHESES

( ) MICROSCOPIC BLOOD VESSELS
( ) THE LARGEST ARTERY
( ) THE LARGEST VEIN ABOVE THE HEART
( ) SMALL ARTERIES
( ) LARGEST VEIN BELOW THE HEART
( ) SMALL VEINS

A - INFERIOR VENA CAVA
B - CAPILLARIES
C - VENULES
D - AORTA
E - SUPERIOR VENA CAVA
F - ARTERIOLES

ORGANS OF THE LYMPHATIC SYSTEM

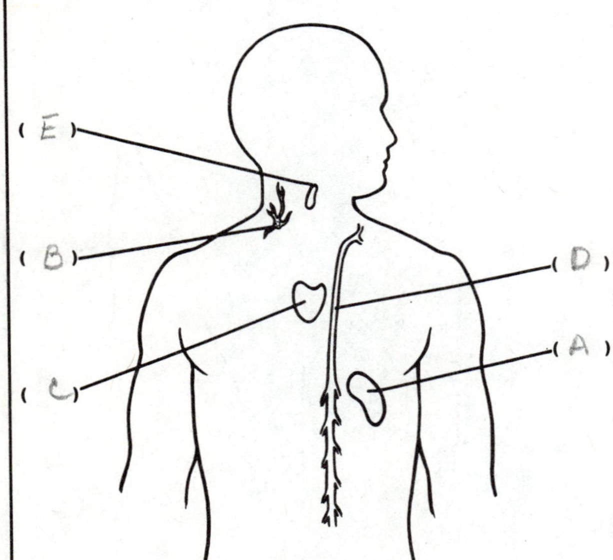

A - SPLEEN
B - RIGHT LYMPHATIC DUCT
C - THYMUS
D - THORACIC DUCT
E - TONSILS

STRUCTURAL RELATIONSHIPS OF LYMPHATIC VESSELS

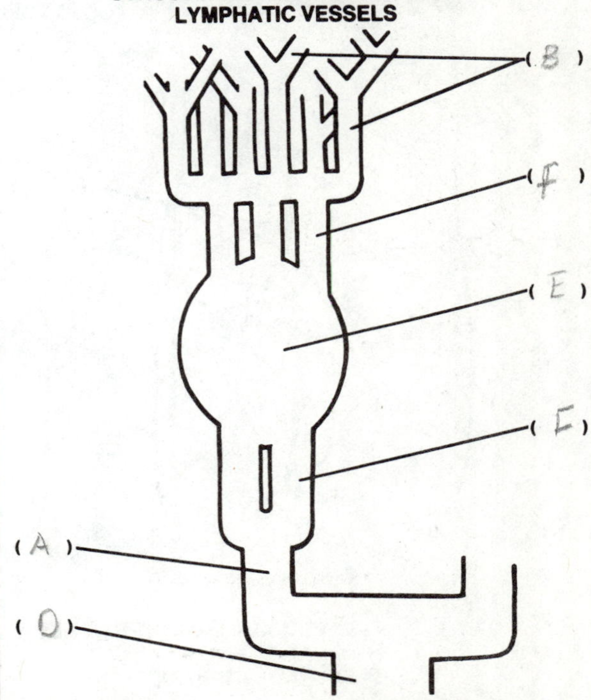

A - (LYMPH) TRUNK
B - (LYMPH) CAPILLARIES
C - (LYMPH) VESSELS
D - (LYMPHATIC) DUCT (EITHER THORACIC OR RIGHT LYMPHATIC)
E - (LYMPH) NODE
F - (LYMPH) VESSELS

PRE TEST
PRINT THE CORRECT LETTER WITHIN THE PARENTHESES

LYMPH NODES

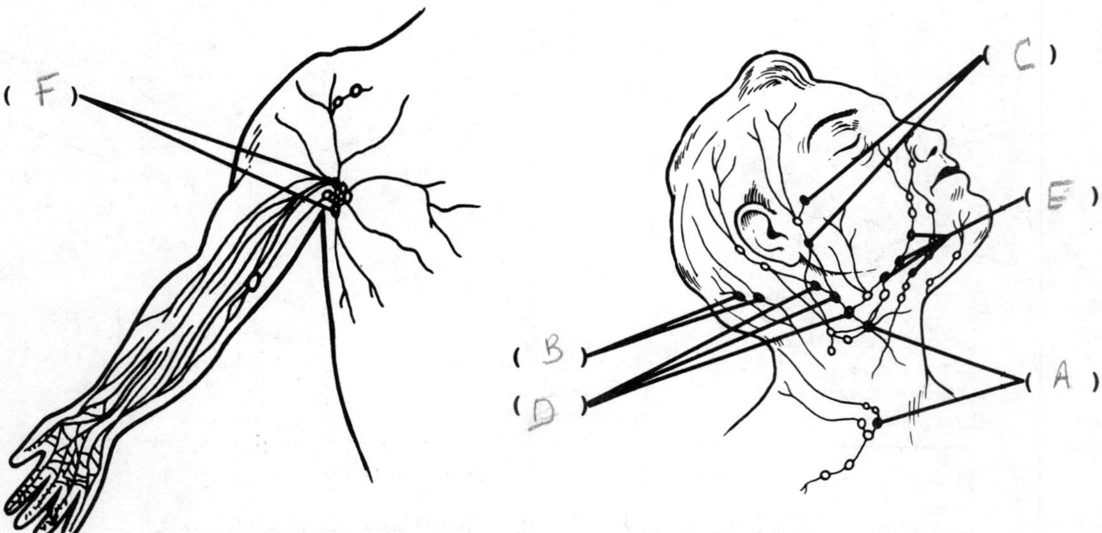

A - DEEP CERVICAL LYMPH NODES

B - OCCIPITAL LYMPH NODES

C - PAROTID LYMPH NODES

D - SUPERFICIAL CERVICAL LYMPH NODES

E - SUBMANDIBULAR CERVICAL LYMPH NODES

F - AXILLARY LYMPH NODES

LYMPH NODES

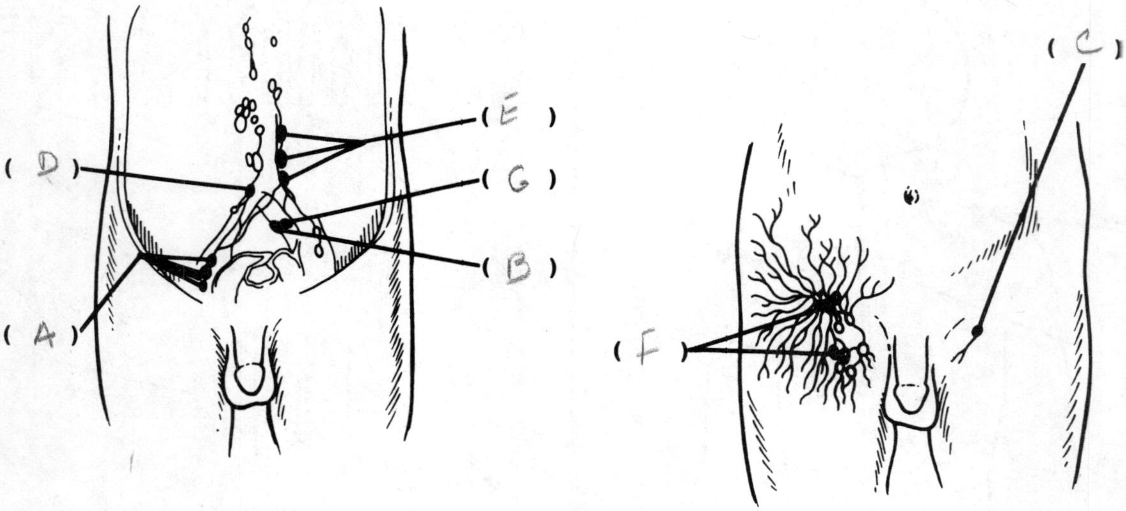

A - EXTERNAL ILIAC LYMPH NODES

B - SACRAL LYMPH NODE

C - DEEP INGUINAL LYMPH NODES

D - COMMON ILIAC LYMPH NODE

E - LUMBAR LYMPH NODES

F - SUPERFICIAL INGUINAL LYMPH NODES

G - INTERNAL ILIAC LYMPH NODE

PRE TEST
PRINT THE CORRECT LETTER WITHIN THE PARENTHESES

GLANDS OF THE ENDOCRINE SYSTEM

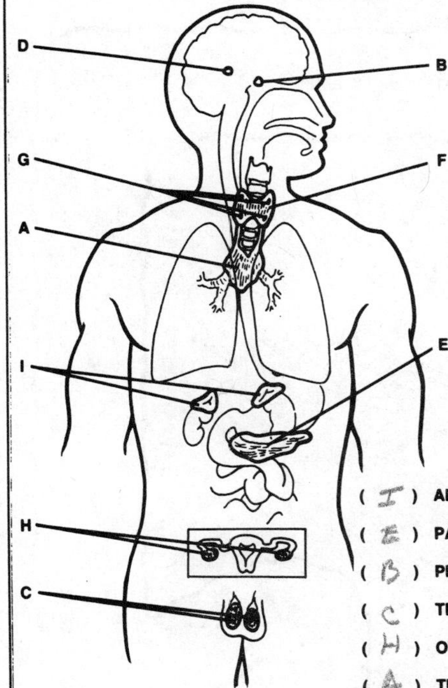

(I) ADRENAL GLANDS
(E) PANCREAS
(B) PITUITARY GLAND
(C) TESTES
(H) OVARIES
(A) THYMUS GLAND
(D) PINEAL GLAND
(G) PARATHYROID GLANDS
(F) THYROID GLAND

ORGANS OF THE URINARY SYSTEM

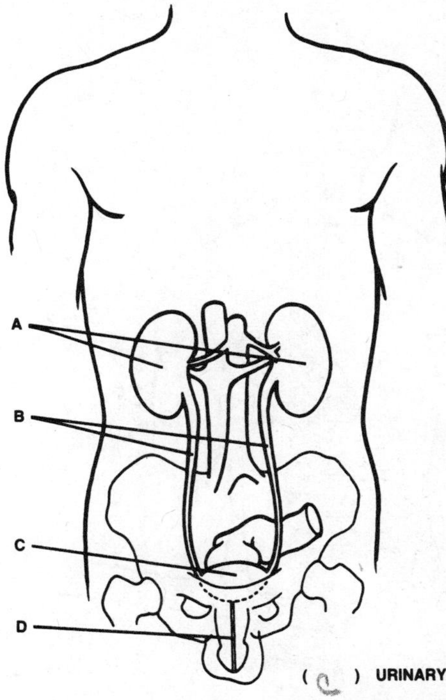

(C) URINARY BLADDER
(B) URETER
(D) URETHRA
(A) KIDNEY

ORGANS OF THE ALIMENTARY CANAL

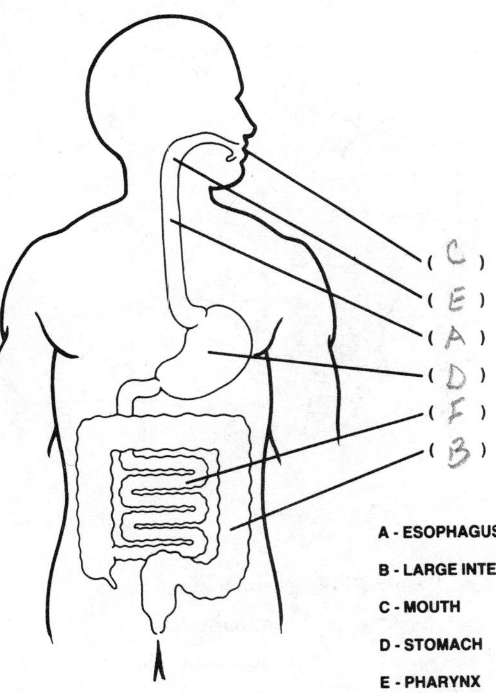

A - ESOPHAGUS
B - LARGE INTESTINE
C - MOUTH
D - STOMACH
E - PHARYNX
F - SMALL INTESTINE

PARTS OF THE SMALL INTESTINE

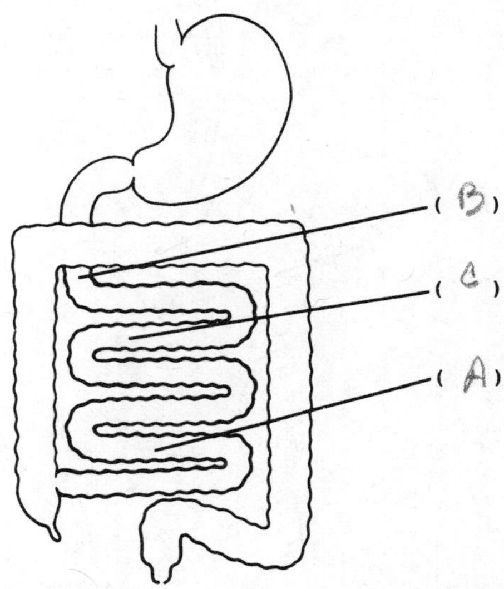

A - ILEUM
B - DUODENUM
C - JEJUNUM

PRE TEST
PRINT THE CORRECT LETTER WITHIN THE PARENTHESES

PARTS OF THE LARGE INTESTINE

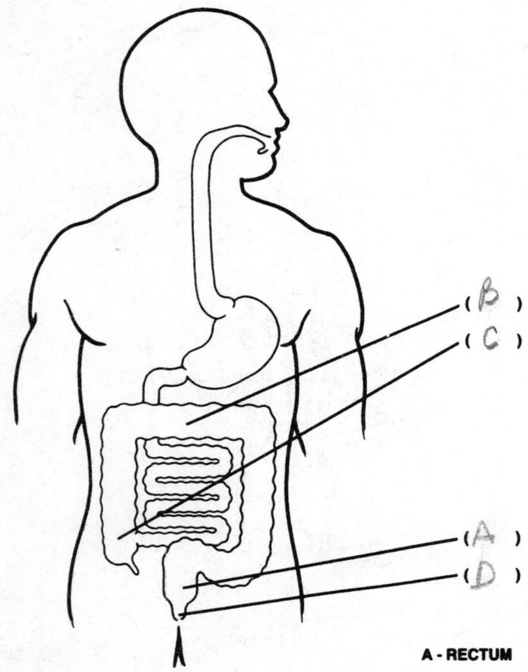

A - RECTUM
B - COLON
C - CECUM
D - ANUS

SEGMENTS OF THE COLON

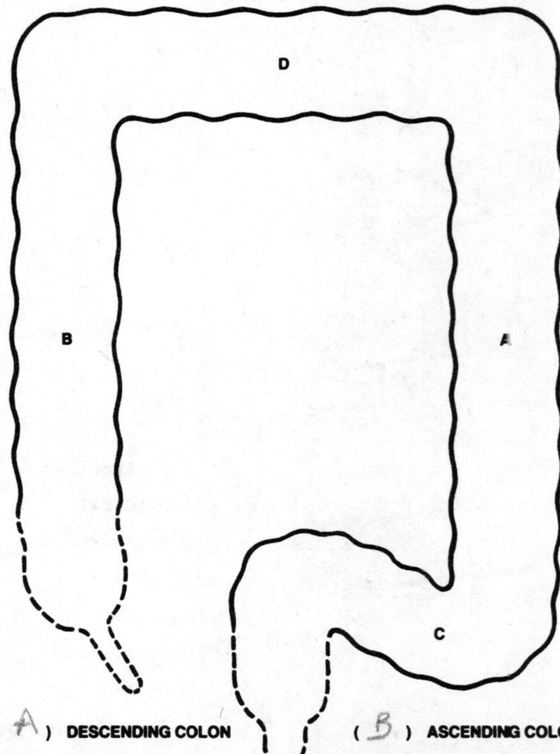

(A) DESCENDING COLON
(D) TRANSVERSE COLON
(B) ASCENDING COLON
(C) SIGMOID COLON

MAJOR ACCESSORY ORGANS

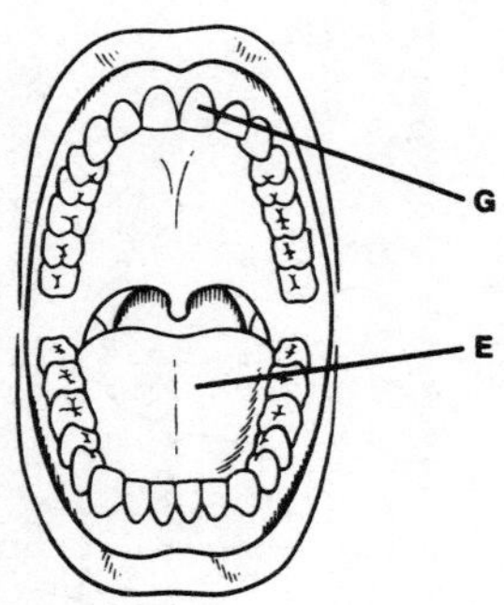

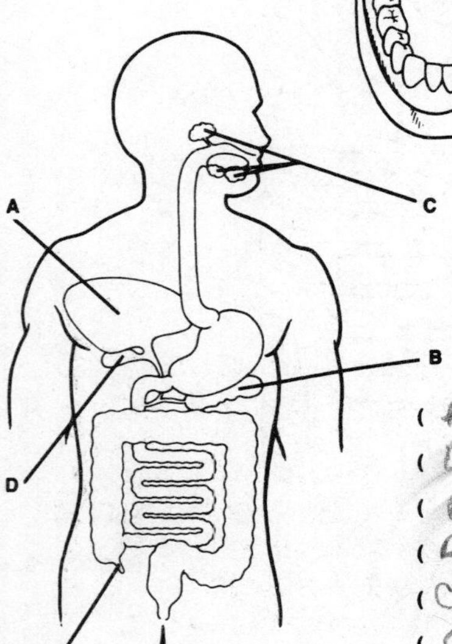

(f) APPENDIX
(D) GALLBLADDER
(B) PANCREAS
(A) LIVER
(C) SALIVARY GLANDS
(G) TEETH
(E) TONGUE

SALIVARY GLANDS

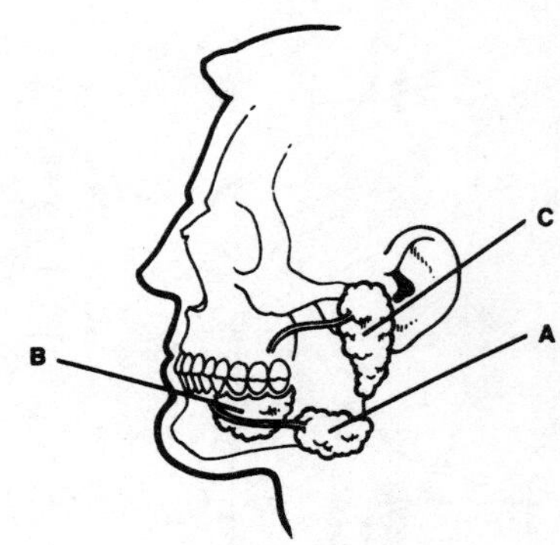

(A) SUBMANDIBULAR GLAND
(C) PAROTID GLAND
(B) SUBLINGUAL GLAND

PRE TEST

Mark an "X" under the appropriate heading to indicate whether the body part is a part of the alimentary canal or is an accessory organ.

ALIMENTARY CANAL		ACCESSORY ORGAN	LOCATION
( )	DESCENDING COLON	( )	( )
( )	CECUM	( )	( )
( )	ASCENDING COLON	( )	( )
( )	ANUS	( )	( )
( )	SUBMANDIBULAR GLAND	( )	( )
( )	TEETH	( )	( )
( )	PANCREAS	( )	( )
( )	GALLBLADDER	( )	( )
( )	APPENDIX	( )	( )
( )	DUODENUM	( )	( )
( )	TRANSVERSE COLON	( )	( )
( )	PHARYNX	( )	( )
( )	LIVER	( )	( )
( )	RECTUM	( )	( )
( )	ILEUM	( )	( )
( )	SIGMOID COLON	( )	( )
( )	SUBLINGUAL GLAND	( )	( )
( )	TONGUE	( )	( )
( )	PAROTID GLAND	( )	( )
( )	JEJUNUM	( )	( )
( )	STOMACH	( )	( )
( )	MOUTH	( )	( )
( )	ESOPHAGUS	( )	( )

PRINT THE CORRECT LETTER WITHIN THE PARENTHESES UNDER THE HEADING - LOCATION

A- LOCATED BETWEEN THE PHARYNX AND STOMACH
B- LOCATED BETWEEN THE DUODENUM AND ILEUM
C- LOCATED BETWEEN THE MOUTH AND ESOPHAGUS
D- LOCATED BETWEEN THE TRANSVERSE AND SIGMOID COLON
E- LOCATED BETWEEN THE JEJUNUM AND ASCENDING COLON
F- LOCATED BETWEEN THE DESCENDING COLON AND RECTUM
G- LOCATED BETWEEN THE STOMACH AND JEJUNUM
H- LOCATED BETWEEN THE ASCENDING AND DESENDING COLON
I- LOCATED BETWEEN THE SIGMOID COLON AND ANUS
J- LOCATED BETWEEN THE ESOPHAGUS AND DUODENUM
K- LOCATED BETWEEN THE ILEUM AND TRANSVERSE COLON
L- A SALIVARY GLAND LOCATED NEAR THE EAR
M- A SALIVARY GLAND LOCATED UNDER THE TONGUE
N- A SALIVARY GLAND LOCATED UNDER THE MANDIBLE
O- THE TERMINAL OPENING OF THE ALIMENTARY CANAL
P- THE BEGINNING OF THE ALIMENTARY CANAL

PRE TEST
PRINT THE CORRECT LETTER WITHIN THE PARENTHESES

ORGANS AND STRUCTURES OF THE MALE REPRODUCTIVE SYSTEM

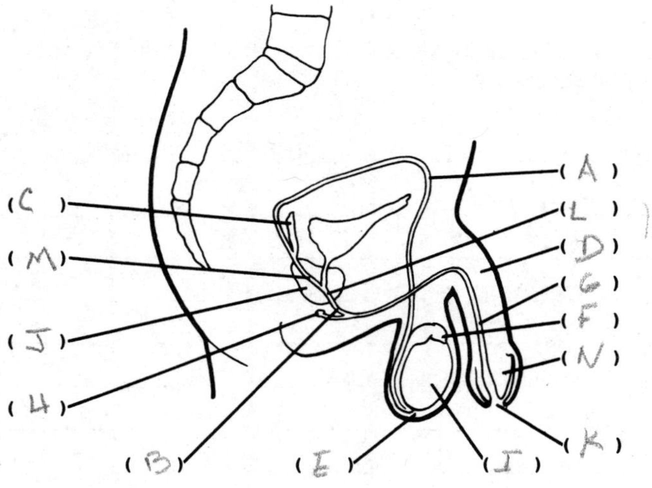

A - DUCTUS DEFERENS
B - MEMBRANOUS URETHRA
C - SEMINAL VESICLE
D - PENIS
E - SCROTUM
F - EPIDIDYMIS
G - SPONGY URETHRA
H - BULBOURETHRAL GLAND
I - TESTIS
J - PROSTATE GLAND
K - URETHRAL ORIFICE
L - PROSTATIC URETHRA
M - EJACULATORY DUCT
N - GLANS PENIS

ORGANS OF THE FEMALE REPRODUCTIVE SYSTEM

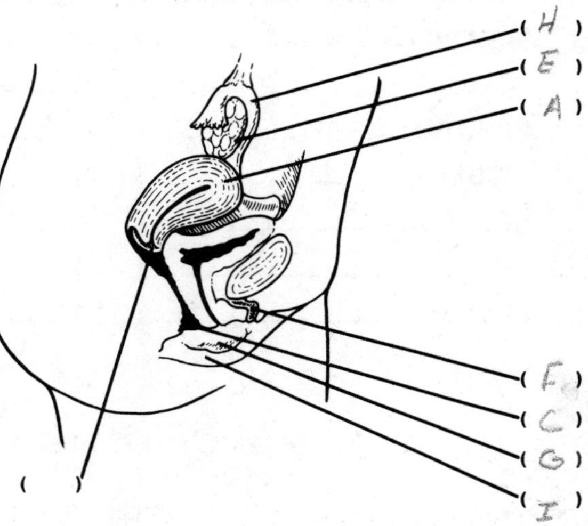

EXTERNAL GENITALIA OF THE FEMALE (   )

BREASTS (   )

A - UTERUS
B - CERVIX
C - VAGINA
D - VULVA
E - OVARY
F - CLITORIS
G - LABIUM MINOR
H - UTERINE TUBE
I - LABIUM MAJOR
J - MAMMARY GLANDS

LESSON 1

INTRODUCTION

PART A

- ANATOMICAL TERMS
- ANATOMICAL LOCATIONS

REMEMBER!

1st ***Pronounce*** *the name of the body part or term*
2nd ***Recall*** *and* ***pronounce*** *the audionym*
3rd ***For body parts: visualize*** *the audionym in place*
For terms: visualize *the association*
4th ***Pronounce*** *the name of the body part or term again.*

LESSON 1 — REVIEW
INTRODUCTION — PART A
ANATOMICAL TERMS AND LOCATIONS

WORD	AUDIONYM	VISUAL IMAGE / ASSOCIATION	MEANING
crani(al)	crane	See the **crane** made of a **skull**!	skull (pertaning to the upper portion of the skull)
cephal	sieve fall	See the **sieve fall**ing with a **head** in it!	head
caudal	cod	See the **cod** with many **tails**!	tail
superior	soup	See the **soup** being held **above** everything!	above
inferior	inn fire (bellows)	See the **inn fire** with a gigantic **bellows** sticking in it!	below
epi	a pea	See **a pea** with many peas **upon** it! There are peas all **over** it!	upon, over
hypo	hippo	See the **hippo under** the table!	under
proximal	peroxide (knee/rust)	See the bottle of **peroxide** with the **knee/rust** sticking out of it!	nearest
distal	distillery (farm)	See the **distillery** with a **far**m on it!	far
ventral	vent	See the **vent** on **front** of the body!	front
anterior	ant	See the **ant** with a **vent** on **front** of it!	front, ventral
dorsal	doors	See the **doors** on **back** of the body!	back
posterior	poster	See the **poster** with **doors** on **back** of the body!	back, dorsal
lateral	ladder	See the **ladder** on the **side** of the body!	side
gastr	gas truck	See the **gas truck** with a **stomach** for a tank!	stomach
renal	rain	See it **rain**ing **kidneys**!	kidney

LESSON 1 — REVIEW
INTRODUCTION — PART A
ANATOMICAL TERMS AND LOCATIONS

WORD	AUDIONYM	VISUAL IMAGE / ASSOCIATION	MEANING
chondr	cone/door (cart of leaves)	See the **cone/door** with a **cart of leaves** coming out of it!	cartilage
axillary	axle	See the **axle** in the **arm pit**!	arm pit
brachial	brake	See the **brake** on the **arm** (between the shoulder and elbow)!	arm
inguinal	indian	See the **indian between the abdomen and thigh**	between the abdomen and thigh
cubital	cube	See the **cube** in **front of the elbow**!	front of elbow
popliteal	puppet/tail	See the **puppet/tail** in **back of the knee**!	back of knee
pulmonary	pool/moon	See the **pool/moon** (a **pool** with the **moon** in it). The **moon** has **lungs** on it!	lung
viscera	visor	See the **visor** with a **vent** on it! The **vent** has **organs** coming out of it!	ventral organs

LESSON 1 — REVIEW
INTRODUCTION — PART A
ANATOMICAL TERMS AND LOCATIONS

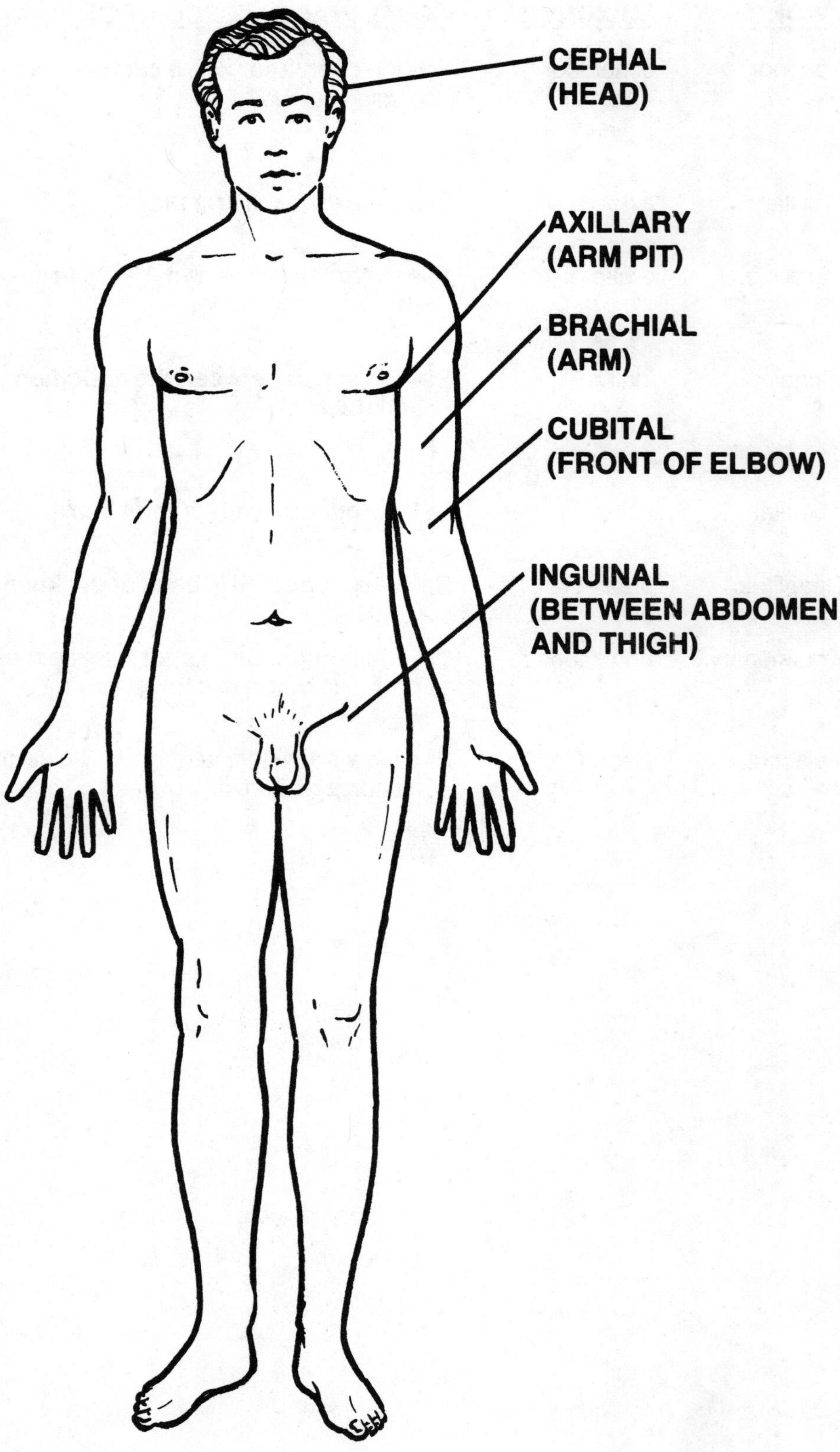

ANTERIOR (FRONT) VIEW

LESSON 1 — REVIEW
INTRODUCTION — PART A
ANATOMICAL TERMS AND LOCATIONS

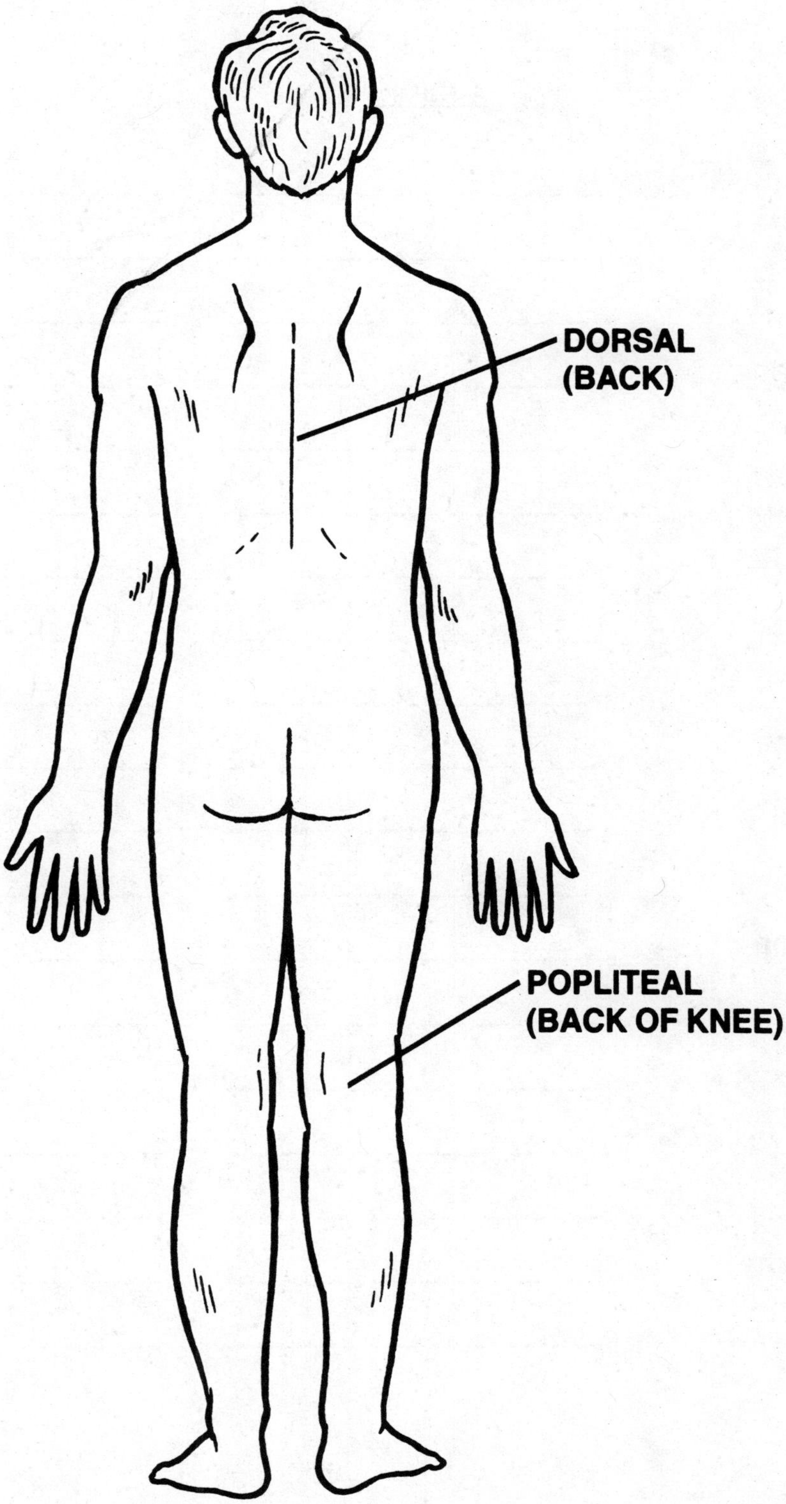

POSTERIOR (BACK) VIEW

LESSON 1 — WORKSHEET
INTRODUCTION — PART A
ANATOMICAL TERMS AND LOCATIONS

COMPLETE THE BLANKS:

WORD	AUDIONYM	MEANING
CRANIAL	Crane	Skull
CEPHAL	Sieve Fall	head
CAUDAL	Cod	Tail
SUPERIOR	Soup	above
INFERIOR	INN Fire	below
EPI	a Pea	upon over
HYPO	hippo	under
PROXIMAL	Peroxide (knee bust)	Nearest
DISTAL	distillery (Farm)	Far
VENTRAL	Vent	Front
ANTERIOR	ant	Front (ventral)
DORSAL	doors	back
POSTERIOR	Poster	back (Dorsal)
LATERAL	Ladder	Side
GASTR	Gas Truck	stomache
RENAL	rain	Kidney
CHONDR	Cone door	Cartillage
PULMONARY	Pool moon	Lung
VISCERA	Visor	Ventral organ

LESSON 1 — WORKSHEET
INTRODUCTION — PART A
ANATOMICAL TERMS AND LOCATIONS

PRINT THE CORRECT LETTER WITHIN THE PARENTHESES

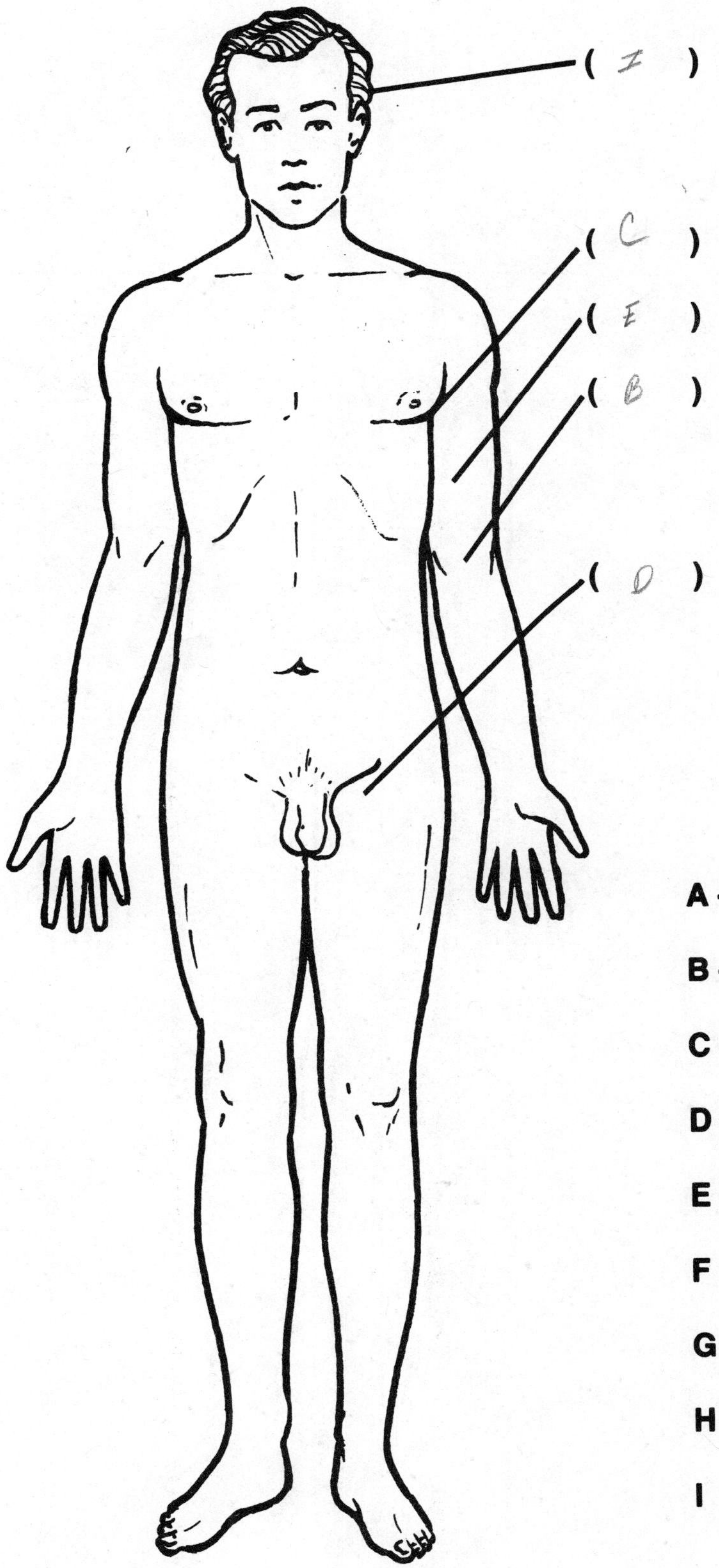

VIEW (Front **)**
Anterior

A - POPLITEAL

B - CUBITAL

C - AXILLARY

D - INGUINAL

E - BRACHIAL

F - POSTERIOR

G - ANTERIOR

H - LATERAL

I - CEPHAL

LESSON 1 — WORKSHEET
INTRODUCTION — PART A
ANATOMICAL TERMS AND LOCATIONS

PRINT THE CORRECT LETTER WITHIN THE PARENTHESES

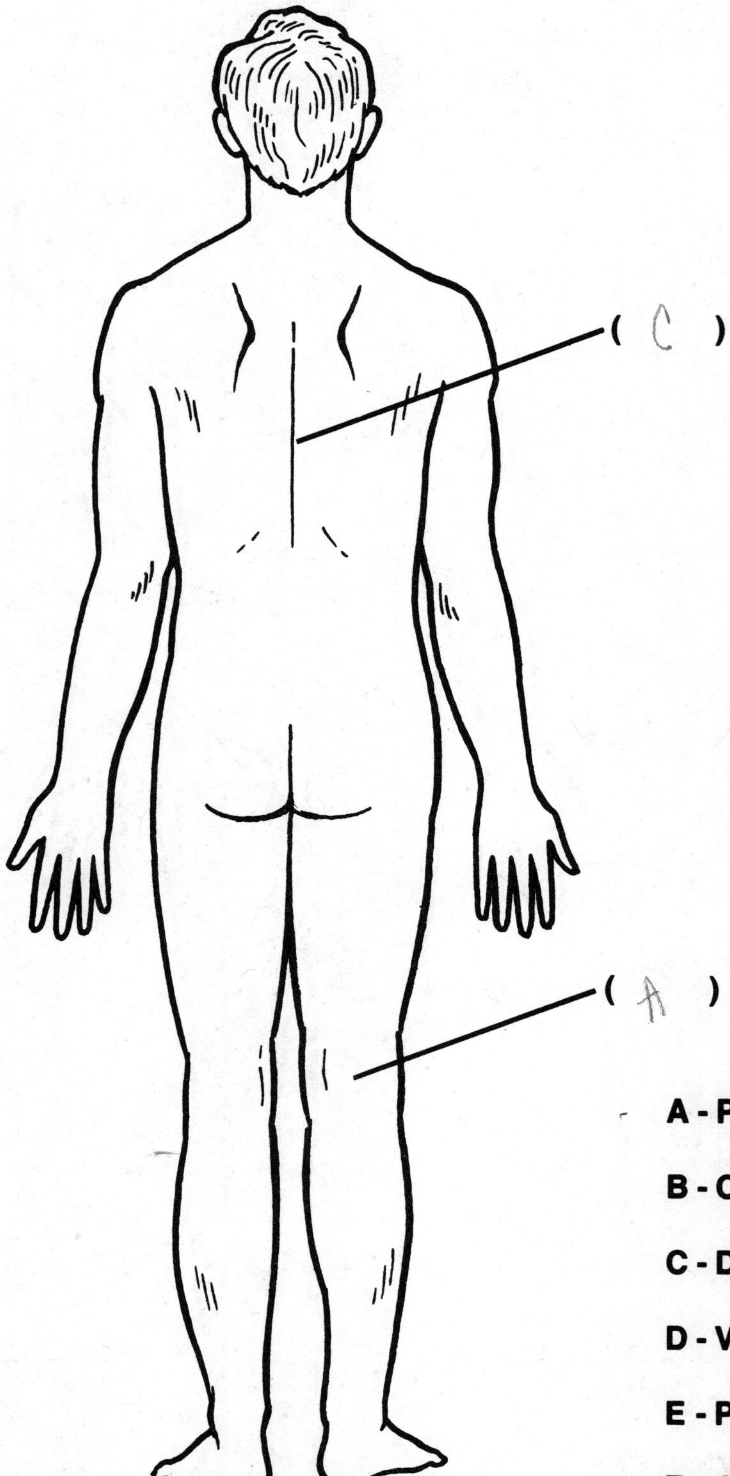

VIEW (Back **)**

A - POPLITEAL

B - CUBITAL

C - DORSAL

D - VENTRAL

E - POSTERIOR

F - ANTERIOR

LESSON 1

INTRODUCTION

PART B

- ANATOMICAL POSITION
- BODY PLANES
- ABDOMINOPELVIC QUADRANTS
- REGIONAL SUBDIVISIONS
- BODY CAVITIES

REMEMBER!

1st **Pronounce** *the name of the body part or term*
2nd **Recall** *and* **pronounce** *the audionym*
3rd **For body parts: visualize** *the audionym in place*
For terms: visualize *the association*
4th **Pronounce** *the name of the body part or term again.*

LESSON 1 — REVIEW
INTRODUCTION — PART B
ANATOMICAL POSITION

1

STANDING ERECT

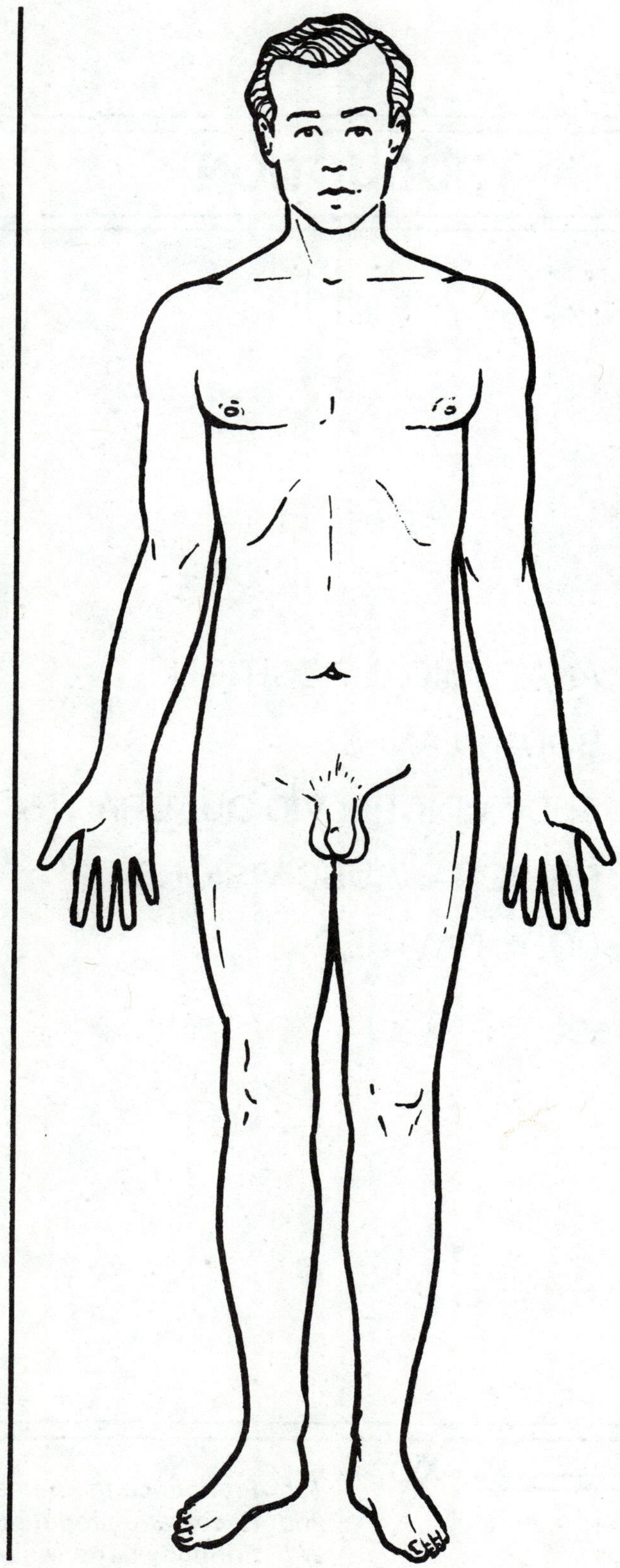

2

FACING FORWARD

3

ARMS HANGING AT SIDES

4

PALMS FORWARD

LESSON 1 — REVIEW
INTRODUCTION — PART B
BODY PLANES
(IMAGINARY FLAT SURFACES)

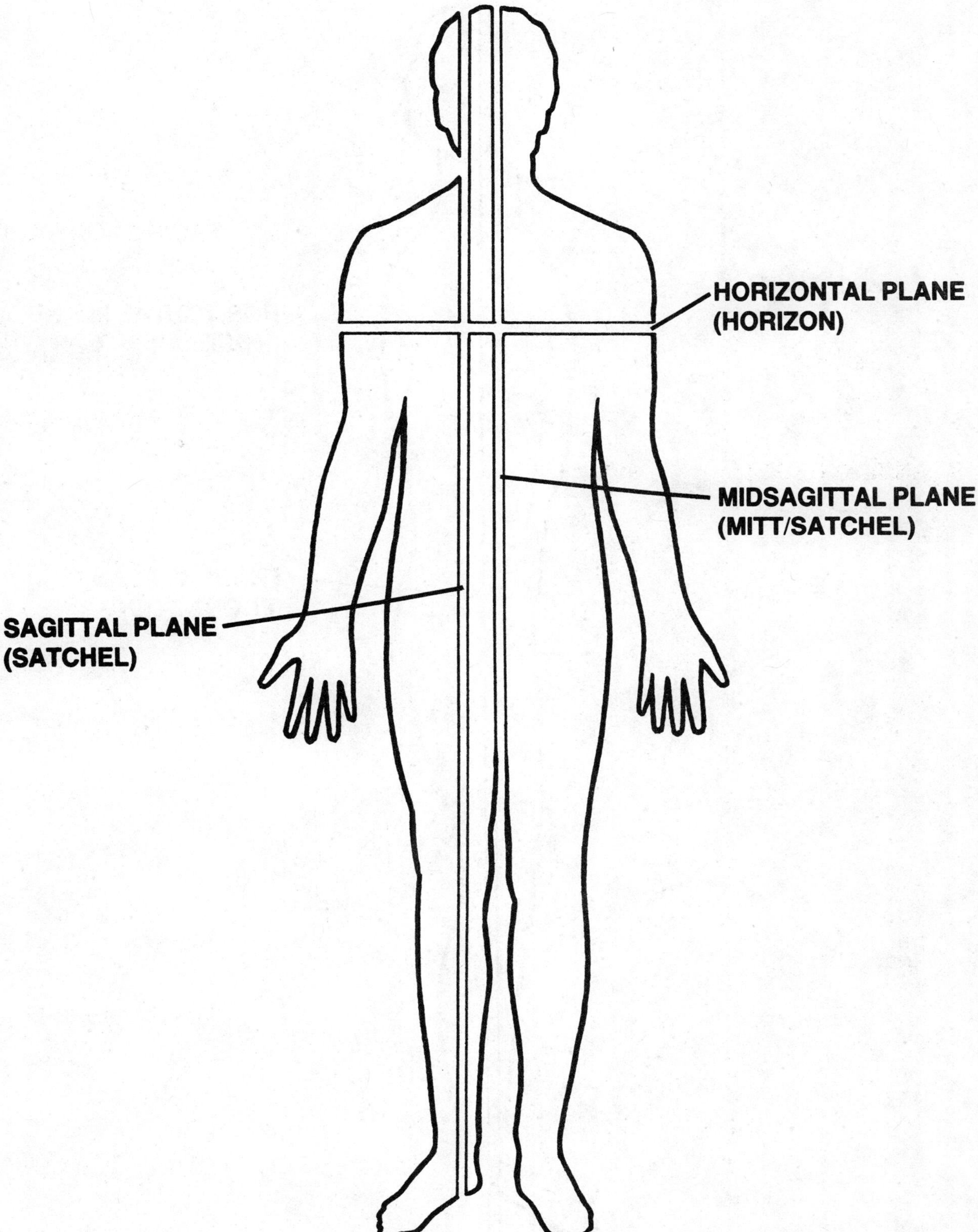

ANTERIOR (FRONT) VIEW

LESSON 1 — REVIEW
INTRODUCTION — PART B
BODY PLANES
(IMAGINARY FLAT SURFACES)

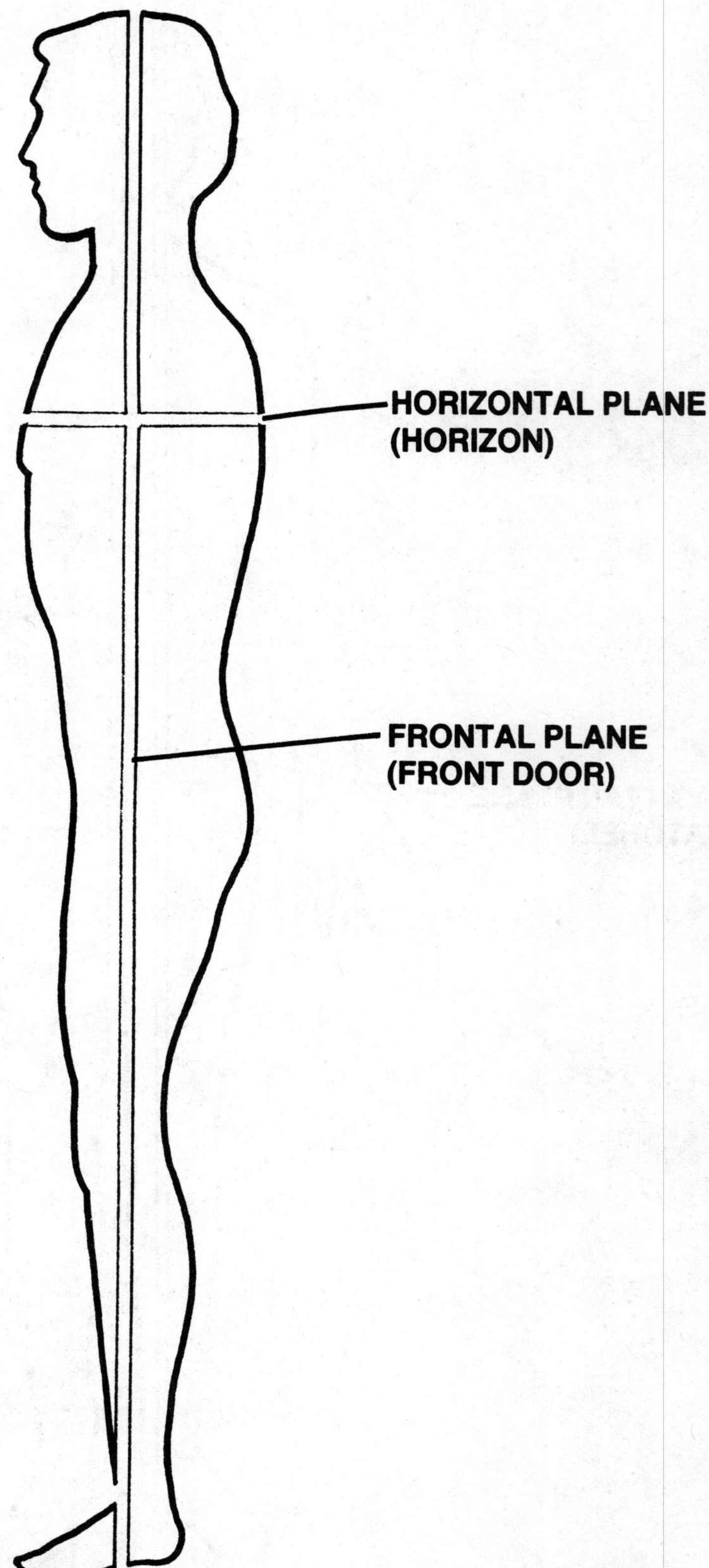

LATERAL (SIDE) VIEW

LESSON 1 — REVIEW
INTRODUCTION — PART B
ABDOMINOPELVIC QUADRANTS

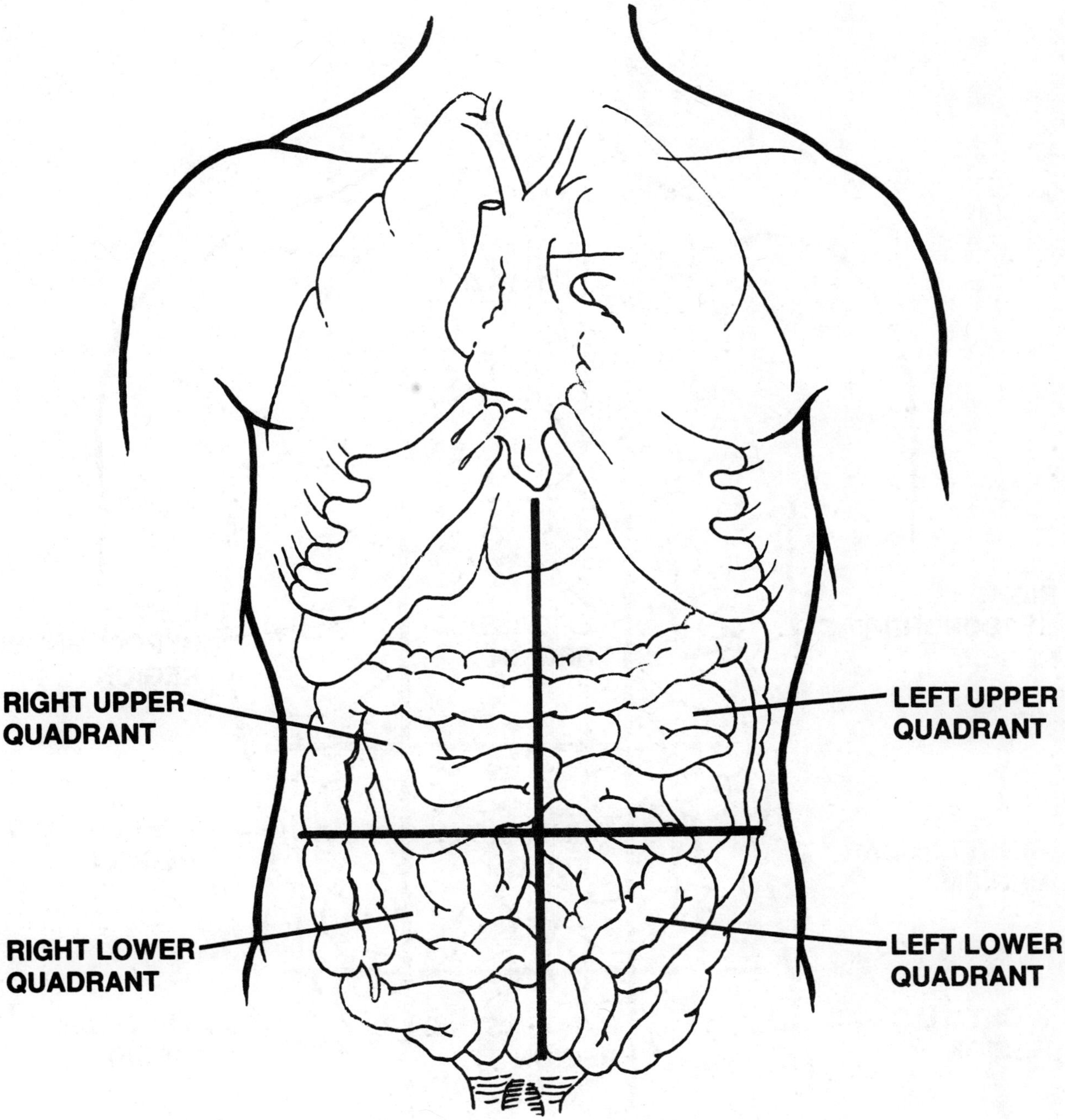

LESSON 1 — REVIEW
INTRODUCTION — PART B
REGIONAL SUBDIVISIONS OF ABDOMINOPELVIC CAVITY

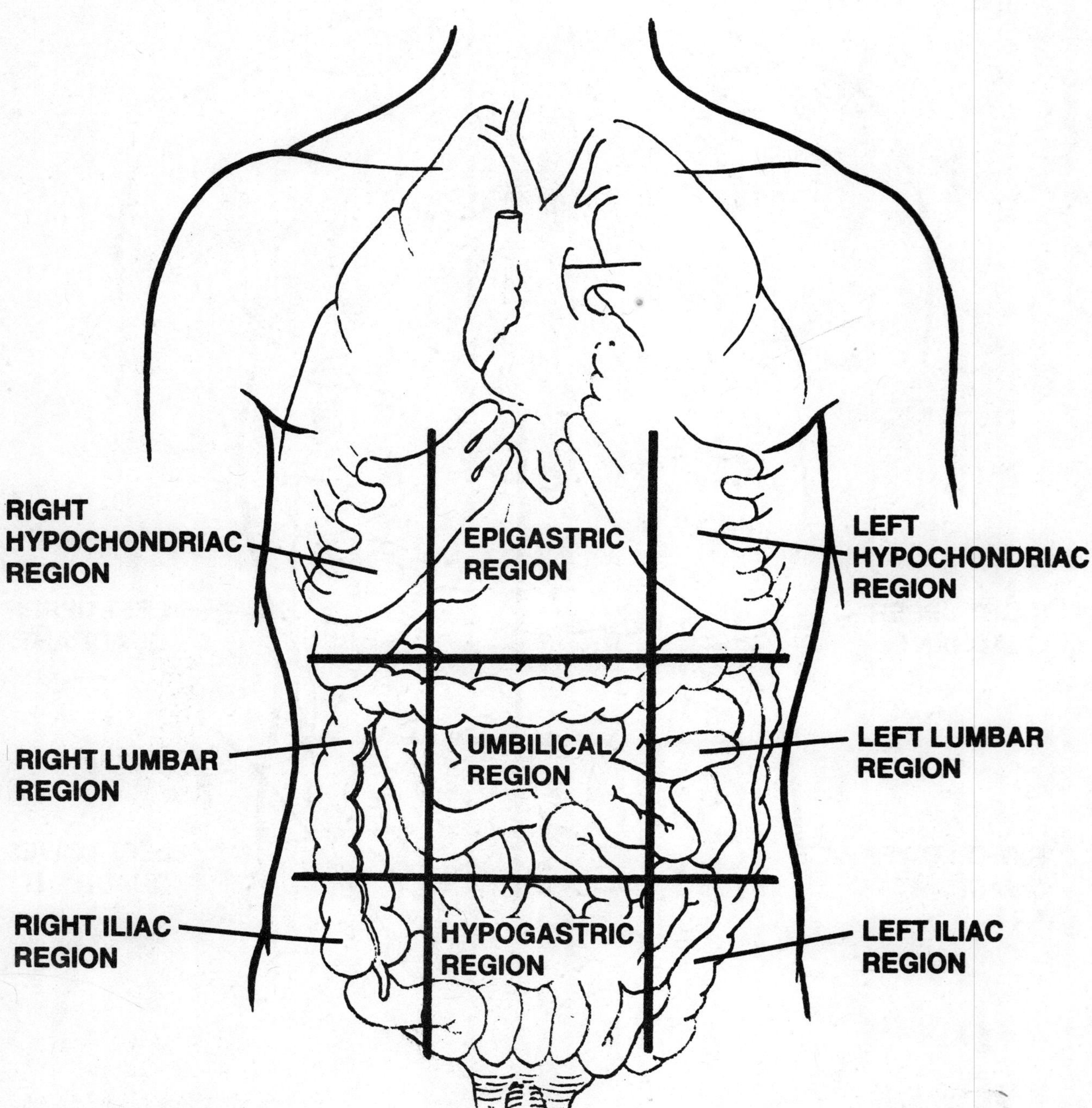

LESSON 1 — REVIEW
INTRODUCTION — PART B
BODY CAVITIES

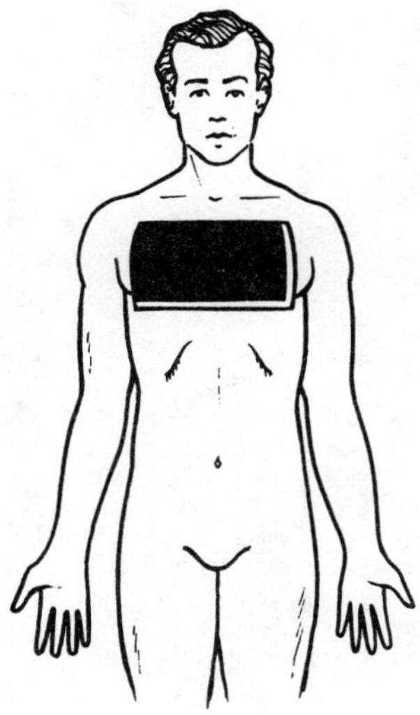

THORACIC CAVITY

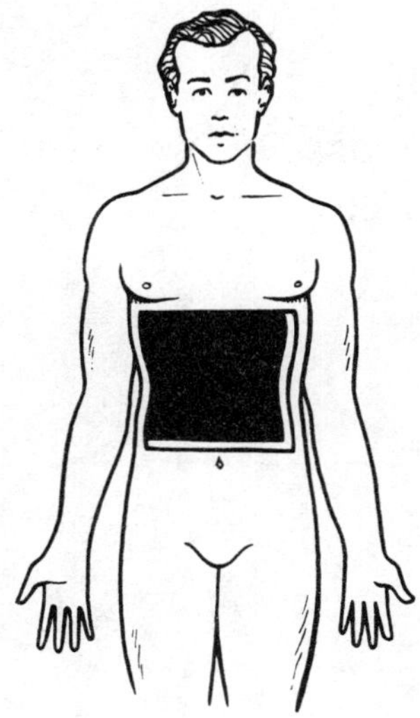

ABDOMINAL CAVITY

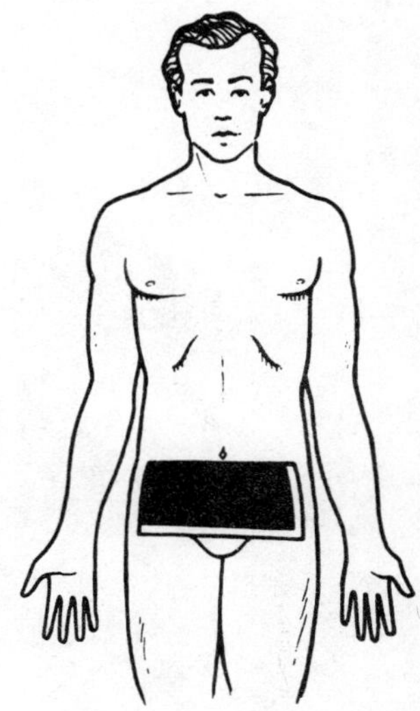

PELVIC CAVITY

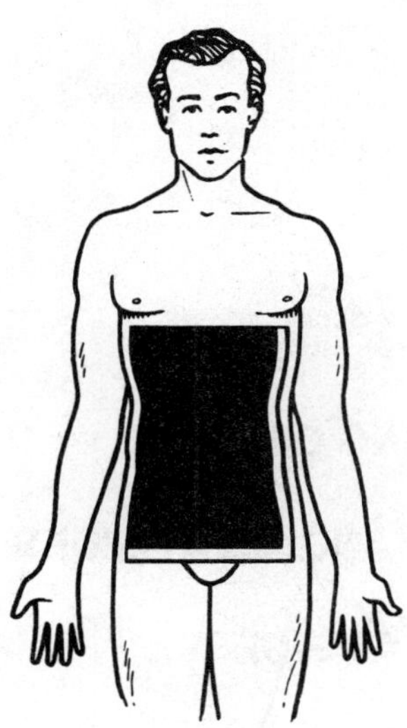

ABDOMINOPELVIC CAVITY

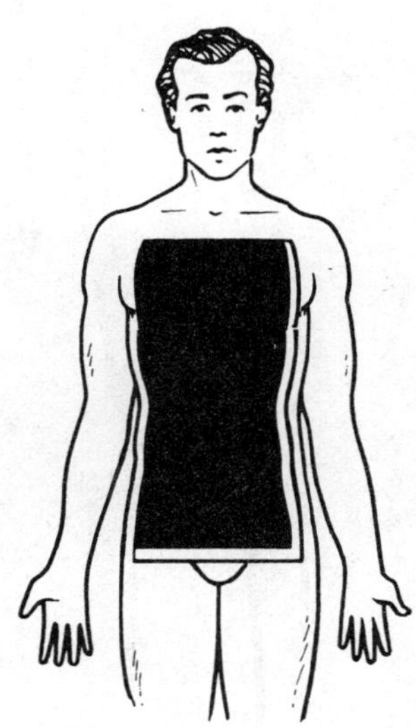

VENTRAL CAVITY

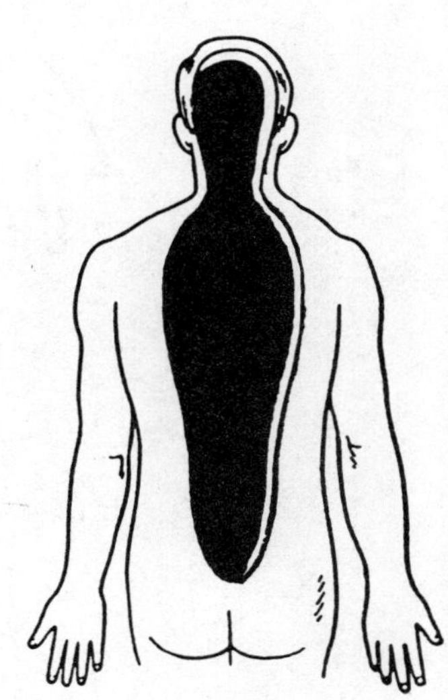

DORSAL CAVITY

LESSON 1 — WORKSHEET
INTRODUCTION — PART B
ANATOMICAL POSITION

PRINT THE CORRECT LETTER WITHIN THE PARENTHESES

1. (E)
2. (H)
3. (B)
4. (G)

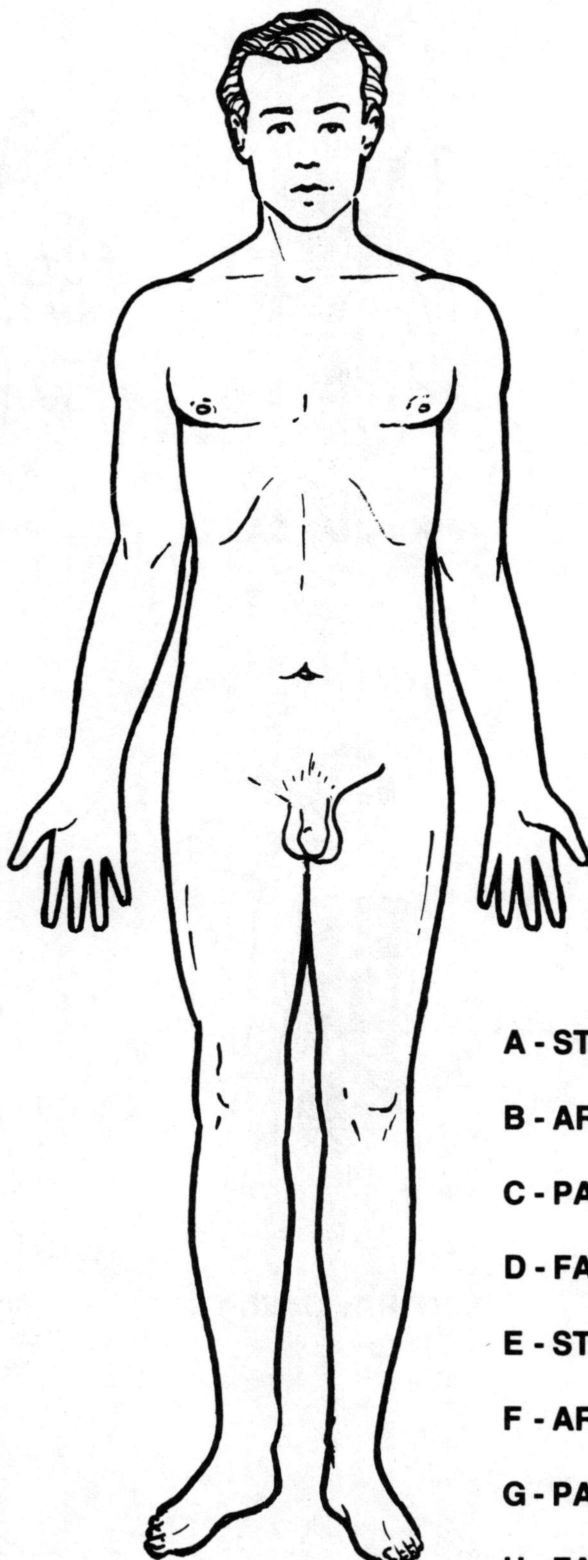

A - STANDING OBLIQUE

B - ARMS HANGING AT SIDES

C - PALMS AT SIDES

D - FACING LATERALLY

E - STANDING ERECT

F - ARMS AT REST

G - PALMS FORWARD

H - FACING FORWARD

LESSON 1 — WORKSHEET
INTRODUCTION — PART B
BODY PLANES

PRINT THE CORRECT LETTER WITHIN THE PARENTHESES

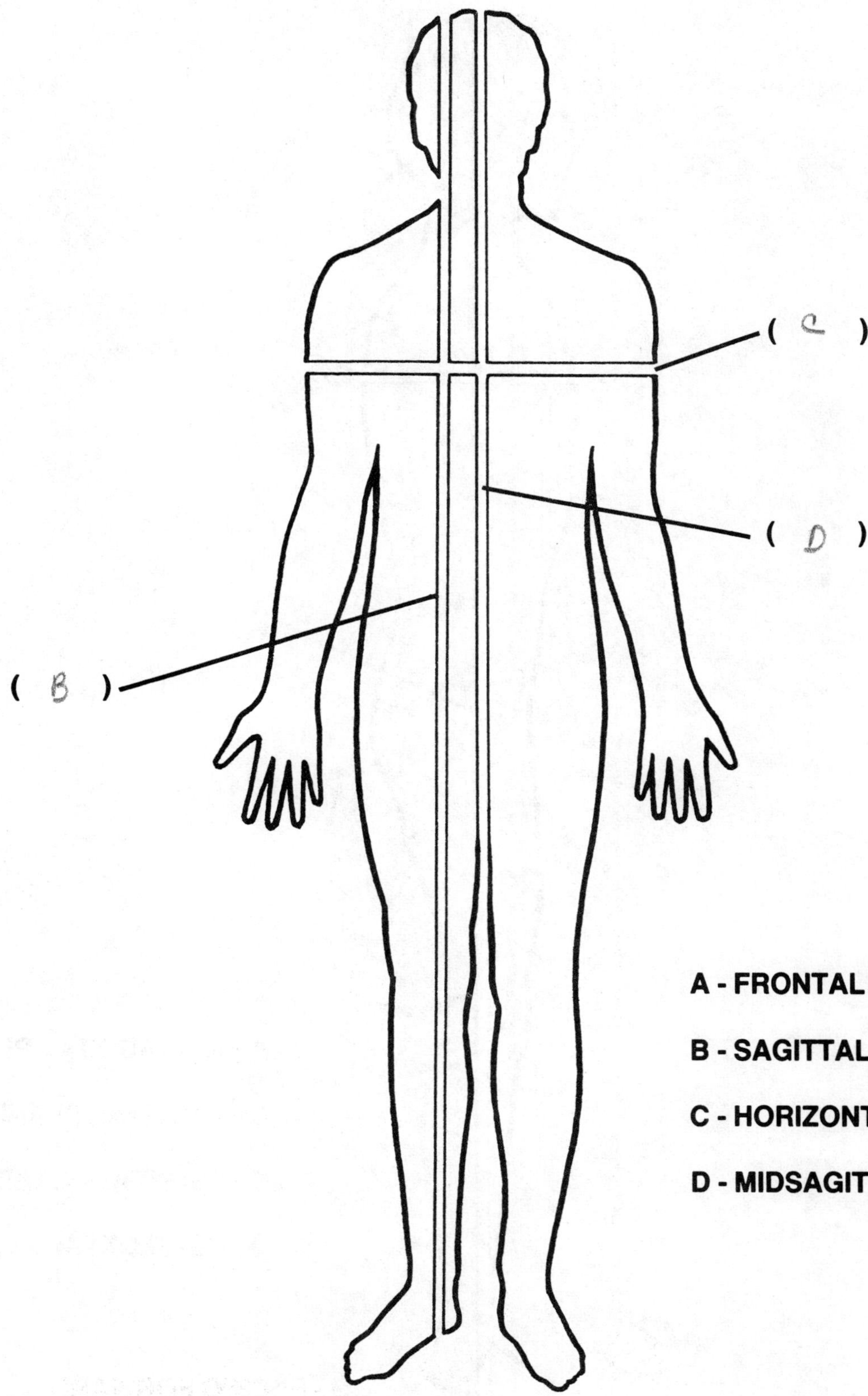

A - FRONTAL PLANE

B - SAGITTAL PLANE

C - HORIZONTAL PLANE

D - MIDSAGITTAL PLANE

LESSON 1 — WORKSHEET
INTRODUCTION — PART B
BODY PLANES

PRINT THE CORRECT LETTER WITHIN THE PARENTHESES

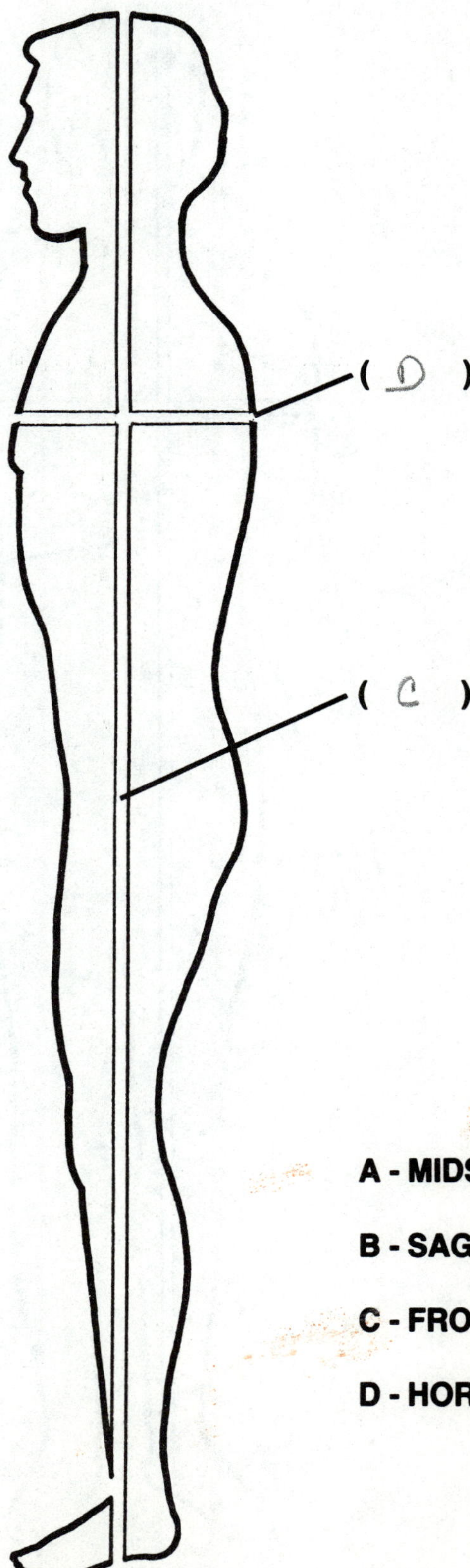

A - MIDSAGITTAL PLANE

B - SAGITTAL PLANE

C - FRONTAL PLANE

D - HORIZONTAL PLANE

LESSON 1 — WORKSHEET
INTRODUCTION — PART B
ABDOMINOPELVIC QUADRANTS

PRINT THE CORRECT LETTER WITHIN THE PARENTHESES

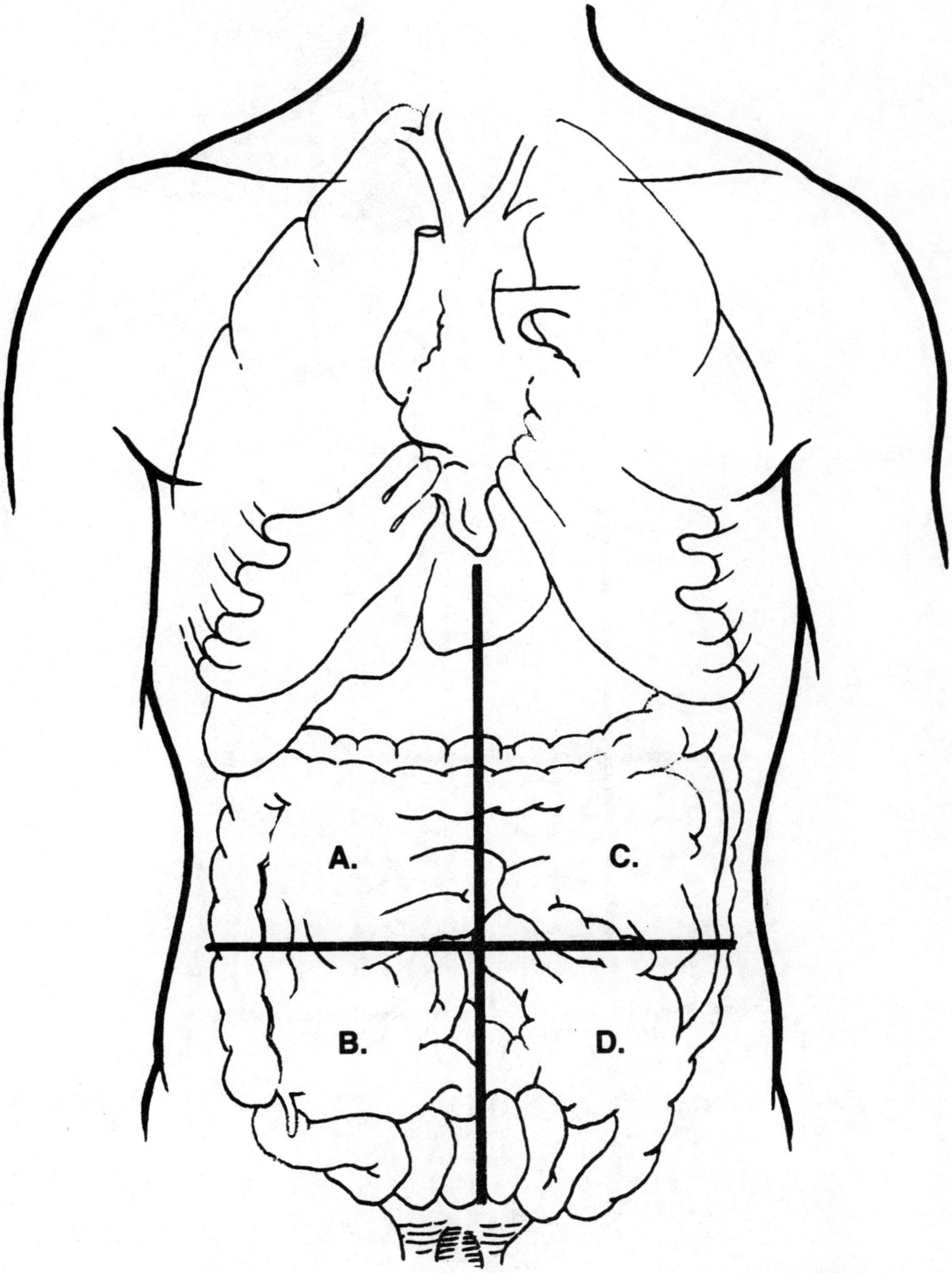

(B) **RIGHT LOWER QUADRANT**

(C) **LEFT UPPER QUADRANT**

(A) **RIGHT UPPER QUADRANT**

(D) **LEFT LOWER QUADRANT**

LESSON 1 — WORKSHEET

INTRODUCTION — PART B

REGIONAL SUBDIVISIONS OF THE ABDOMINOPELVIC CAVITY

PRINT THE CORRECT LETTER WITHIN THE PARENTHESES

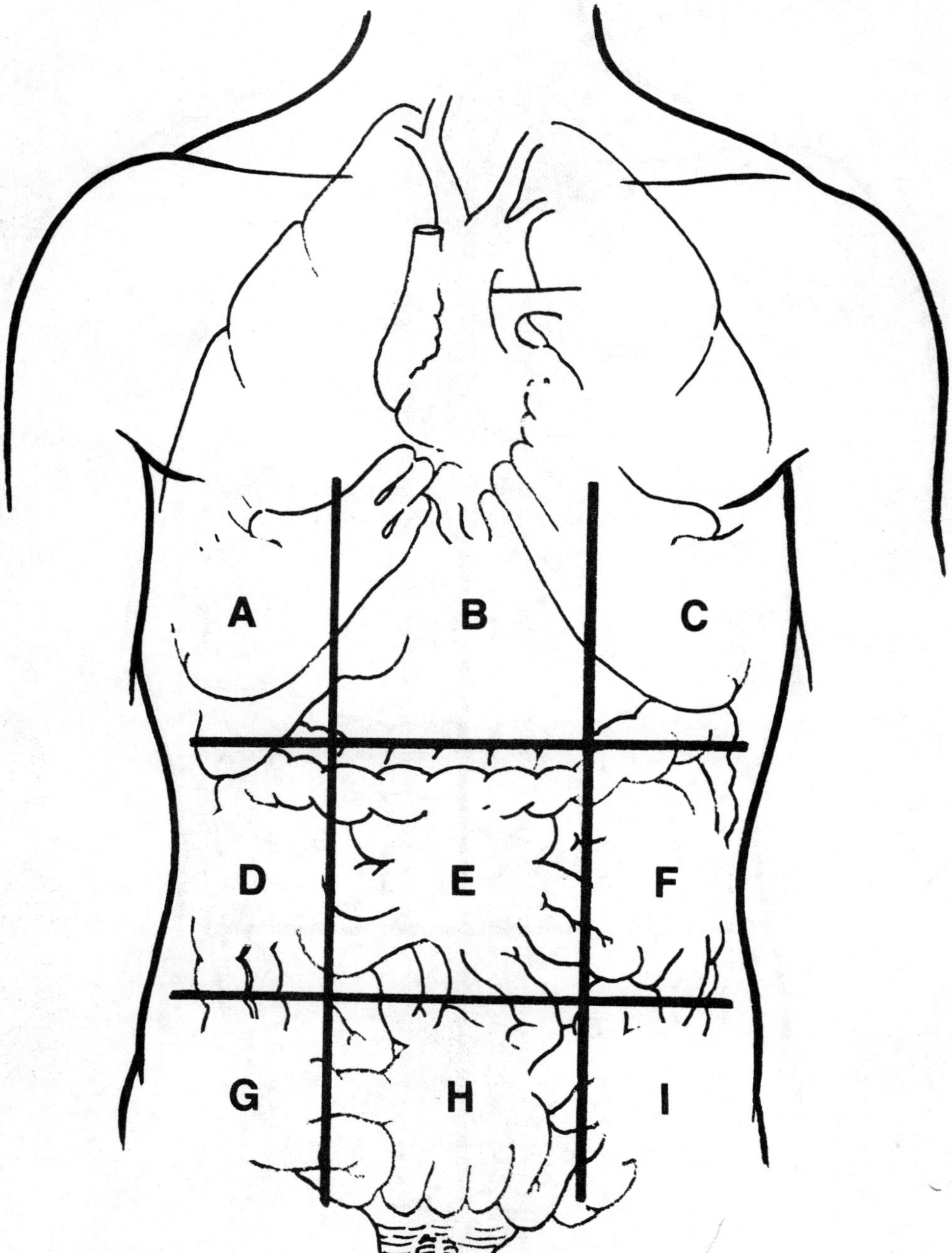

(F) **LEFT LUMBAR REGION**

(A) **RIGHT HYPOCHONDRIAC REGION**

(E) **UMBILICAL REGION**

(B) **EPIGASTRIC REGION**

(G) **LEFT ILIAC REGION**

(C) **LEFT HYPOCHONDRIAC REGION**

(I) **RIGHT ILIAC REGION**

(H) **HYPOGASTRIC REGION**

(D) **RIGHT LUMBAR REGION**

LESSON 1 — WORKSHEET
INTRODUCTION — PART B
BODY CAVITIES

PRINT THE CORRECT LETTER WITHIN THE PARENTHESES

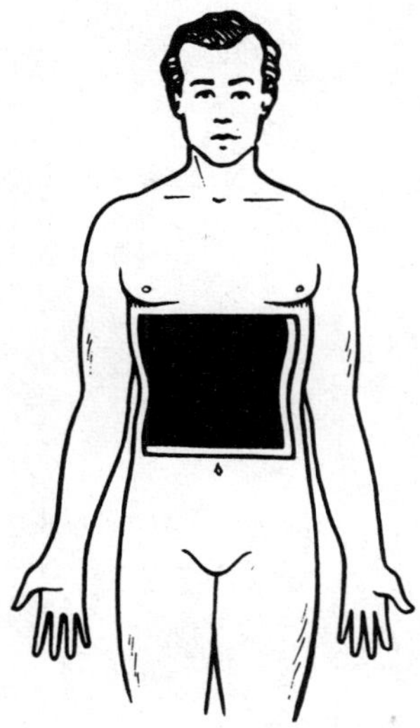

(B)

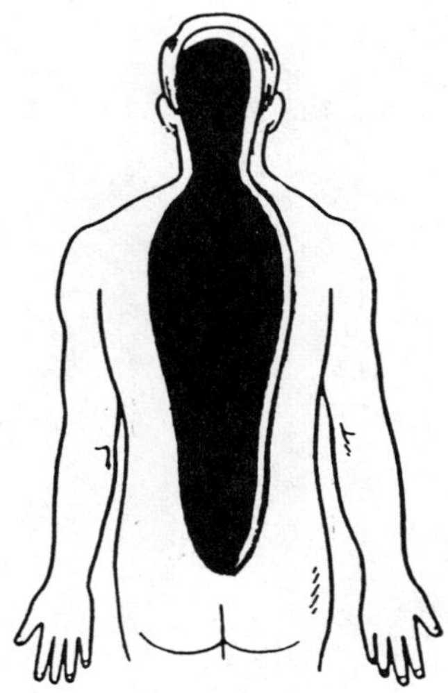

(E)

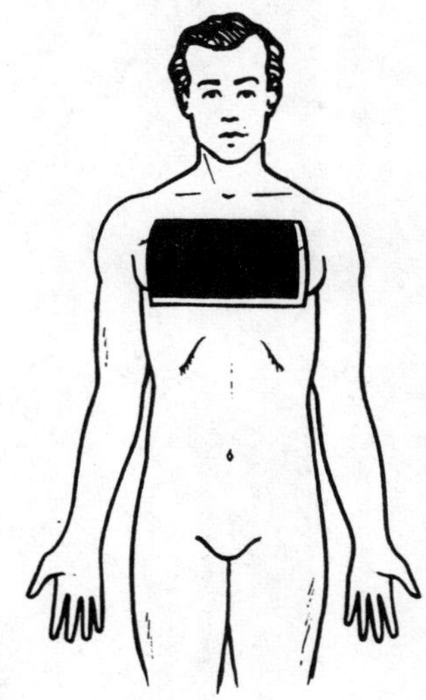

(C)

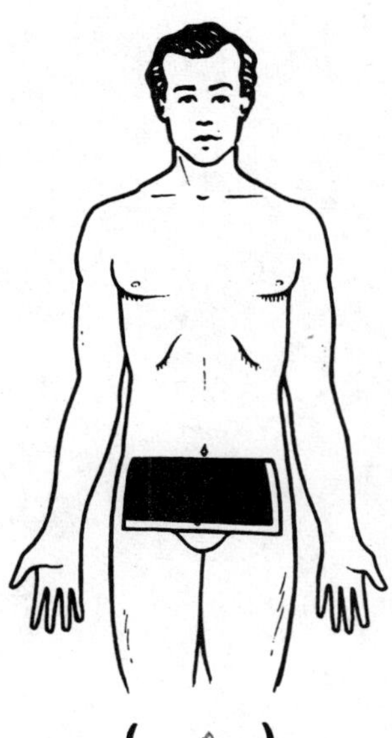

(A)

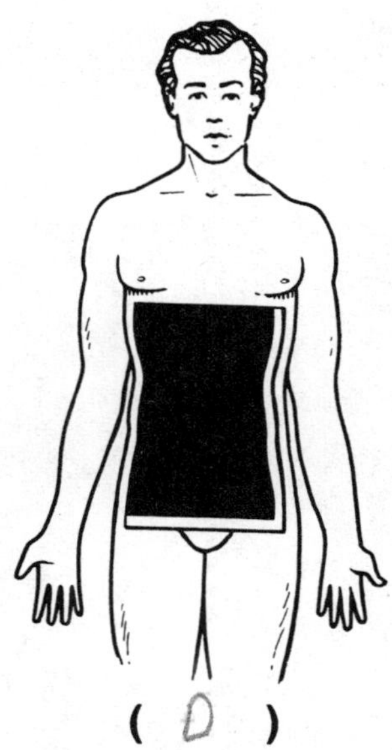

(D)

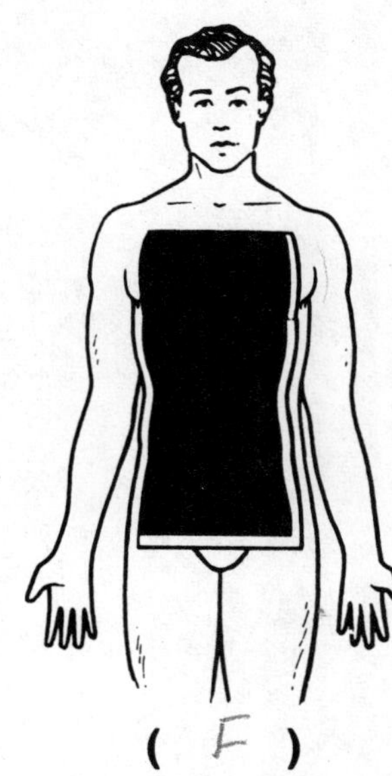

(F)

A - PELVIC CAVITY

B - ABDOMINAL CAVITY

C - THORACIC CAVITY

D - ABDOMINOPELVIC CAVITY

E - DORSAL CAVITY

F - VENTRAL CAVITY

LESSON 2

THE SKELETAL SYSTEM

CRANIUM AND FACE (SKULL)

22 bones

● CRANIUM

8 bones

BONE NAME	NUMBER
FRONTAL	1
PARIETAL	2
OCCIPITAL	1
TEMPORAL	2
SPHENOID	1
ETHMOID	1

● FACE

14 bones

BONE NAME	NUMBER
ZYGOMATIC/MALAR	2
LACRIMAL	2
NASAL	2
VOMER	1
CONCHA	2
PALATINE	2
MAXILLA	2
MANDIBLE	1

REMEMBER!

1st ***Pronounce*** *the name of the body part or term*
2nd ***Recall*** *and* ***pronounce*** *the audionym*
3rd ***For body parts: visualize*** *the audionym in place*
For terms: visualize *the association*
4th ***Pronounce*** *the name of the body part or term again.*

LESSON 2 — REVIEW
THE SKELETAL SYSTEM
THE SKULL
BONES OF THE CRANIUM AND FACE
(22 BONES)

CRANIUM
(8)

BONE	AUDIONYM
FRONTAL	FRONT DOLL
PARIETAL	PARROT
OCCIPITAL	OX
TEMPORAL	TEMPLE
SPHENOID	SPHINX
ETHMOID	A THUMB OILED

FACE
(14)

BONE	AUDIONYM
ZYGOMATIC/MALAR	CYCLEMATIC/MAIL
LACRIMAL	LAKE RIM
NASAL	NASAL SPRAY
VOMER	FOAM
CONCHA	CONE KEY
PALATINE	PILE OF TIN
MAXILLA	MACK TRUCK
MANDIBLE	MAN ON THE BULL

LESSON 2 — REVIEW
THE SKELETAL SYSTEM
THE SKULL
BONES OF THE CRANIUM

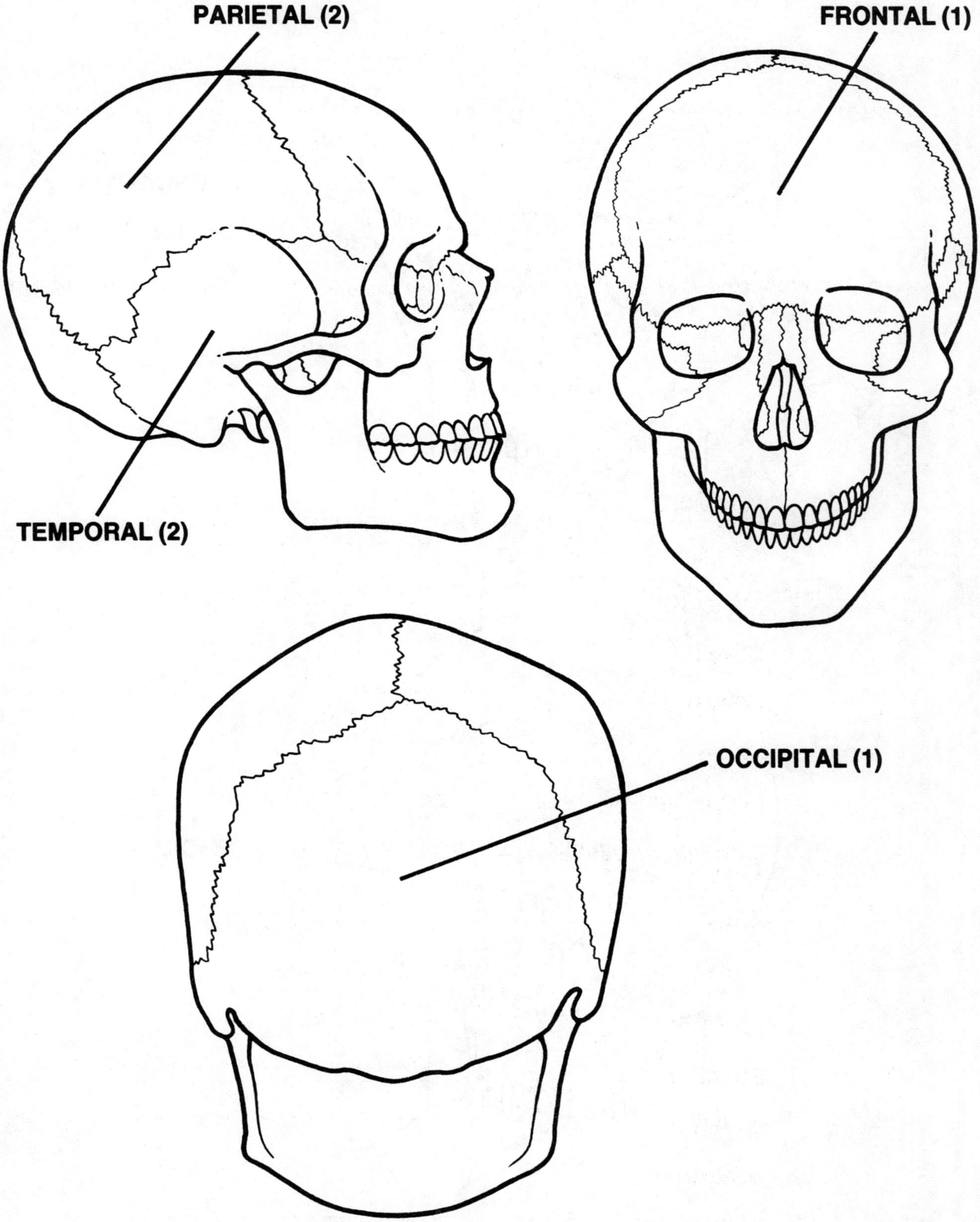

LESSON 2 — REVIEW
THE SKELETAL SYSTEM
THE SKULL
BONES OF THE CRANIUM

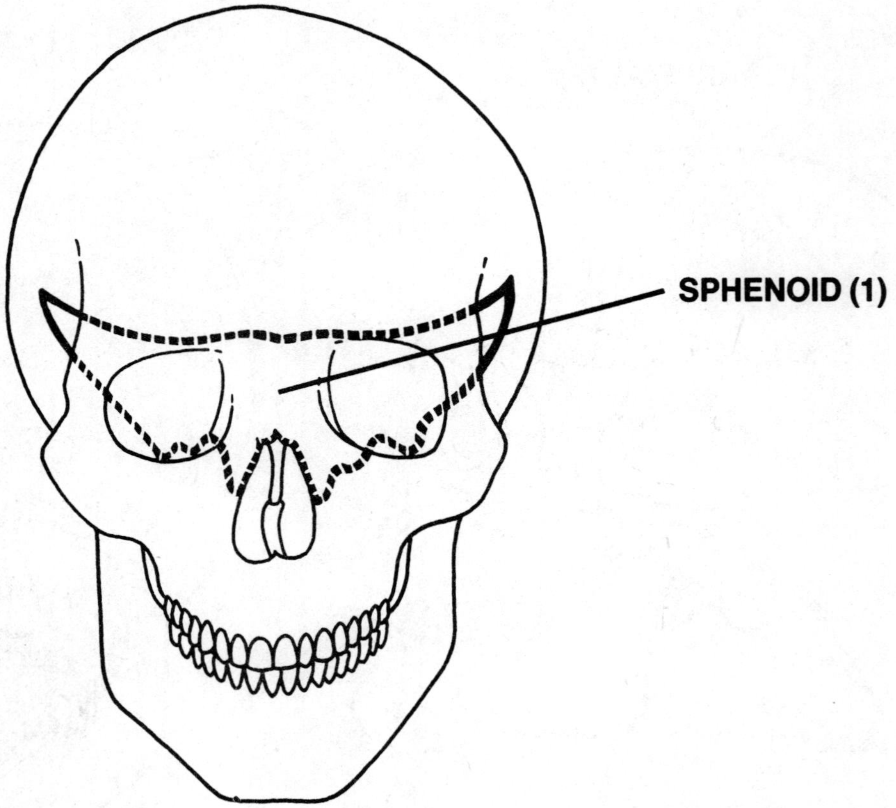

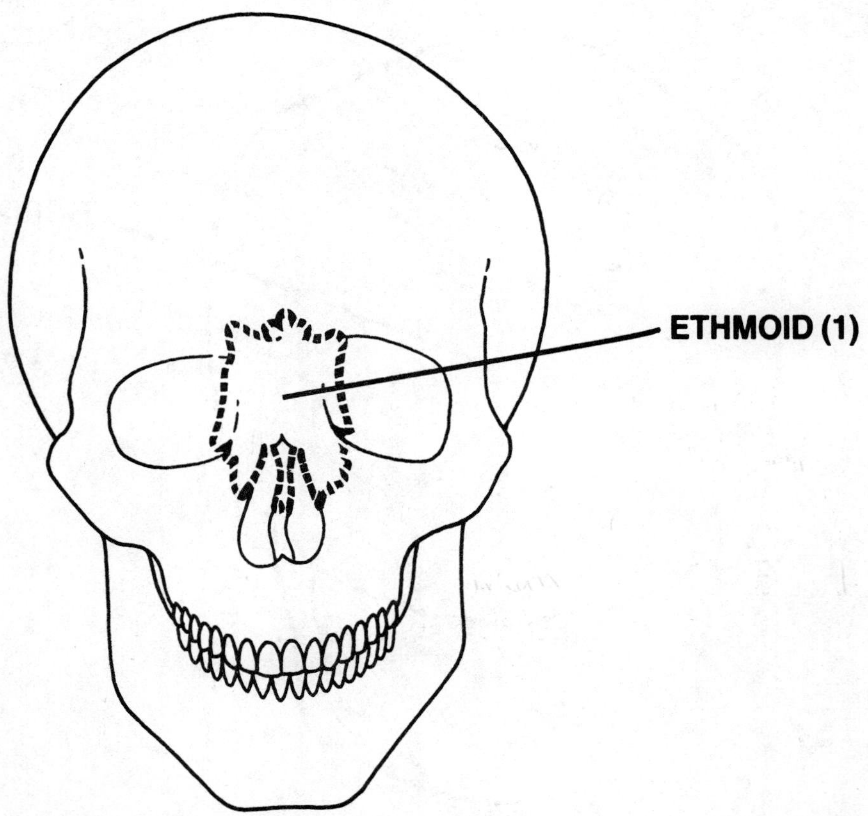

LESSON 2 — REVIEW
THE SKELETAL SYSTEM
THE SKULL
BONES OF THE FACE

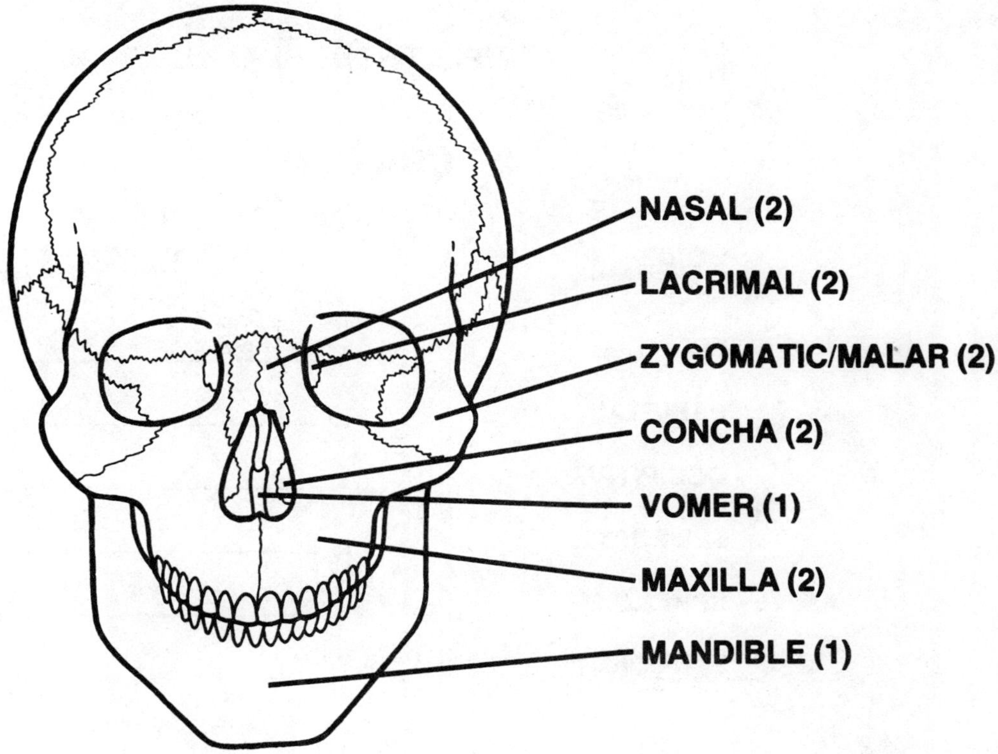

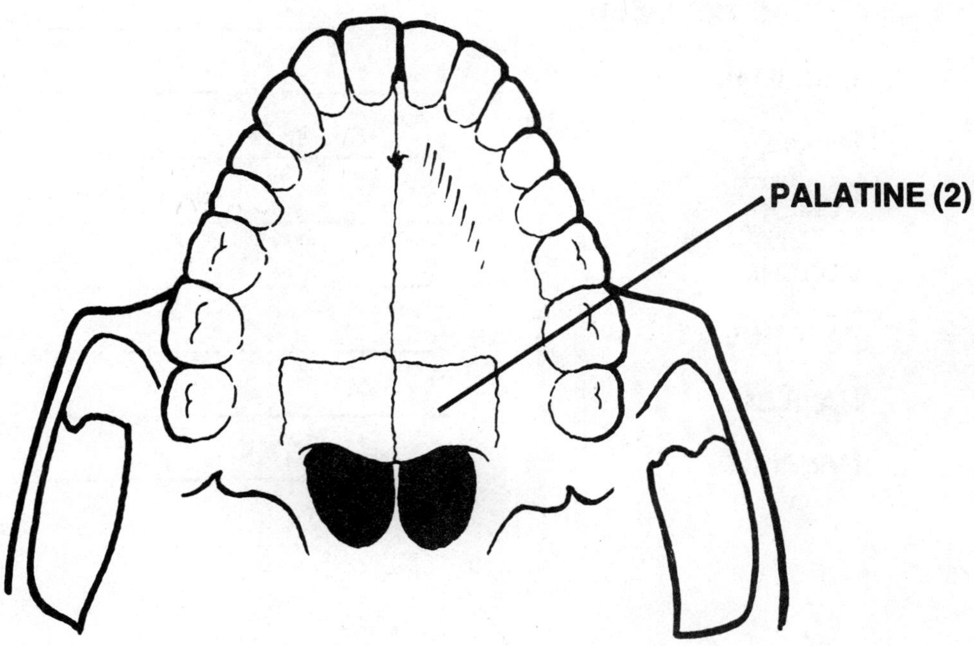

LESSON 2 — WORKSHEET
SKELETAL SYSTEM
CRANIUM AND FACE

COMPLETE THE BLANKS

CRANIUM

BONE	AUDIONYM
FRONTAL	Front doll
PARIETAL	Parrot
OCCIPITAL	ox
TEMPORAL	Temple
SPHENOID	spHinx
ETHMOID	A Thumb oiled

FACE

BONE	AUDIONYM
ZYGOMATIC/MALAR	Cyclematic/Mail
LACRIMAL	Lake Rim
NASAL	Nasel spray
VOMER	Foam
CONCHA	Cone Key
PALATINE	Pile OF Tin
MAXILLA	mack Truck
MANDIBLE	Man on The Bull

LESSON 2 — WORKSHEET
THE SKELETAL SYSTEM
THE SKULL
BONES OF THE CRANIUM

PRINT THE CORRECT LETTER WITHIN THE PARENTHESES

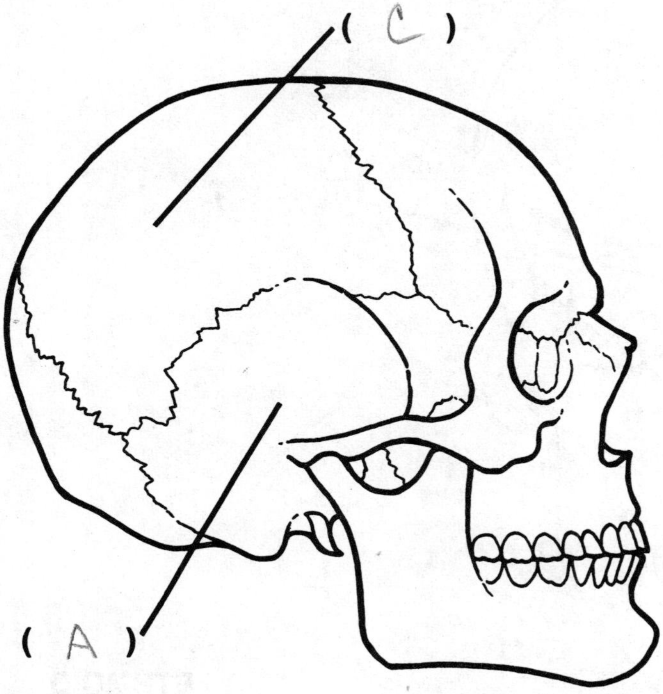

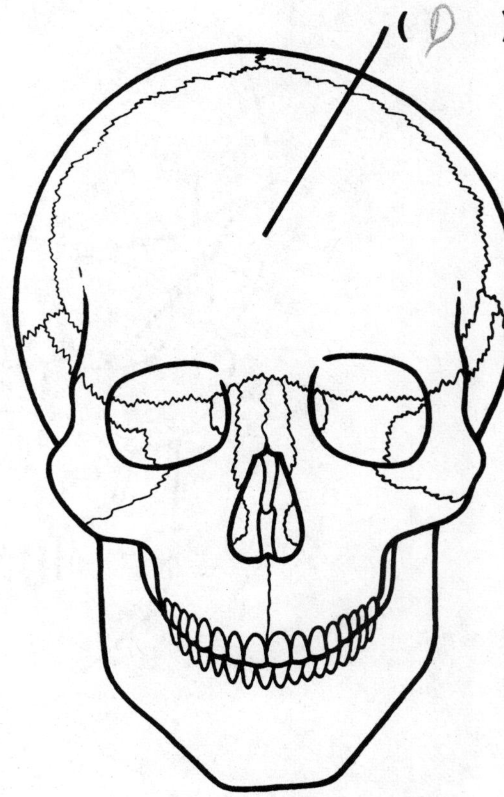

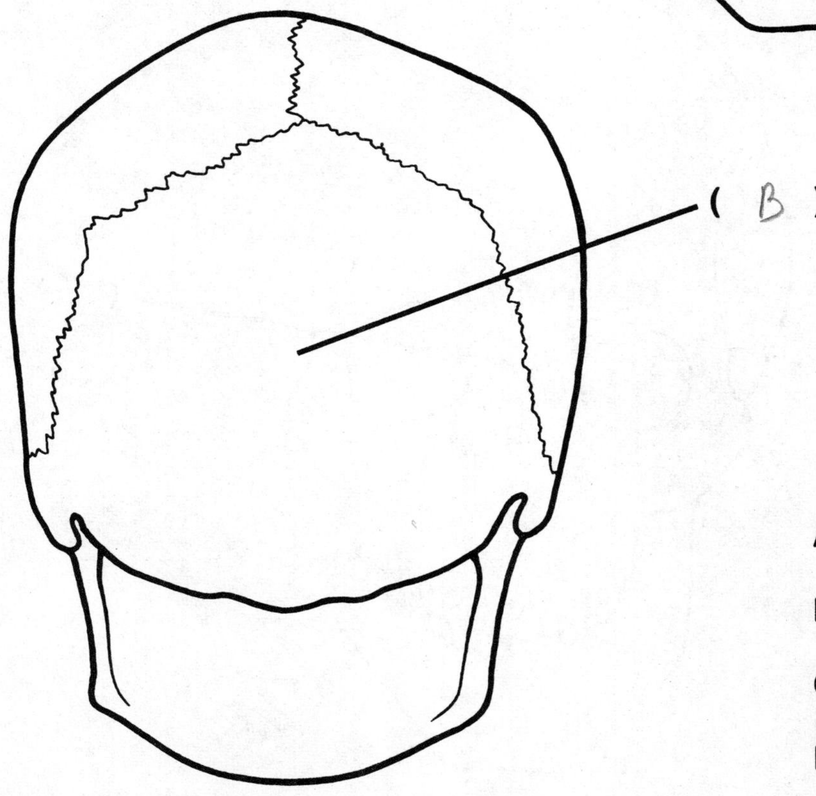

A - TEMPORAL

B - OCCIPITAL

C - PARIETAL

D - FRONTAL

LESSON 2 — WORKSHEET
THE SKELETAL SYSTEM
THE SKULL
BONES OF THE CRANIUM

PRINT THE CORRECT LETTER WITHIN THE PARENTHESES

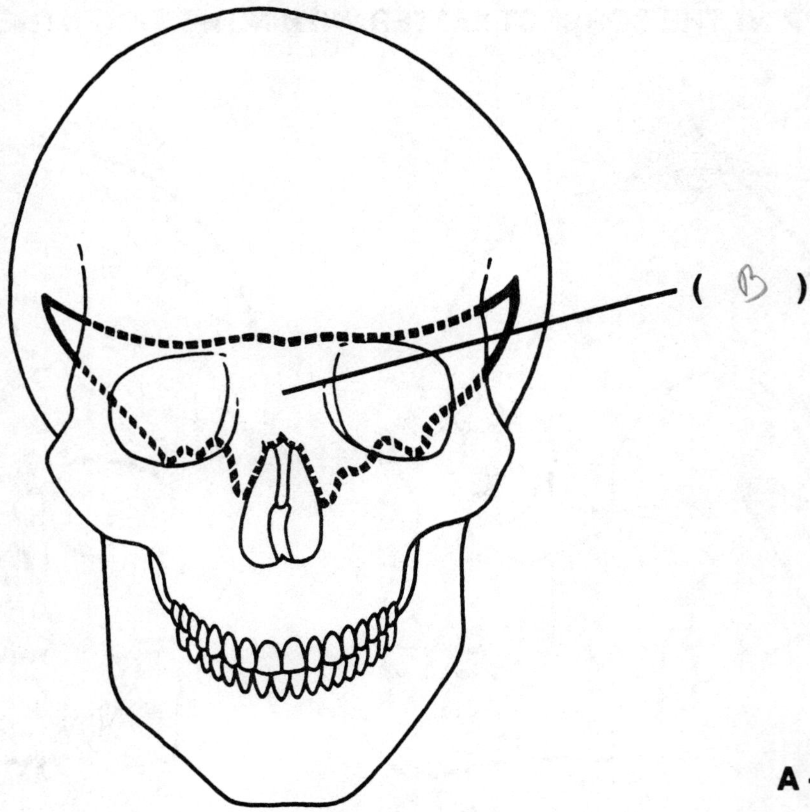

A - ETHMOID

B - SPHENOID

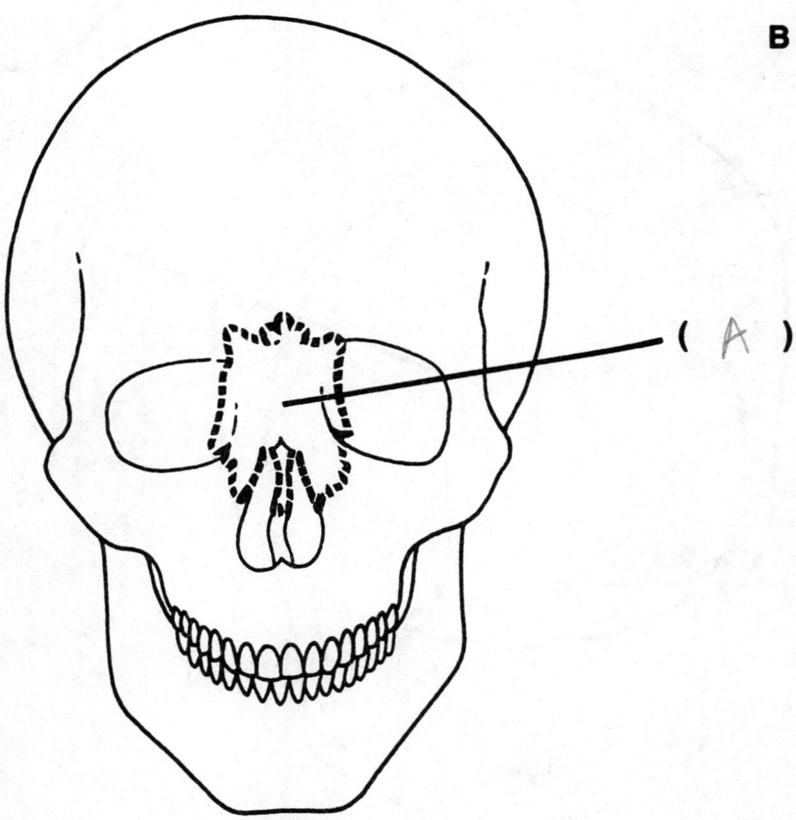

LESSON 2 — WORKSHEET
THE SKELETAL SYSTEM
THE SKULL
BONES OF THE FACE

PRINT THE CORRECT LETTER WITHIN THE PARENTHESES

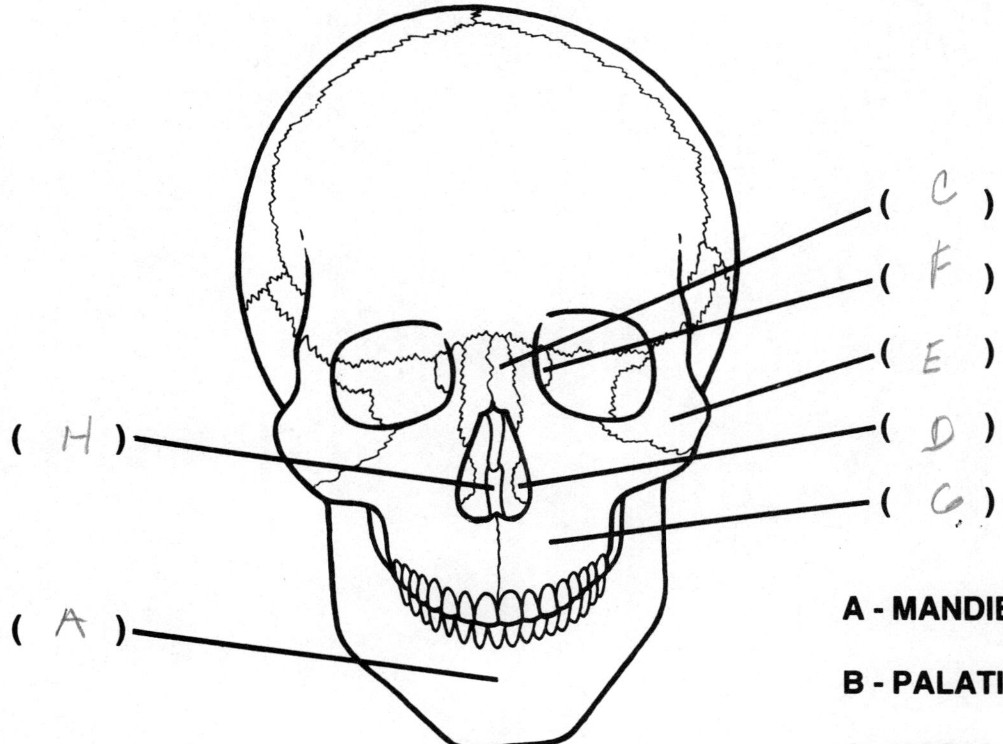

A - MANDIBLE

B - PALATINE

C - NASAL

D - CONCHA

E - ZYGOMATIC/MALAR

F - LACRIMAL

G - MAXILLA

H - VOMER

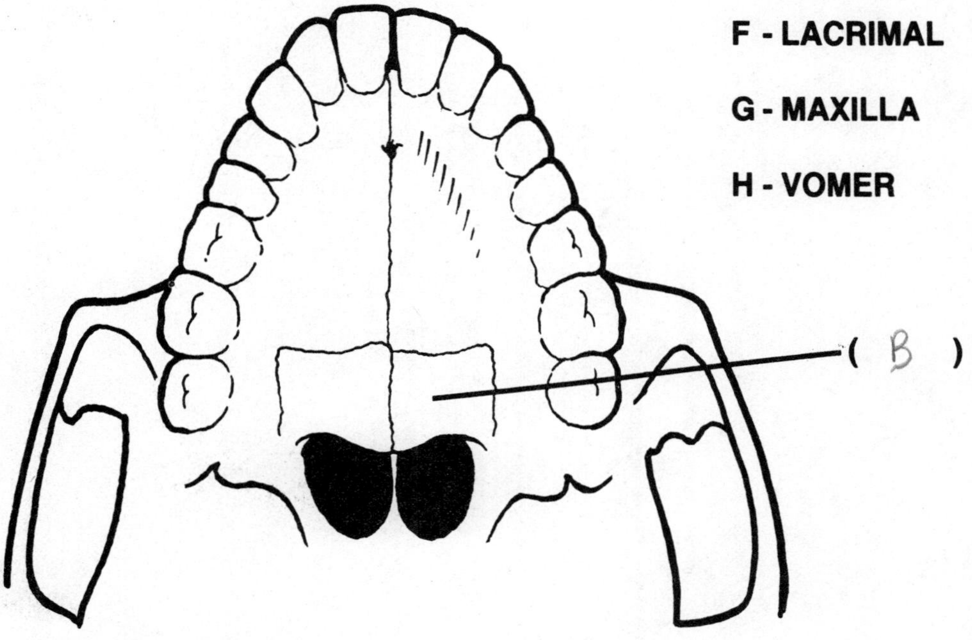

LESSON 3

THE SKELETAL SYSTEM

EAR, NECK, TRUNK

58 bones

EAR

6 bones

BONE NAME	NUMBER (left)	NUMBER (right)
MALLEUS	1	1
INCUS	1	1
STAPES	1	1

NECK

1 bone

BONE NAME	NUMBER
HYOID	1

TRUNK

51 bones

BONE NAME	NUMBER
SEVEN CERVICAL (VERTEBRAE)	7
TWELVE THORACIC (VERTEBRAE)	12
FIVE LUMBAR (VERTEBRAE)	5
SACRUM	1
COCCYX	1
RIBS	24 (12 pairs)
STERNUM	1

REMEMBER!

1st ***Pronounce*** *the name of the body part or term*
2nd ***Recall*** *and* ***pronounce*** *the audionym*
3rd ***For body parts: visualize*** *the audionym in place*
For terms: visualize *the association*
4th ***Pronounce*** *the name of the body part or term again.*

LESSON 3 — REVIEW
THE SKELETAL SYSTEM
EAR, NECK, TRUNK

EAR

COMMON NAME	VISUAL IMAGE/ASSOCIATION	BONE
HAMMER	MOLASSES	MALLEUS
ANVIL	INKS	INCUS
STIRRUP	STAPLES	STAPES

NECK

BONE	AUDIONYM
HYOID	HIDE

TRUNK

BONE	AUDIONYM
SEVEN CERVICAL	SEVEN-UP/SURF BOARD
TWELVE THORACIC	TWO ELVES - DRAWER/AX
FIVE LUMBAR	FIFE LUMBER
SACRUM	SACK OF RUM
COCCYX	COGS
RIBS	RIBS
STERNUM	STEERING WHEEL

LESSON 3 — REVIEW
THE SKELETAL SYSTEM
BONES OF THE EAR

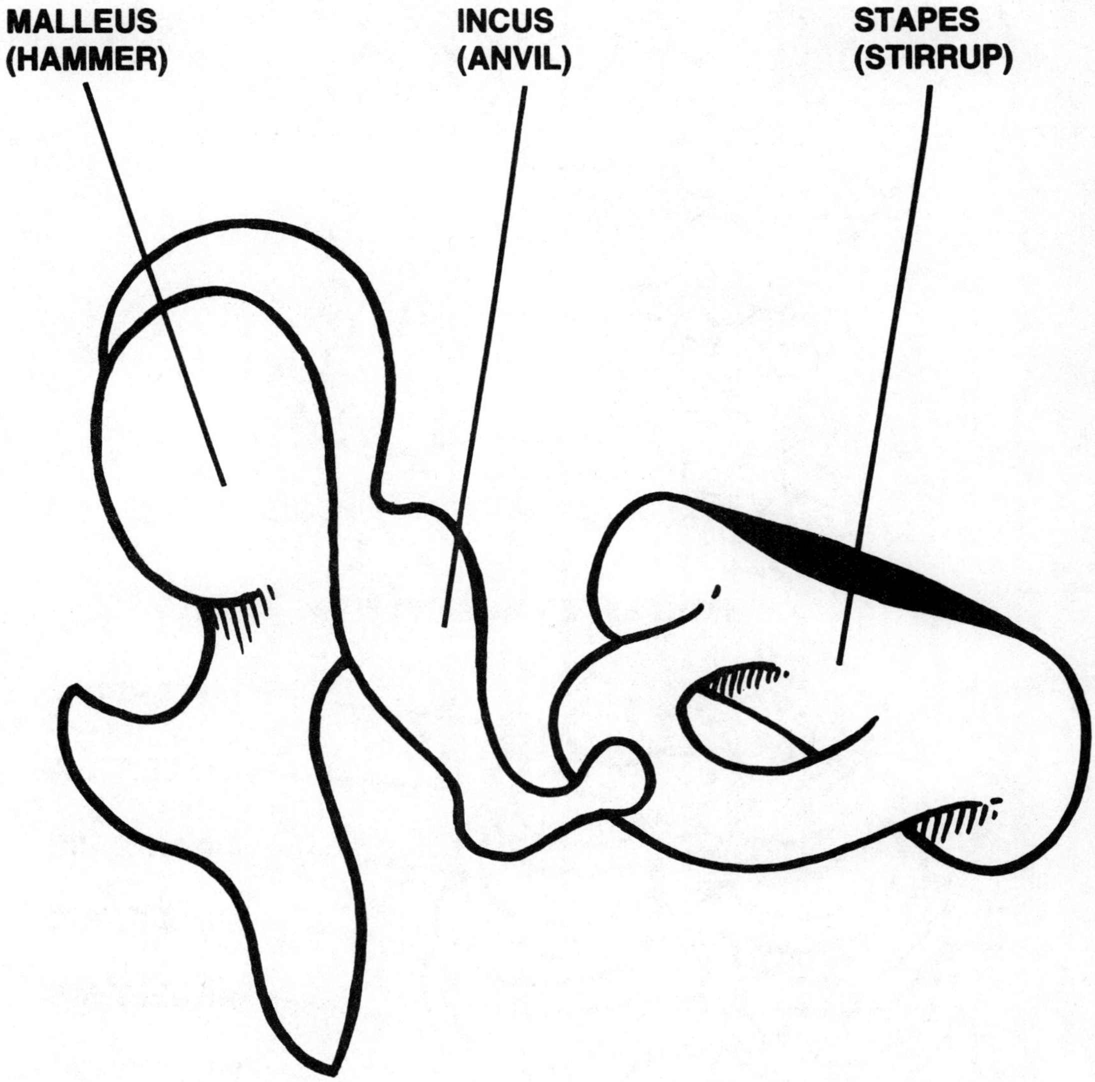

LESSON 3 — REVIEW
THE SKELETAL SYSTEM
BONES OF THE NECK AND TRUNK

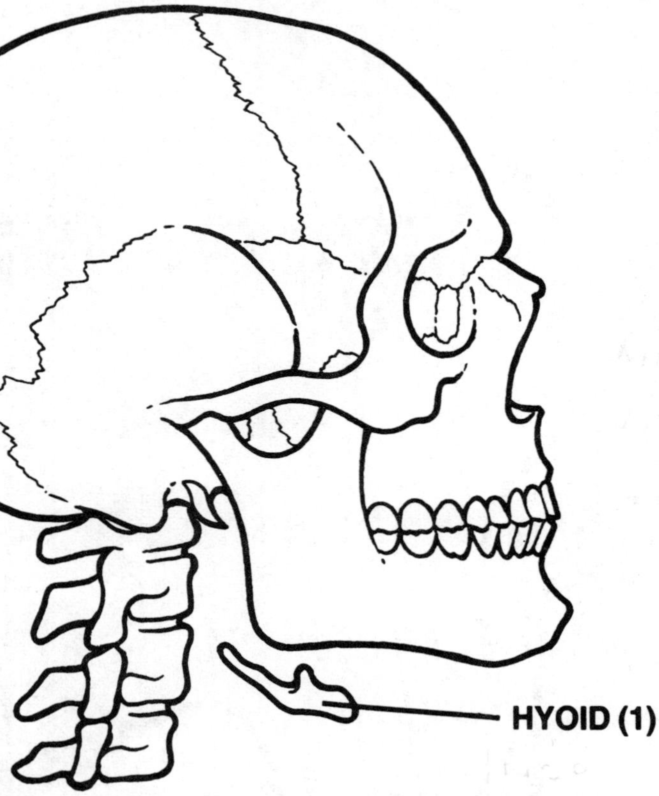

RIGHT LATERAL (SIDE) VIEW

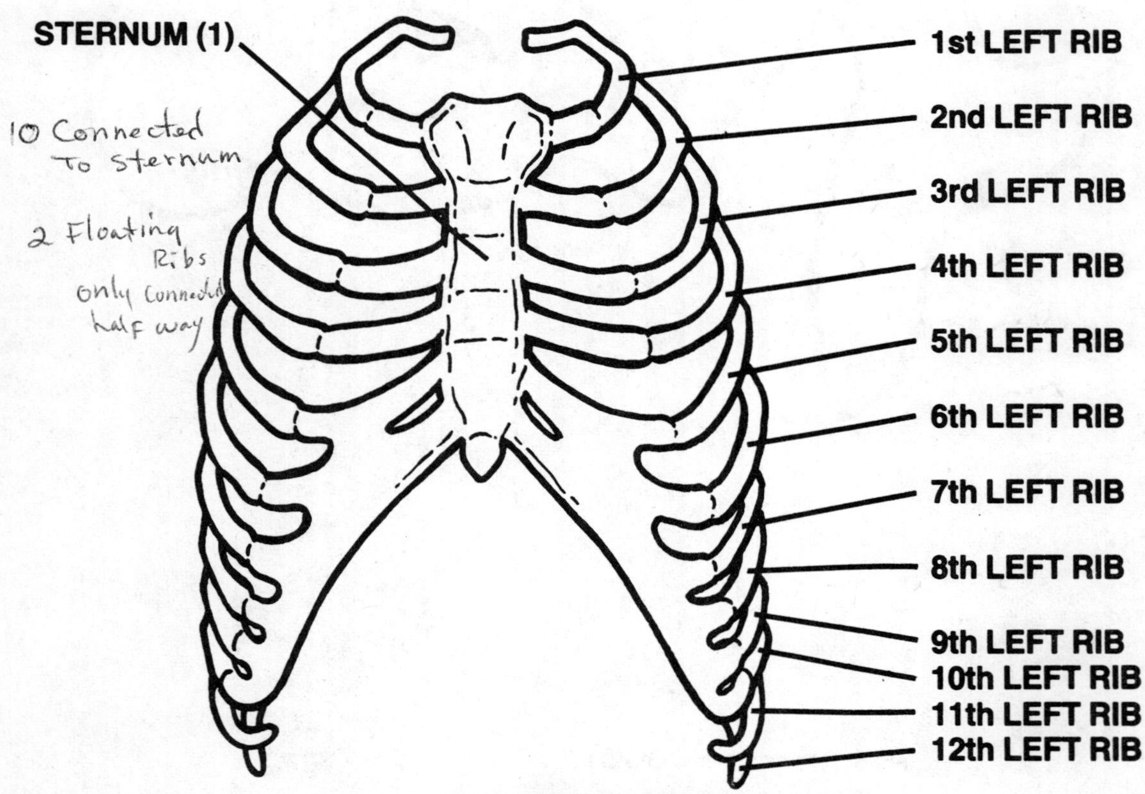

ANTERIOR (FRONT) VIEW

LESSON 3 — REVIEW
THE SKELETAL SYSTEM
BONES OF THE TRUNK
THE VERTEBRAL COLUMN
(THE SPINAL VERTEBRAE)

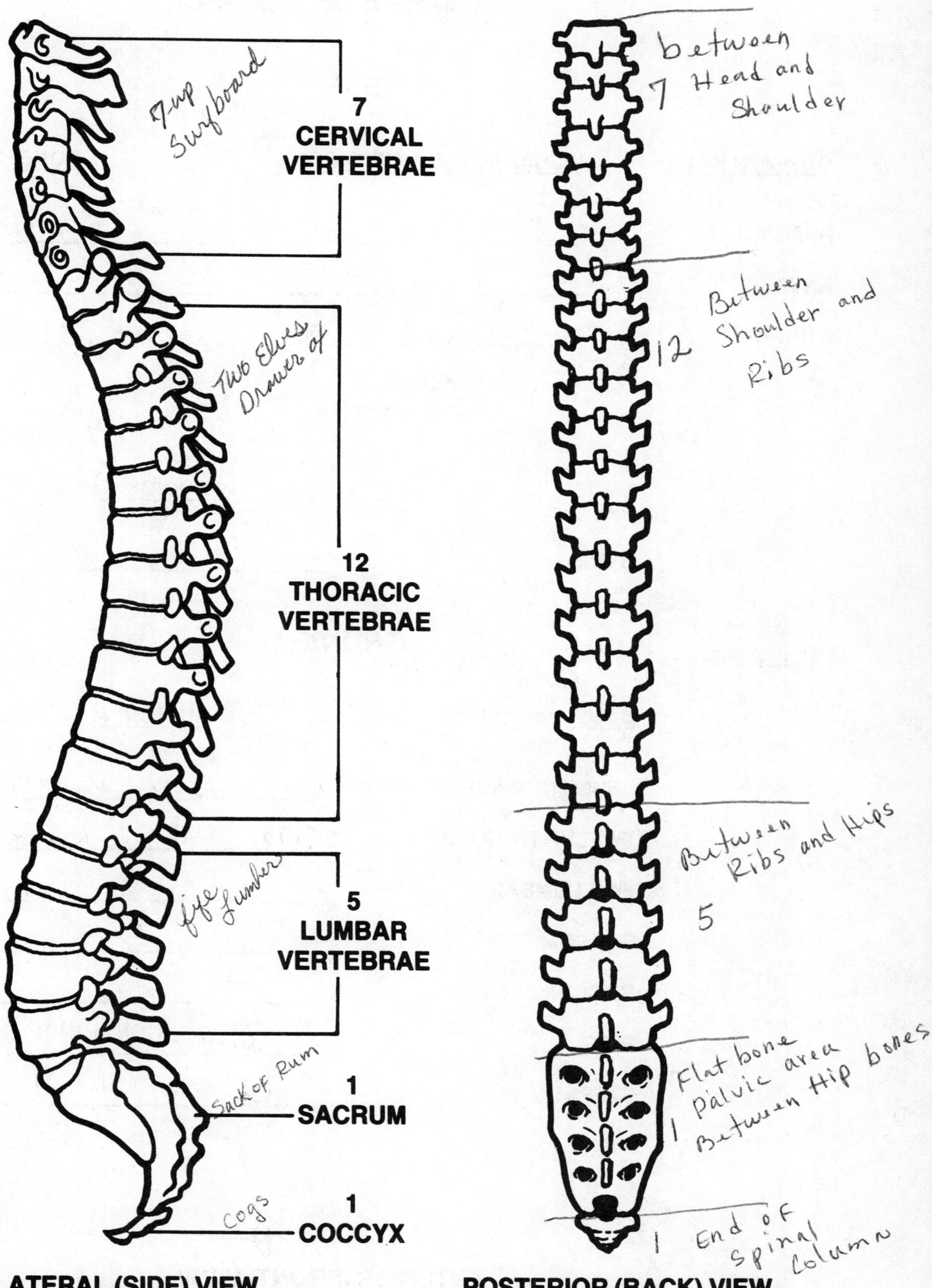

LATERAL (SIDE) VIEW **POSTERIOR (BACK) VIEW**

ME

LESSON 3 — WORKSHEET
THE SKELETAL SYSTEM
EAR, NECK, TRUNK

COMPLETE THE BLANKS

EAR

COMMON NAME	VISUAL IMAGE (AUDIONYM)	BONE
HAMMER	Molasses	Malleus
ANVIL	inks	Incus
STIRRUP	Staples	stapes

NECK

BONE	AUDIONYM
HYOID	Hide

TRUNK

BONE	AUDIONYM
SEVEN CERVICAL	Seven up/ Surf board
TWELVE THORACIC	Two Elves Drawer ax
FIVE LUMBAR	Fife Lumber
SACRUM	Sack of Rum
COCCYX	Cogs
RIBS	Ribs (COMMON TERM)
STERNUM	Steering wheel

LESSON 3 — WORKSHEET
THE SKELETAL SYSTEM
BONES OF THE EAR

PRINT THE CORRECT LETTER WITHIN THE PARENTHESES

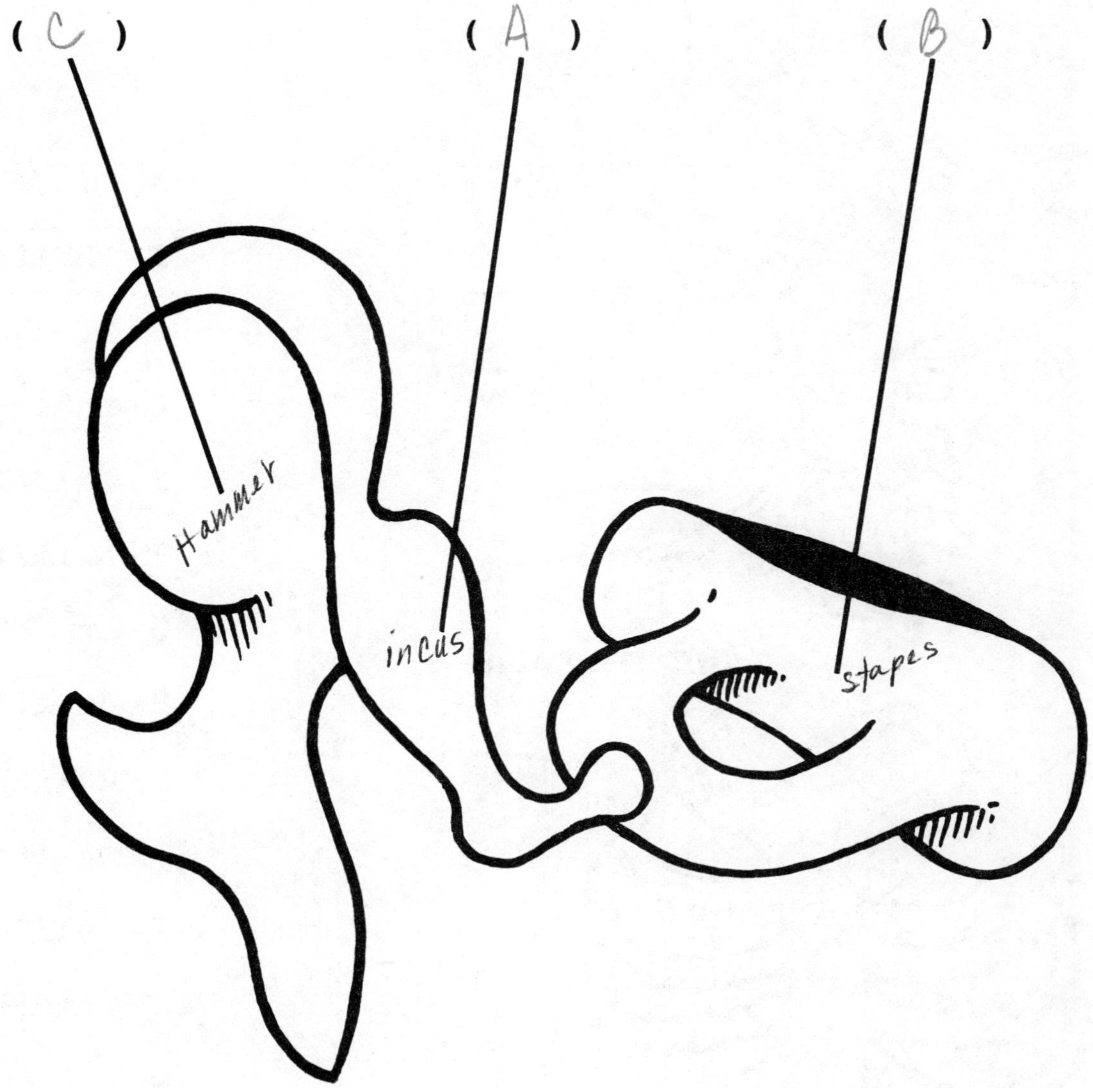

A - INCUS (ANVIL)

B - STAPES (STIRRUP)

C - MALLEUS (HAMMER)

LESSON 3 — WORKSHEET
THE SKELETAL SYSTEM
BONES OF THE NECK AND TRUNK

PRINT THE CORRECT LETTER WITHIN THE PARENTHESES

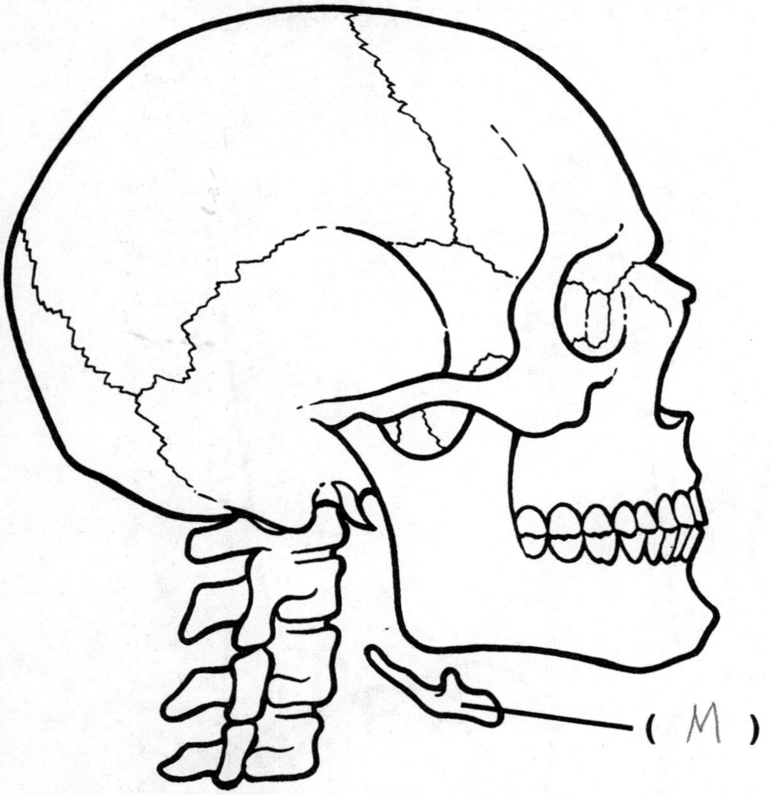

RIGHT LATERAL (SIDE) VIEW

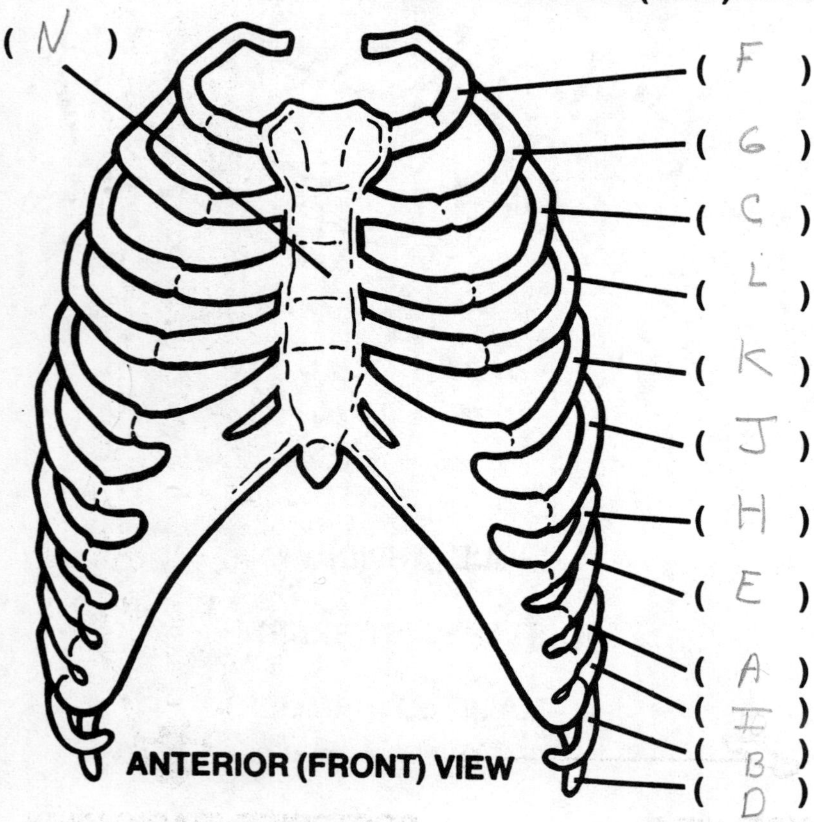

ANTERIOR (FRONT) VIEW

- A - 9th LEFT RIB
- B - 11th LEFT RIB
- C - 3rd LEFT RIB
- D - 12th LEFT RIB
- E - 8th LEFT RIB
- F - 1st LEFT RIB
- G - 2nd LEFT RIB
- H - 7th LEFT RIB
- I - 10th LEFT RIB
- J - 6th LEFT RIB
- K - 5th LEFT RIB
- L - 4th LEFT RIB
- M - HYOID
- N - STERNUM

LESSON 3 — WORKSHEET
THE SKELETAL SYSTEM
BONES OF THE TRUNK
THE VERTEBRAL COLUMN
(THE SPINAL VERTEBRAE)

PRINT THE CORRECT LETTER WITHIN THE PARENTHESES

(D) — COCCYX

(C) — CERVICAL VERTEBRAE

(B) — SACRUM

(E) — LUMBAR VERTEBRAE

(A) — THORACIC VERTEBRAE

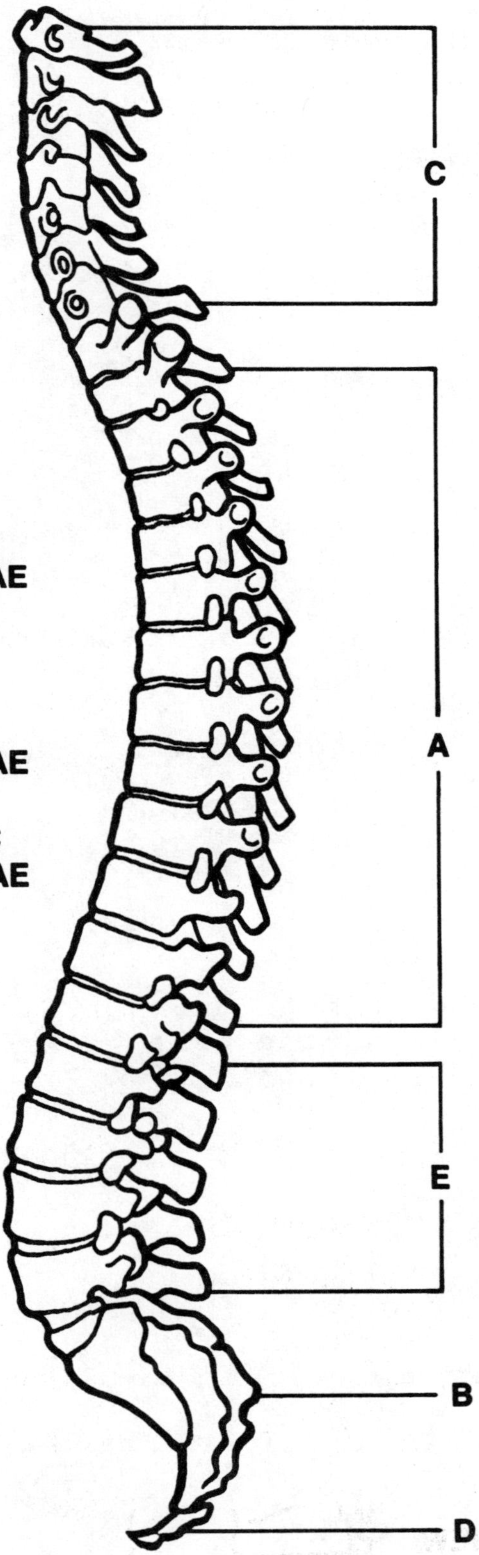

LATERAL (SIDE) VIEW

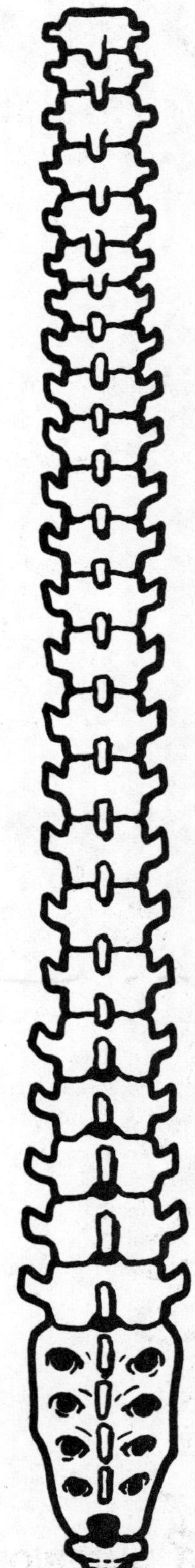

POSTERIOR (BACK) VIEW

LESSON 4

THE SKELETAL SYSTEM

UPPER AND LOWER EXTREMITIES

126 BONES

- **UPPER EXTREMITIES**

  64 bones

BONE NAME	NUMBER (left)	(right)
CLAVICLE	1	1
SCAPULA	1	1
HUMERUS	1	1
ULNA	1	1
RADIUS	1	1
CARPALS	8	8
METACARPALS	5	5
PHALANGES	14	14

- **LOWER EXTREMITIES**

  62 bones

BONE NAME	NUMBER (left)	(right)
HIP	1	1
FEMUR	1	1
PATELLA	1	1
TIBIA	1	1
FIBULA	1	1
TARSALS	7	7
METATARSALS	5	5
PHALANGES	14	14

IMPORTANT:

AN OPTIONAL INDIVIDUALIZED INSTRUCTION SECTION THAT TEACHES THE NAMES AND LOCATIONS OF THE INDIVIDUAL CARPAL AND TARSAL BONES APPEARS AT THE BACK OF THIS WORKBOOK.

REMEMBER!

1st ***Pronounce*** *the name of the body part or term*
2nd ***Recall*** *and* ***pronounce*** *the audionym*
3rd ***For body parts: visualize*** *the audionym in place*
For terms: visualize *the association*
4th ***Pronounce*** *the name of the body part or term again.*

LESSON 4 — REVIEW
THE SKELETAL SYSTEM
UPPER AND LOWER EXTREMITIES
(126 BONES)

UPPER
(64 BONES)

BONE	AUDIONYM
CLAVICLE	CLAY VEHICLE
SCAPULA	SKI CAP
HUMERUS	HAMMER
ULNA	ALL NUTS
RADIUS	RADIO
CARPALS	CARPETS
METACARPALS	METAL CARPETS
PHALANGES	FOIL HINGES

LOWER
(62 BONES)

BONE	AUDIONYM
HIP	HIP
FEMUR	FEMALE
PATELLA	PAD "L"
TIBIA	TEEPEE
FIBULA	FIBERGLASS
TARSALS	TAR SOLES
METATARSALS	METAL TAR SOLES
PHALANGES	FOIL HINGES

LESSON 4 — REVIEW
THE SKELETAL SYSTEM
BONES OF THE UPPER AND LOWER EXTREMITIES

RIGHT **LEFT**

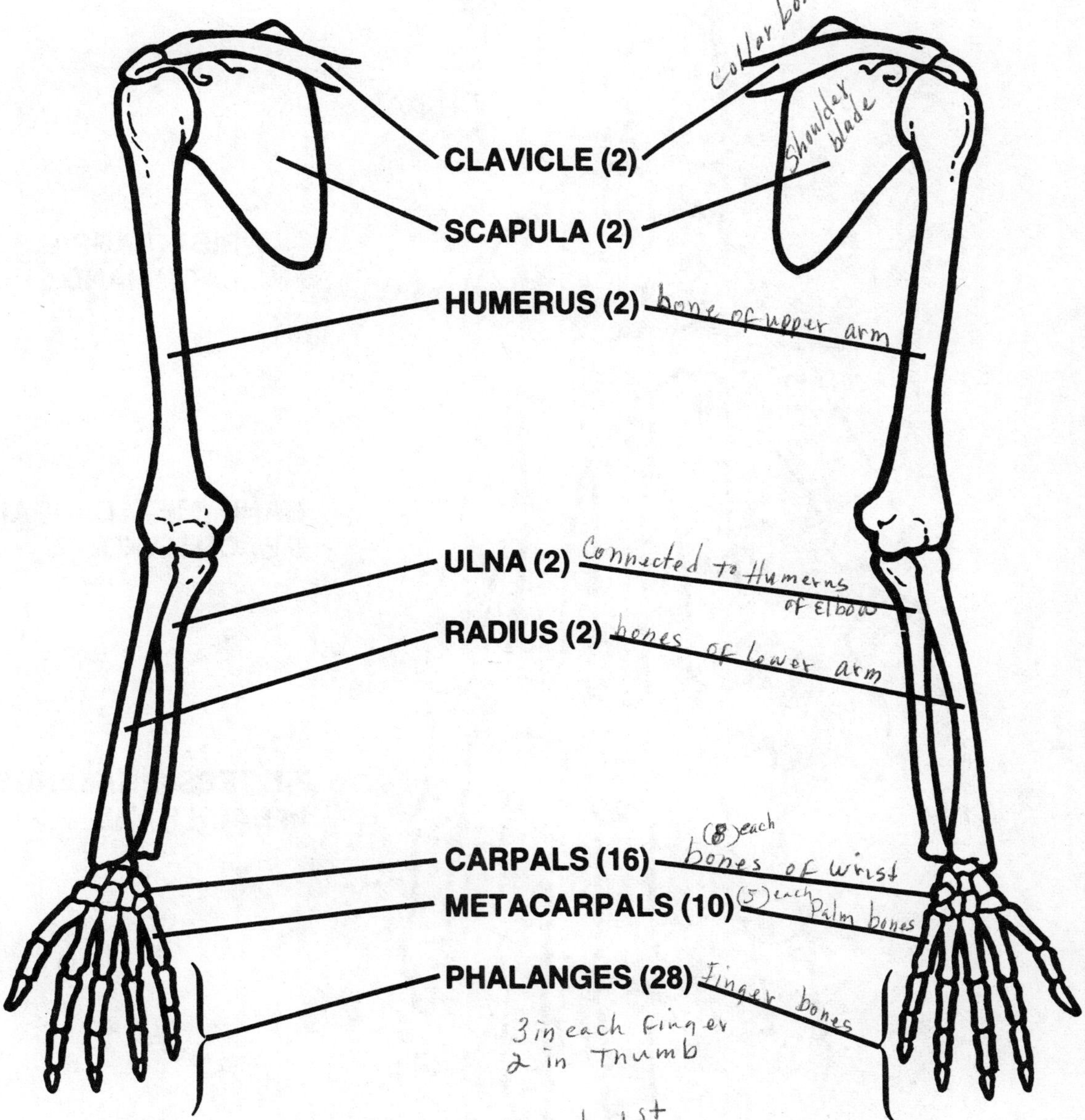

32 (RIGHT) **32 (LEFT)**

TOTAL 64 BONES

ANTERIOR (FRONT) VIEW

LESSON 4 — REVIEW
THE SKELETAL SYSTEM
BONES OF THE WRIST, HAND, AND FINGERS

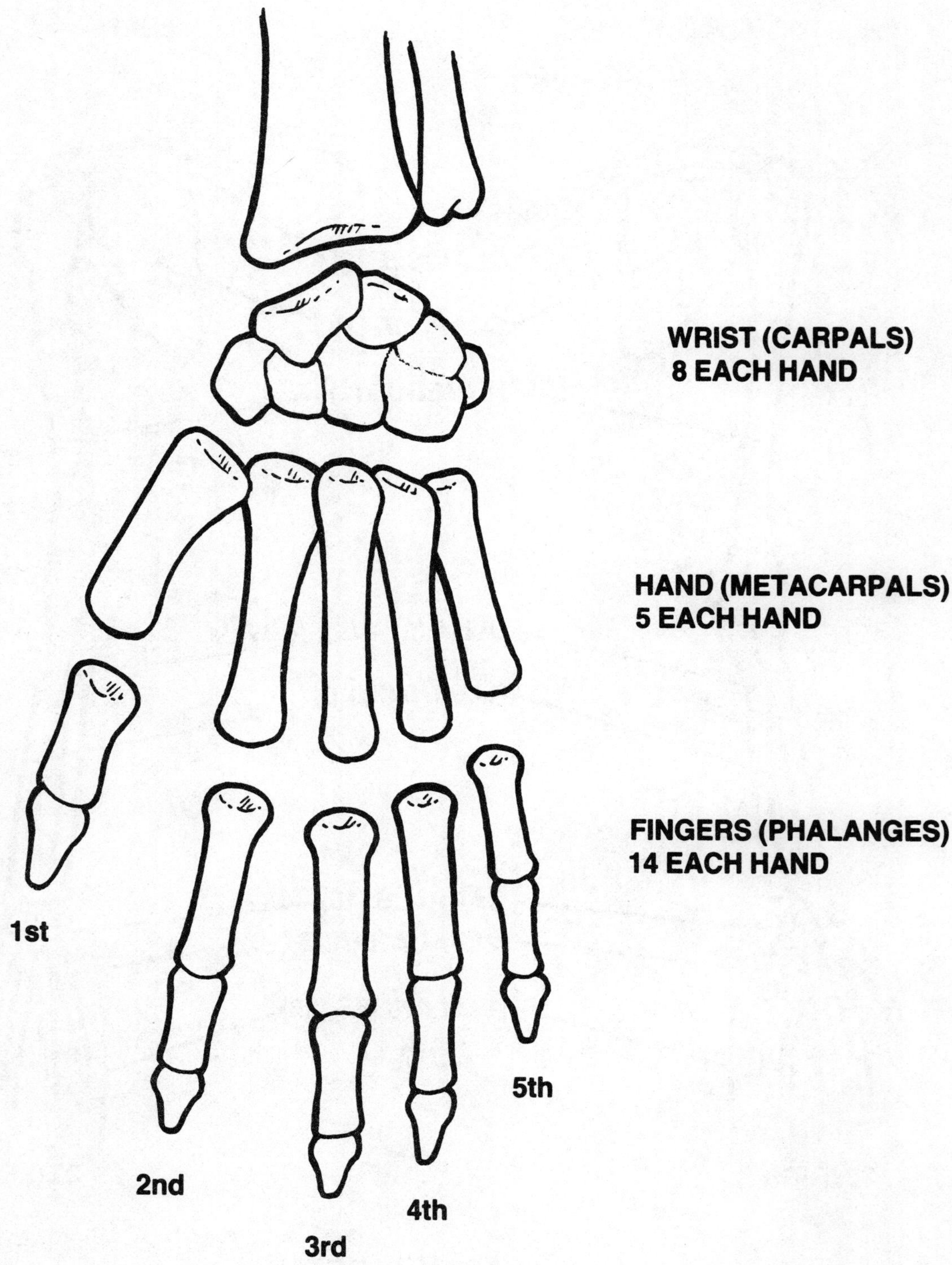

RIGHT HAND

Note: The metacarpals and phalanges are numbered from the thumb side to the side of the little finger as the 1st through the 5th.

LESSON 4 — REVIEW
THE SKELETAL SYSTEM
BONES OF THE WRIST, HAND, AND FINGERS

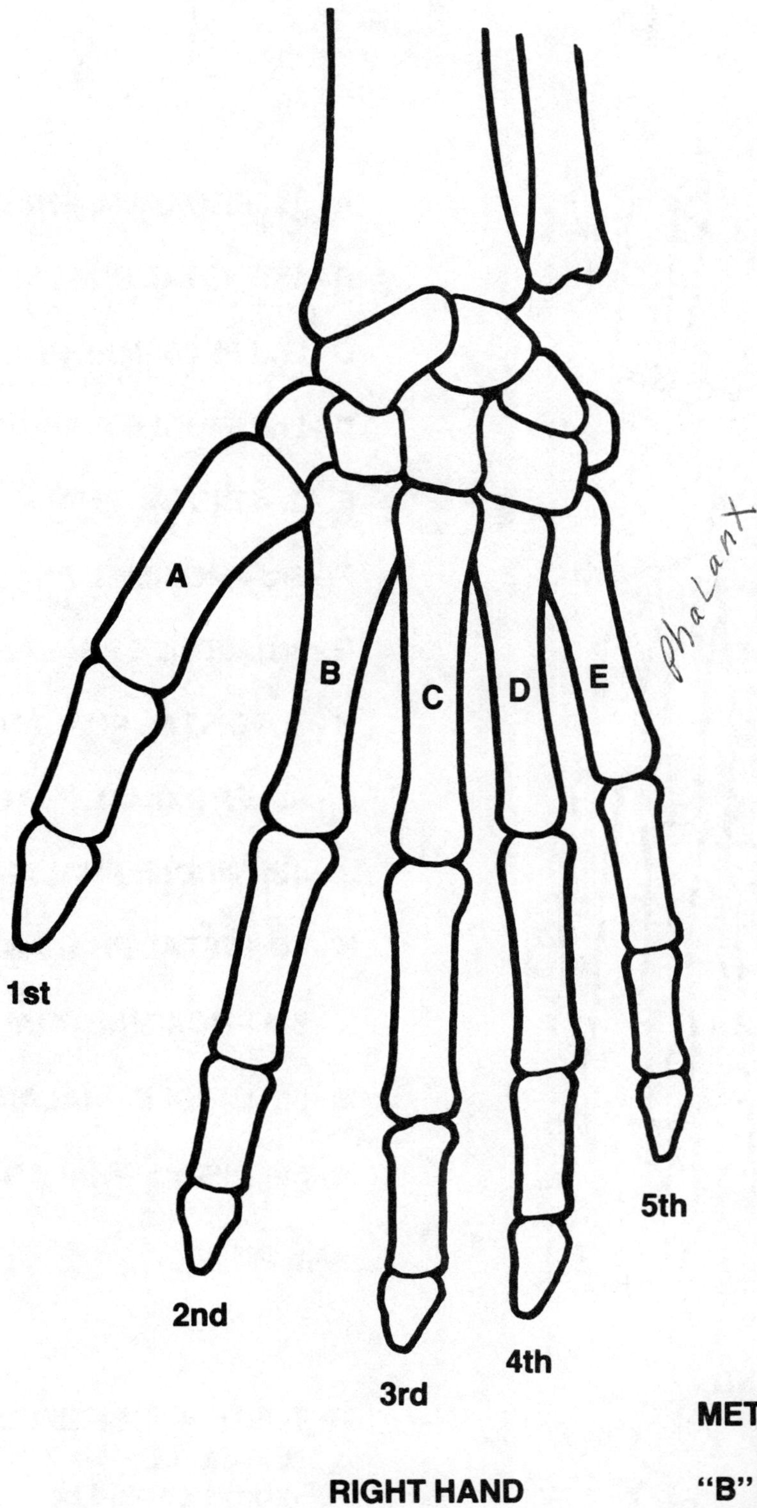

RIGHT HAND

A - 1st METACARPAL

B - 2nd METACARPAL

C - 3rd METACARPAL

D - 4th METACARPAL

E - 5th METACARPAL

METHOD OF IDENTIFICATION
EXAMPLE:
"B" above should be identified as "the 2nd metacarpal of the right hand"

LESSON 4 — REVIEW
THE SKELETAL SYSTEM
BONES OF THE WRIST, HAND, AND FINGERS

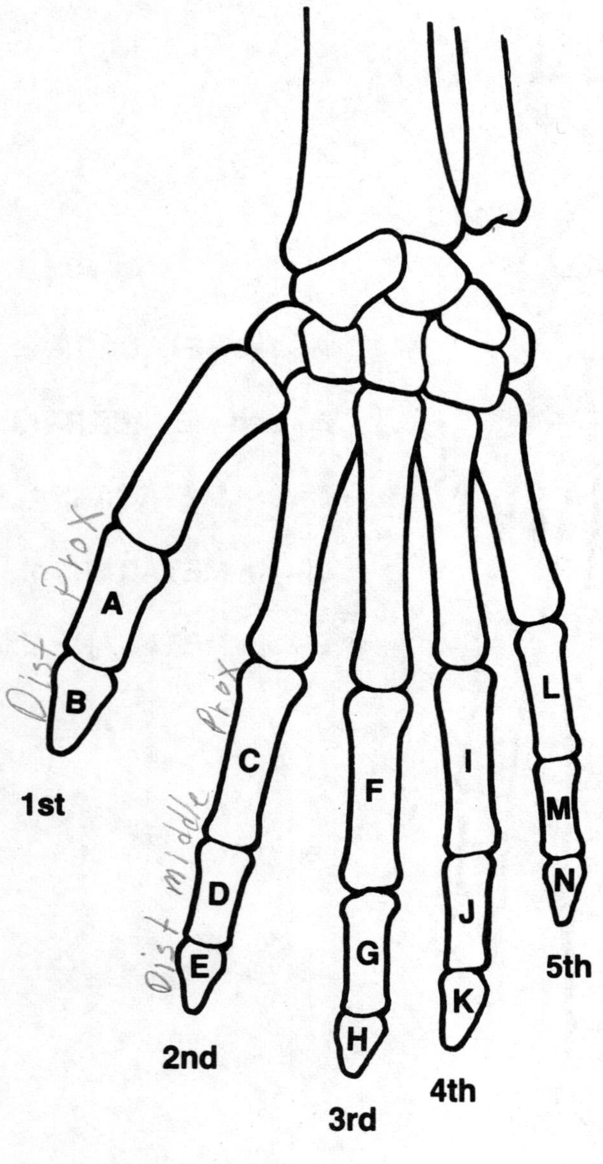

RIGHT HAND

A - 1st PROXIMAL PHALANX

B - 1st DISTAL PHALANX

C - 2nd PROXIMAL PHALANX

D - 2nd MIDDLE PHALANX

E - 2nd DISTAL PHALANX

F - 3rd PROXIMAL PHALANX

G - 3rd MIDDLE PHALANX

H - 3rd DISTAL PHALANX

I - 4th PROXIMAL PHALANX

J - 4th MIDDLE PHALANX

K - 4th DISTAL PHALANX

L - 5th PROXIMAL PHALANX

M - 5th MIDDLE PHALANX

N - 5th DISTAL PHALANX

METHOD OF IDENTIFICATION EXAMPLE:
"D" above should be identified as "the 2nd middle phalanx of the right hand"

LESSON 4 — REVIEW
THE SKELETAL SYSTEM
BONES OF THE LOWER EXTREMITIES

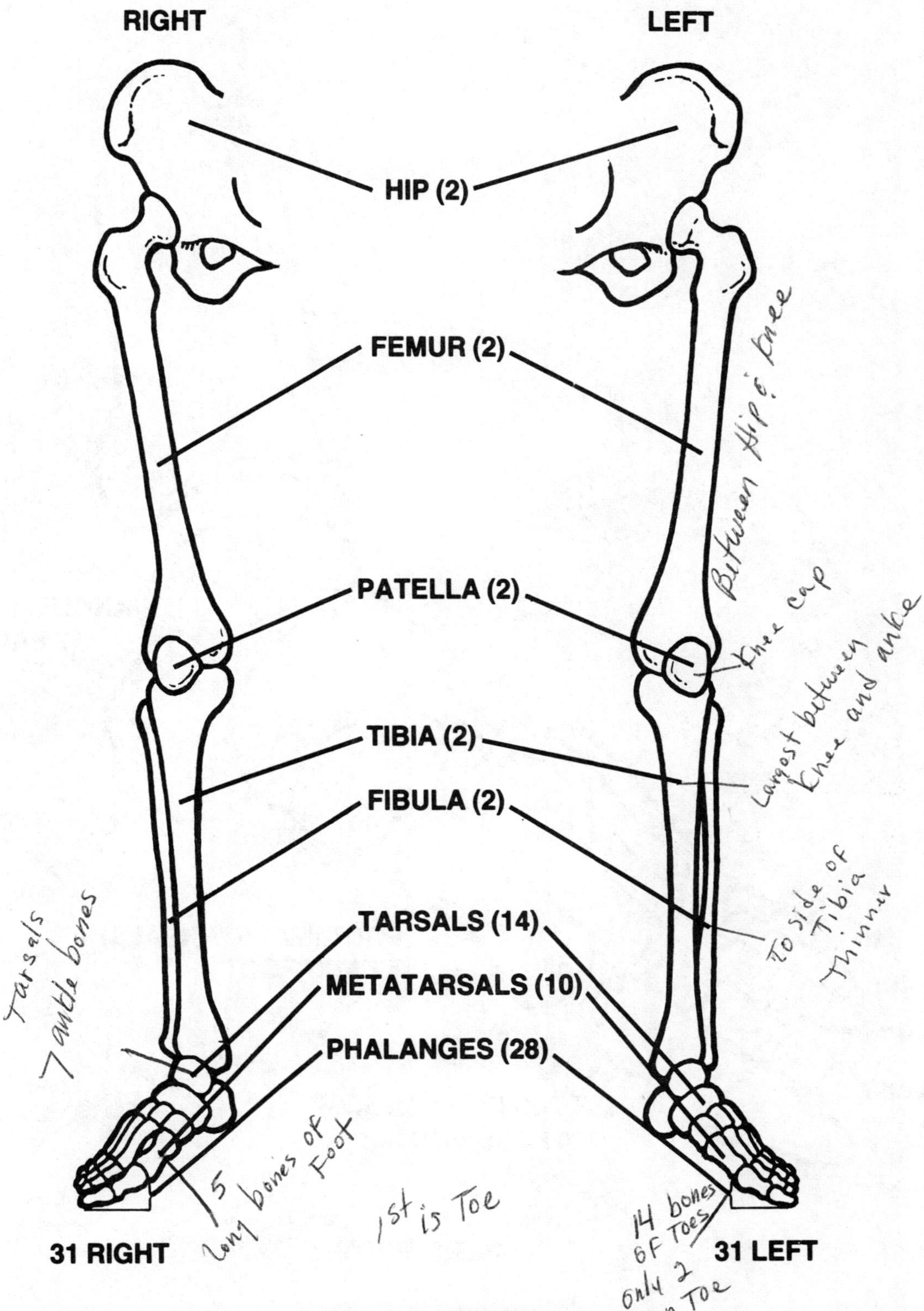

TOTAL 62 BONES

ANTERIOR (FRONT) VIEW

LESSON 4 — REVIEW
THE SKELETAL SYSTEM
BONES OF THE ANKLE, FOOT, AND TOES

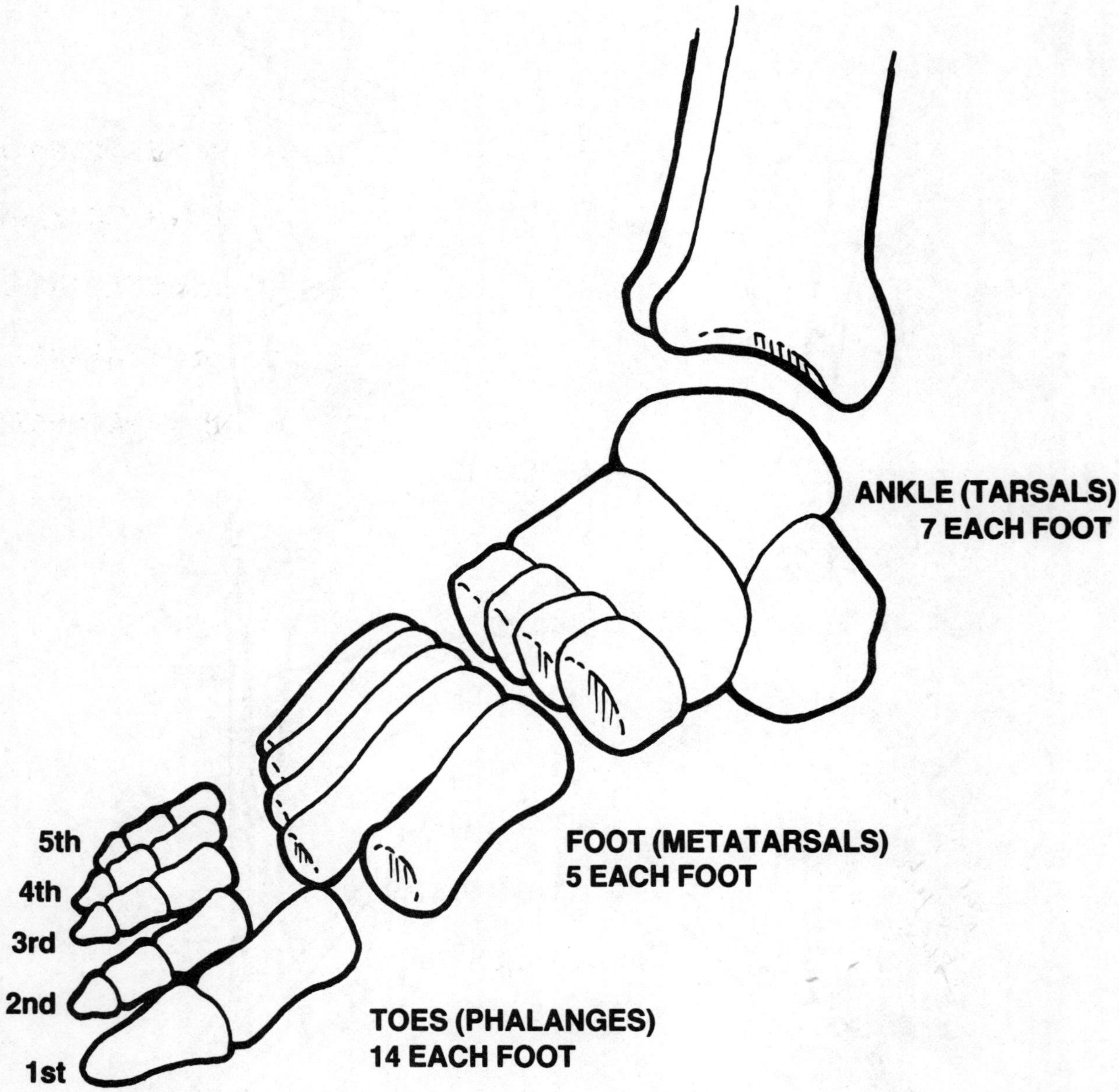

RIGHT FOOT

Note: The metatarsals and phalanges are numbered from the large toe side to the side of the little toe as the 1st through the 5th.

LESSON 4 — REVIEW
THE SKELETAL SYSTEM
BONES OF THE ANKLE, FOOT, AND TOES

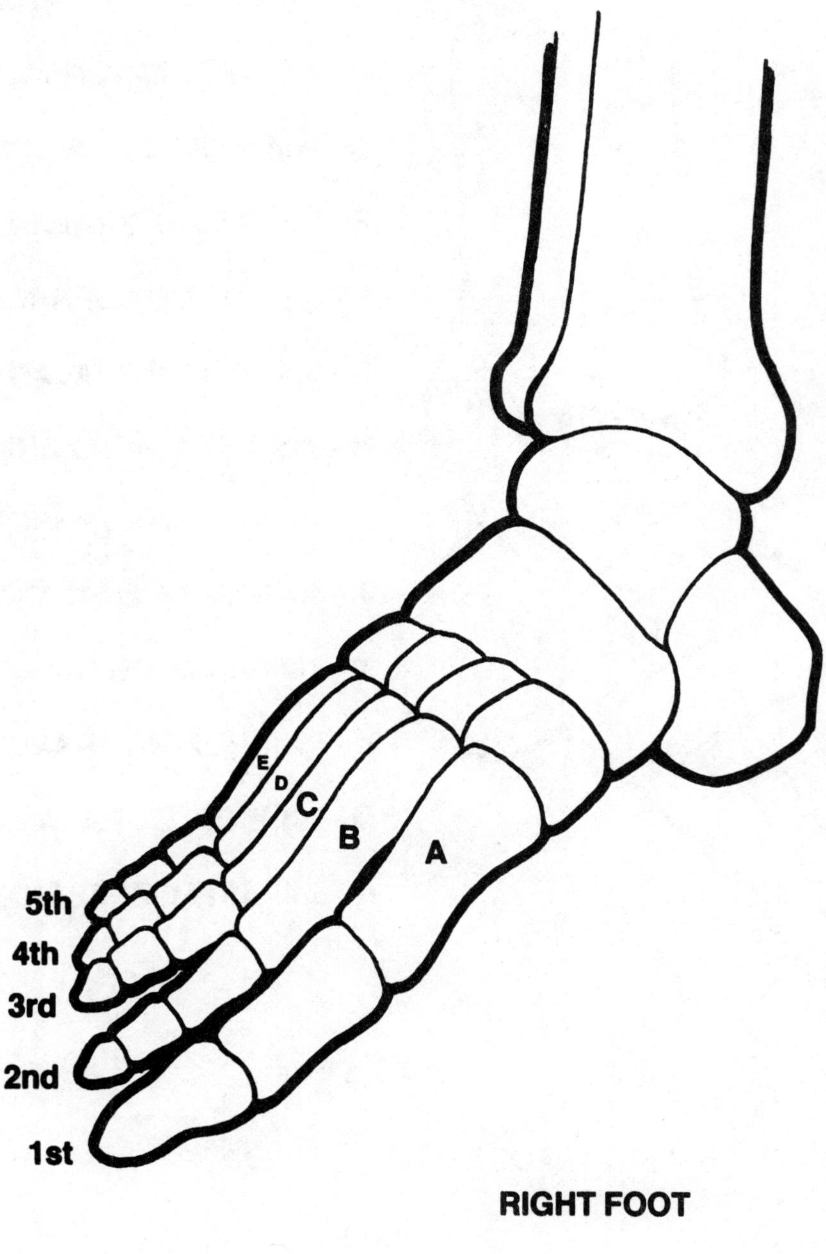

A - 1st METATARSAL

B - 2nd METATARSAL

C - 3rd METATARSAL

D - 4th METATARSAL

E - 5th METATARSAL

RIGHT FOOT

METHOD OF IDENTIFICATION
EXAMPLE:
"B" above should be identified as "the 2nd metatarsal of the right foot"

LESSON 4 — REVIEW
THE SKELETAL SYSTEM
BONES OF THE ANKLE, FOOT, AND TOES

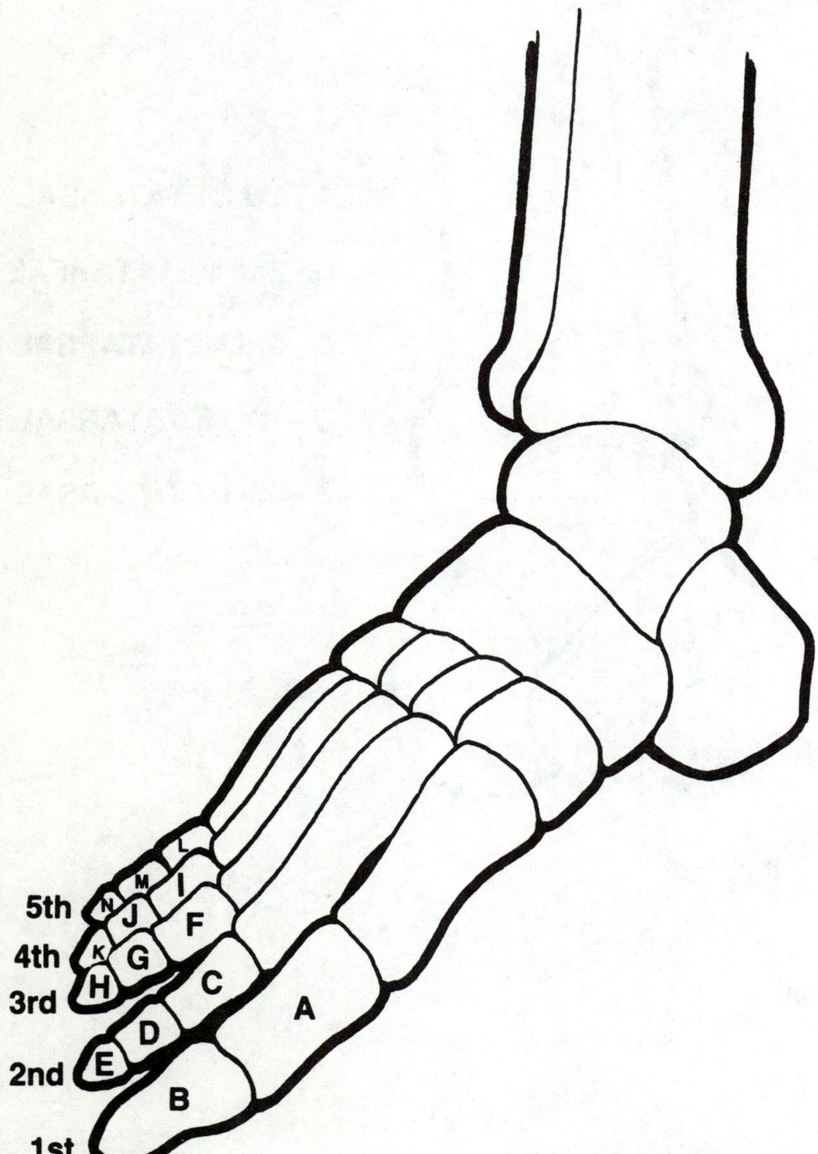

RIGHT FOOT

A - 1st PROXIMAL PHALANX

B - 1st DISTAL PHALANX

C - 2nd PROXIMAL PHALANX

D - 2nd MIDDLE PHALANX

E - 2nd DISTAL PHALANX

F - 3rd PROXIMAL PHALANX

G - 3rd MIDDLE PHALANX

H - 3rd DISTAL PHALANX

I - 4th PROXIMAL PHALANX

J - 4th MIDDLE PHALANX

K - 4th DISTAL PHALANX

L - 5th PROXIMAL PHALANX

M - 5th MIDDLE PHALANX

N - 5th DISTAL PHALANX

METHOD OF IDENTIFICATION
EXAMPLE:
"E" above should be identified as "the 2nd distal phalanx of the right foot"

LESSON 4 — WORKSHEET
SKELETEL SYSTEM
UPPER AND LOWER EXTREMITIES

COMPLETE THE BLANKS

UPPER

BONE	AUDIONYM
CLAVICLE	Clay Vehicle
SCAPULA	Ski cap
HUMERUS	Hammer
ULNA	all nuts
RADIUS	Radio
CARPALS	Carpet
METACARPALS	Metal Carpet
PHALANGES	Foil Hinges

LOWER

BONE	AUDIONYM
HIP	Rt - Lt (COMMON NAME)
FEMUR	Female
PATELLA	Pad L
TIBIA	Tee Pee
FIBULA	Fiber glass
TARSALS	Tar sole
METATARSALS	Metal Tar Sole
PHALANGES	Foil Hinges

LESSON 4 — WORKSHEET
THE SKELETAL SYSTEM
BONES OF THE UPPER EXTREMITIES

PRINT THE CORRECT LETTER WITHIN THE PARENTHESES

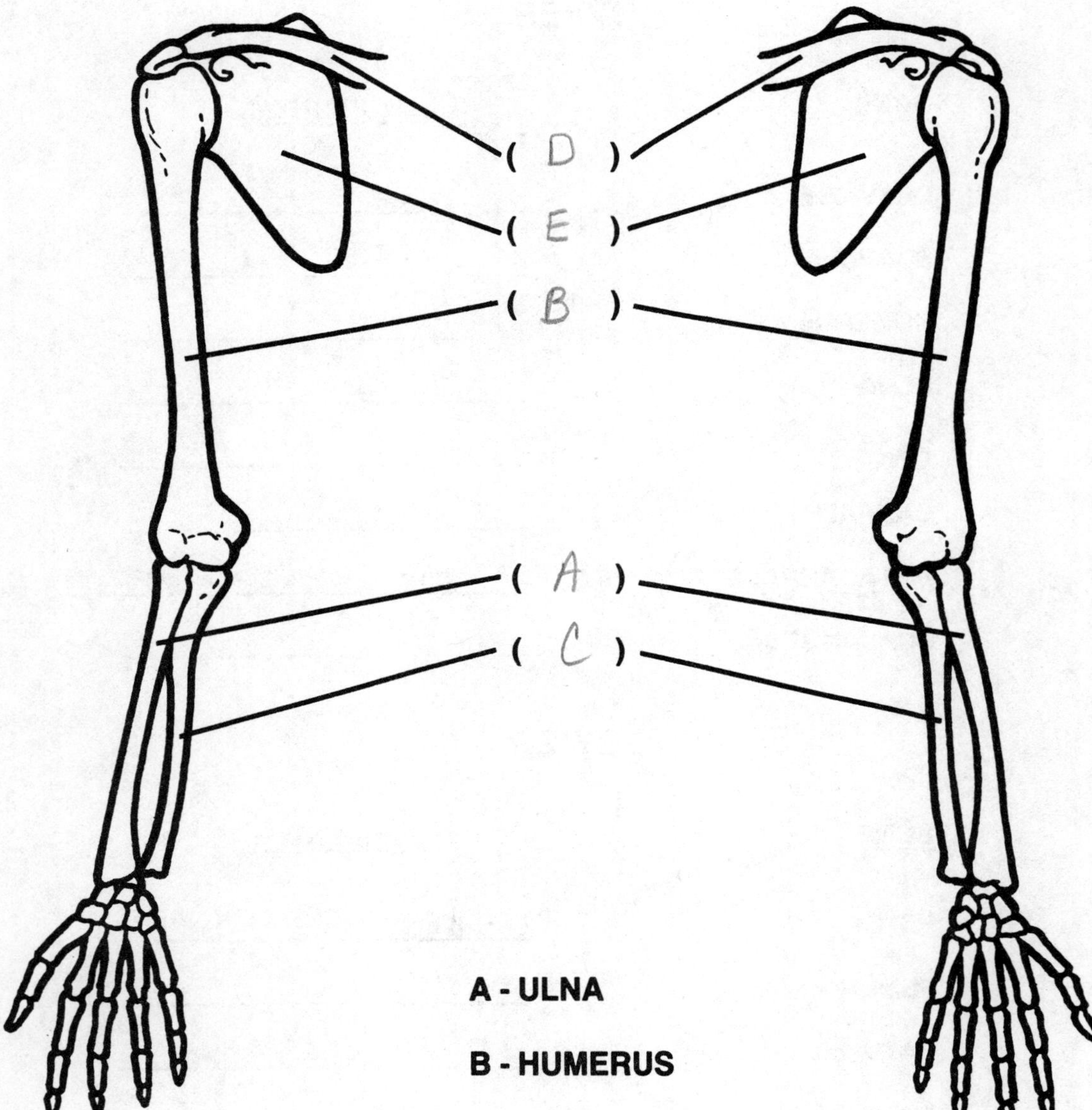

A - ULNA

B - HUMERUS

C - RADIUS

D - CLAVICLE

E - SCAPULA

ANTERIOR (FRONT) VIEW

LESSON 4 — WORKSHEET
THE SKELETAL SYSTEM
BONES OF THE WRIST, HAND, AND FINGERS

PRINT THE CORRECT LETTER WITHIN THE PARENTHESES

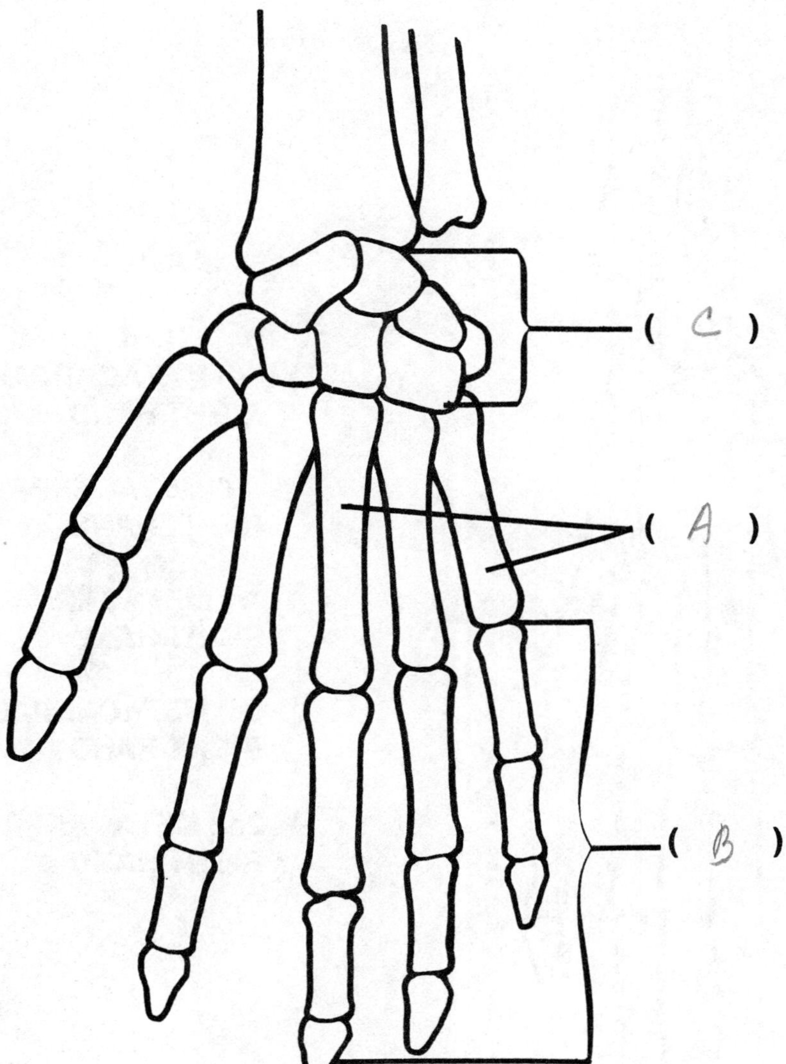

RIGHT HAND

A - METACARPALS

B - PHALANGES

C - CARPALS

LESSON 4 — WORKSHEET
THE SKELETAL SYSTEM
BONES OF THE WRIST, HAND, AND FINGERS

PRINT THE CORRECT LETTER WITHIN THE PARENTHESES

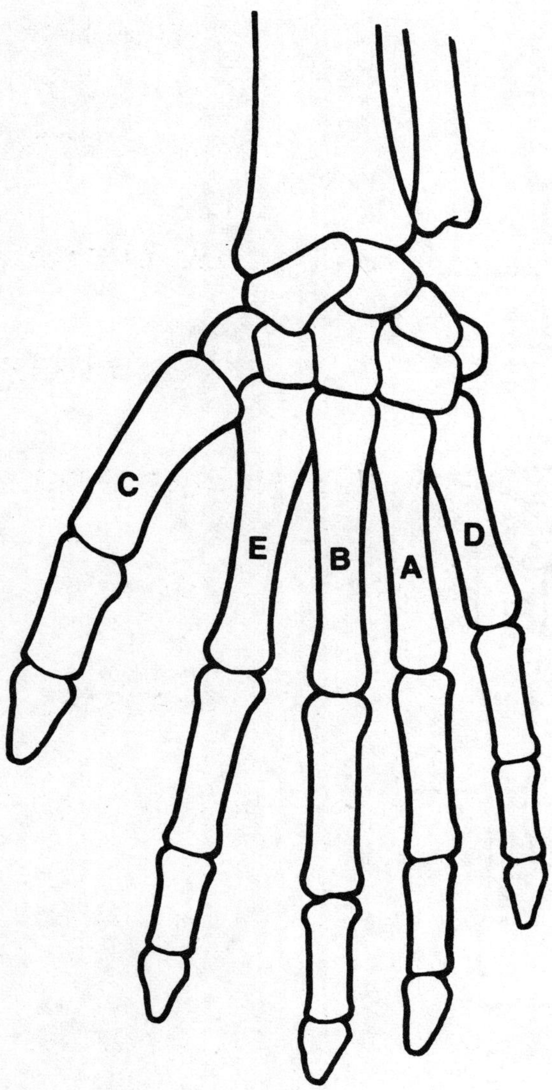

RIGHT HAND

(A) - 4th METACARPAL OF THE RIGHT HAND

(B) - 3rd METACARPAL OF THE RIGHT HAND

(C) - 1st METACARPAL OF THE RIGHT HAND

(D) - 5th METACARPAL OF THE RIGHT HAND

(E) - 2nd METACARPAL OF THE RIGHT HAND

LESSON 4 — WORKSHEET
THE SKELETAL SYSTEM
BONES OF THE WRIST, HAND, AND FINGERS

PRINT THE CORRECT LETTER WITHIN THE PARENTHESES

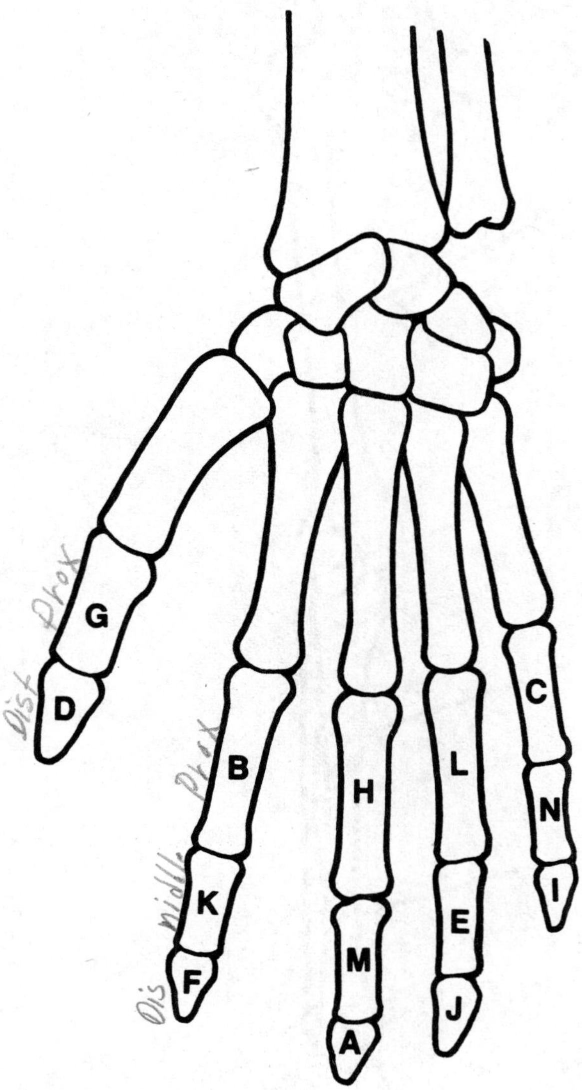

RIGHT HAND

(F) - **2nd DISTAL PHALANX OF THE RIGHT HAND**

(A) - **3rd DISTAL PHALANX OF THE RIGHT HAND**

(G) - **1st PROXIMAL PHALANX OF THE RIGHT HAND**

(K) - **2nd MIDDLE PHALANX OF THE RIGHT HAND**

(C) - **5th PROXIMAL PHALANX OF THE RIGHT HAND**

(E) - **4th MIDDLE PHALANX OF THE RIGHT HAND**

(I) - **5th DISTAL PHALANX OF THE RIGHT HAND**

(D) - **1st DISTAL PHALANX OF THE RIGHT HAND**

(M) - **3rd MIDDLE PHALANX OF THE RIGHT HAND**

(B) - **2nd PROXIMAL PHALANX OF THE RIGHT HAND**

(N) - **5th MIDDLE PHALANX OF THE RIGHT HAND**

(H) - **3rd PROXIMAL PHALANX OF THE RIGHT HAND**

(J) - **4th DISTAL PHALANX OF THE RIGHT HAND**

(L) - **4th PROXIMAL PHALANX OF THE RIGHT HAND**

LESSON 4 — WORKSHEET
THE SKELETAL SYSTEM
BONES OF THE LOWER EXTREMITIES

PRINT THE CORRECT LETTER WITHIN THE PARENTHESES

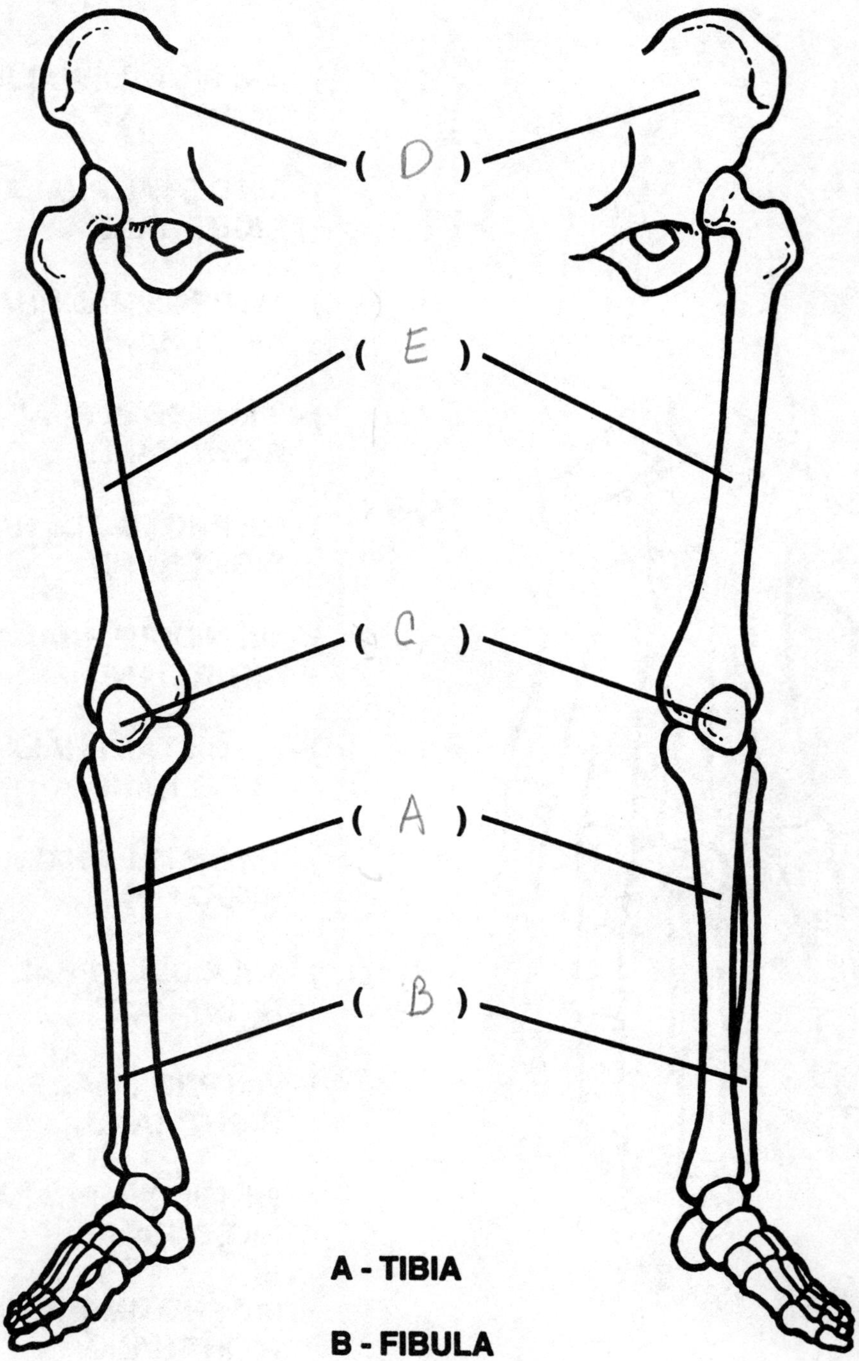

A - TIBIA

B - FIBULA

C - PATELLA

D - HIP

E - FEMUR

LESSON 4 — WORKSHEET
THE SKELETAL SYSTEM
BONES OF THE ANKLE, FOOT, AND TOES

PRINT THE CORRECT LETTER WITHIN THE PARENTHESES

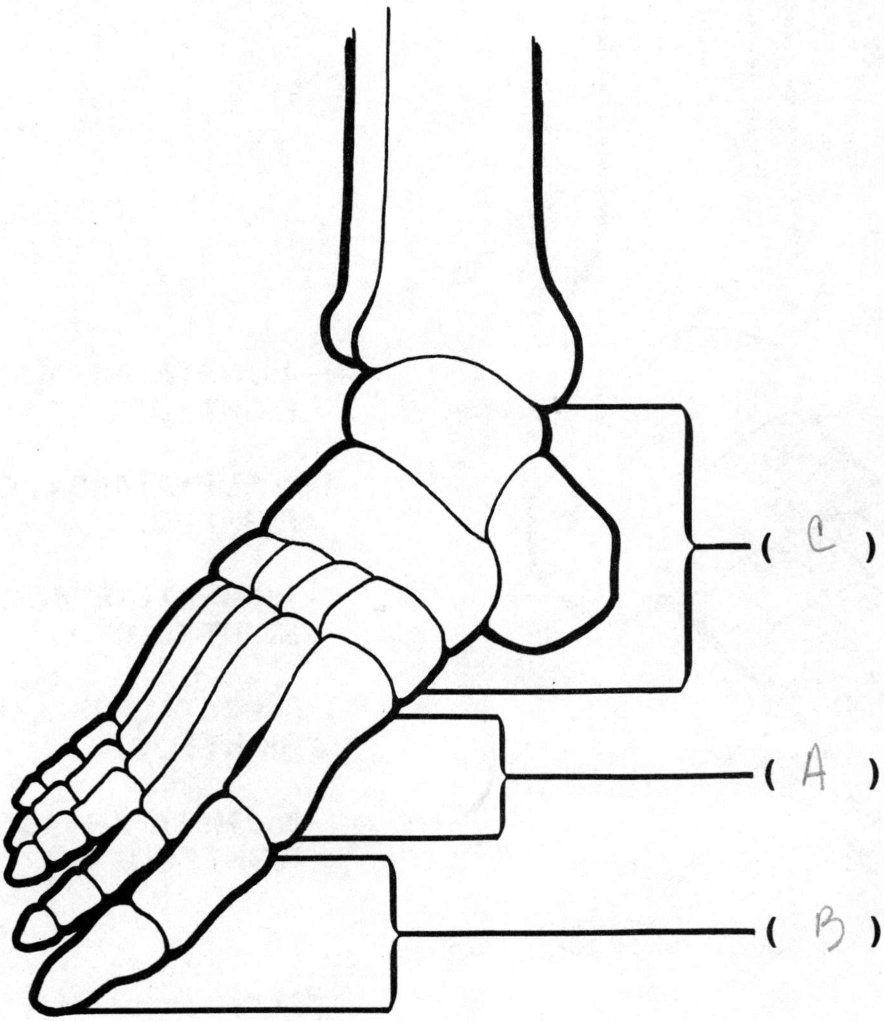

A - METATARSALS

B - PHALANGES

C - TARSALS

LESSON 4 — WORKSHEET
THE SKELETAL SYSTEM
BONES OF THE ANKLE, FOOT, AND TOES

PRINT THE CORRECT LETTER WITHIN THE PARENTHESES

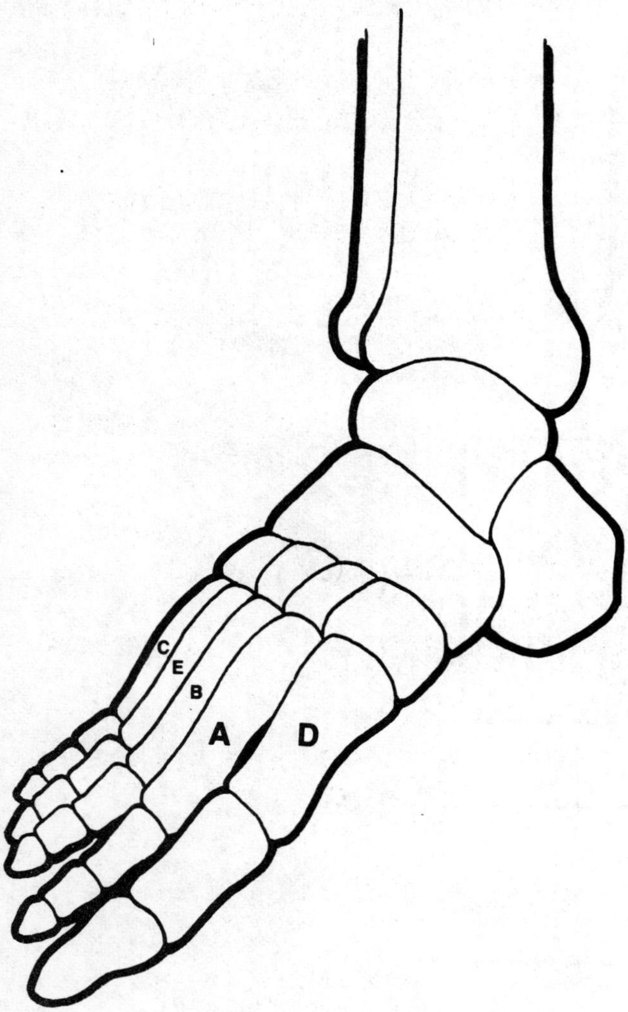

RIGHT FOOT

(E) - 4th METATARSAL OF THE RIGHT FOOT

(B) - 3rd METATARSAL OF THE RIGHT FOOT

(D) - 1st METATARSAL OF THE RIGHT FOOT

(C) - 5th METATARSAL OF THE RIGHT FOOT

(A) - 2nd METATARSAL OF THE RIGHT FOOT

LESSON 4 — WORKSHEET
THE SKELETAL SYSTEM
BONES OF THE ANKLE, FOOT, AND TOES

PRINT THE CORRECT LETTER WITHIN THE PARENTHESES

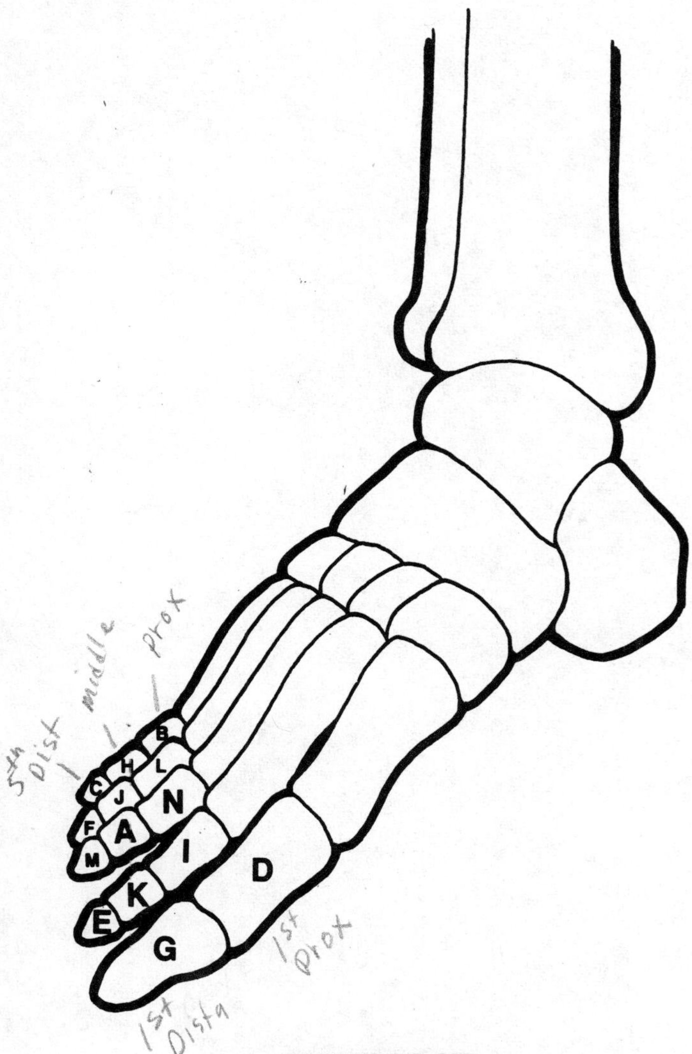

RIGHT FOOT

(K) - **2nd MIDDLE PHALANX OF THE RIGHT FOOT**

(G) - **1st DISTAL PHALANX OF THE RIGHT FOOT**

(A) - **3rd MIDDLE PHALANX OF THE RIGHT FOOT**

(C) - **5th DISTAL PHALANX OF THE RIGHT FOOT**

(J) - **4th MIDDLE PHALANX OF THE RIGHT FOOT**

(D) - **1ST PROXIMAL PHALANX OF THE RIGHT FOOT**

(E) - **2nd DISTAL PHALANX OF THE RIGHT FOOT**

(I) - **2nd PROXIMAL PHALANX OF THE RIGHT FOOT**

(N) - **3rd PROXIMAL PHALANX OF THE RIGHT FOOT**

(H) - **5th MIDDLE PHALANX OF THE RIGHT FOOT**

(M) - **3rd DISTAL PHALANX OF THE RIGHT FOOT**

(L) - **4th PROXIMAL PHALANX OF THE RIGHT FOOT**

(F) - **4th DISTAL PHALANX OF THE RIGHT FOOT**

(B) - **5th PROXIMAL PHALANX OF THE RIGHT FOOT**

LESSON 5

THE MUSCULAR SYSTEM

HOW MUSCLES ARE NAMED

- DIRECTION
- LOCATION
- SIZE
- NUMBER
- SHAPE
- ORIGIN AND INSERTION
- ACTION

REMEMBER!

1st **Pronounce** *the name of the body part or term*
2nd **Recall** *and* **pronounce** *the audionym*
3rd **For body parts: visualize** *the audionym in place*
For terms: visualize *the association*
4th **Pronounce** *the name of the body part or term again.*

LESSON 5 — REVIEW
THE MUSCULAR SYSTEM
HOW MUSCLES ARE NAMED
(THE LINK SYSTEM)

To remember how muscles are named, just see a **name plate** with **muscles**. Then, use the link system to recall each audionym in sequence:

VISUAL IMAGE / ASSOCIATION	MUSCLES ARE NAMED BY:
See a **name plate** with **muscles**, then:	
1. See the **name plate with muscles** with a **book of directions** hanging on it!	Direction (of fibers)
2. See the **book of directions** with a **locomotive** bursting out of it!	Location
3. See the **locomotive** with **"S" eyes** coming out of it!	Size
4. See the **"S" eyes** with **numbers** bursting out of it!	Number (of origins)
5. See the **numbers** with a (milk) **shake** coming out of it!	Shape
6. See the (milk) **shake** with an **orange/ant in short sleeves** bursting out of it!	Origin and Insertion
7. See the **orange/ant in short sleeves** holding an **ax**!	Action

WORD	AUDIONYM
1. DIRECTION	(BOOK OF) DIRECTIONS
2. LOCATION	LOCOMOTIVE
3. SIZE	"S" EYES
4. NUMBER	NUMBERS
5. SHAPE	SHAKE
6. ORIGIN AND INSERTION	ORANGE/ANT IN SHORT SLEEVES
7. ACTION	AX

LESSON 5 — REVIEW
THE MUSCULAR SYSTEM
HOW MUSCLES ARE NAMED

1. MUSCLES NAMED BY DIRECTION (OF FIBERS)

WORD	AUDIONYM	VISUAL IMAGE / ASSOCIATION	MEANING
rectus	wreck	See the **wreck** in **straight** jackets!	straight
trans	trains	See the **trains** going **through a cross**!	through, across
oblique	—	(A common term)	diagonal

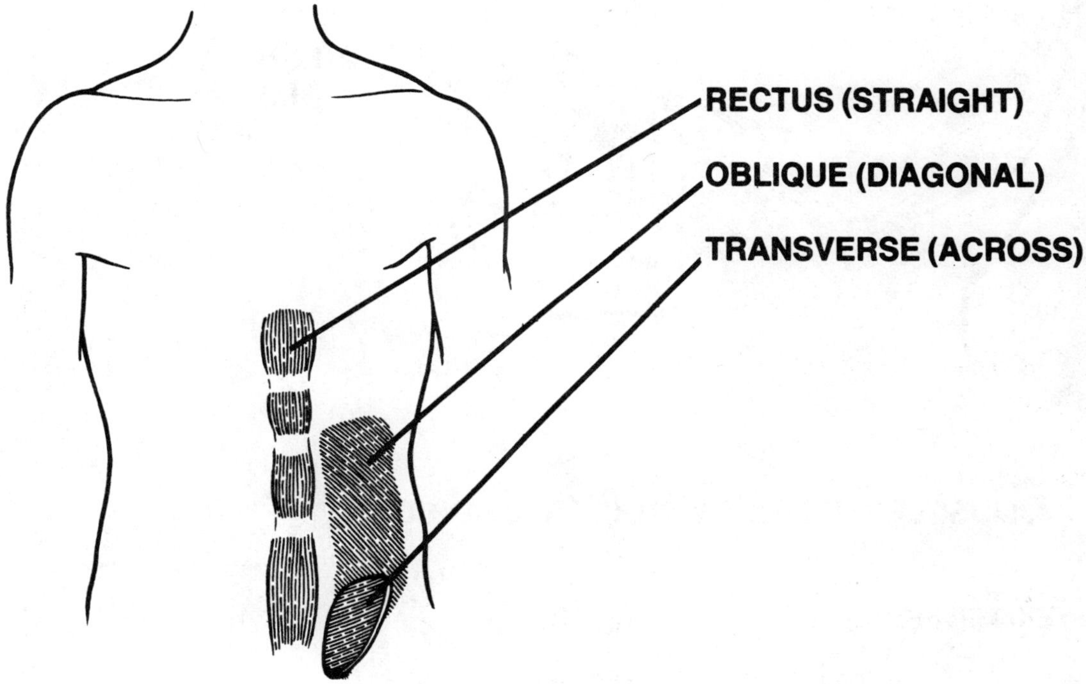

2. MUSCLES NAMED BY LOCATION

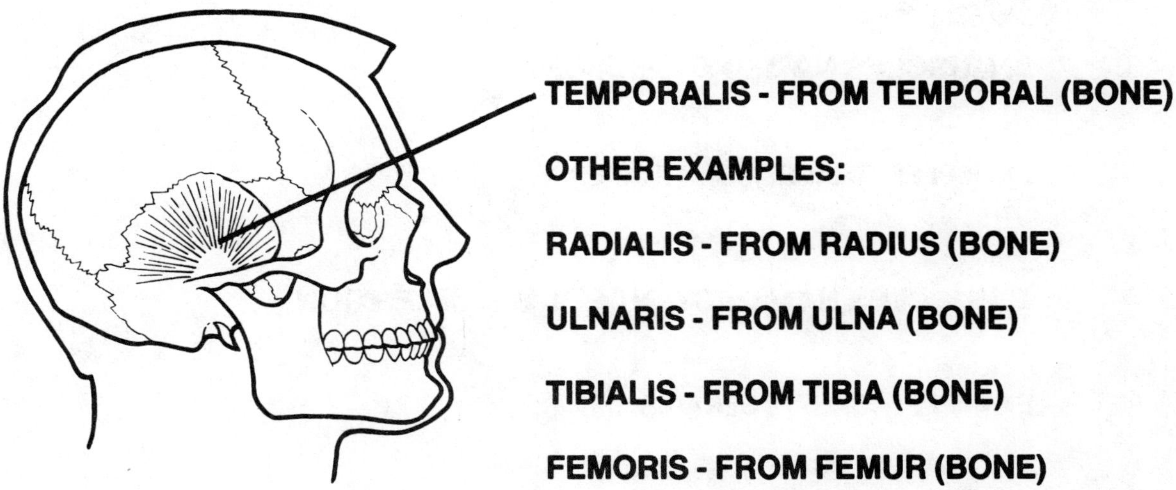

OTHER EXAMPLES:

RADIALIS - FROM RADIUS (BONE)

ULNARIS - FROM ULNA (BONE)

TIBIALIS - FROM TIBIA (BONE)

FEMORIS - FROM FEMUR (BONE)

LESSON 5 — REVIEW
THE MUSCULAR SYSTEM
HOW MUSCLES ARE NAMED

3. MUSCLES NAMED BY SIZE

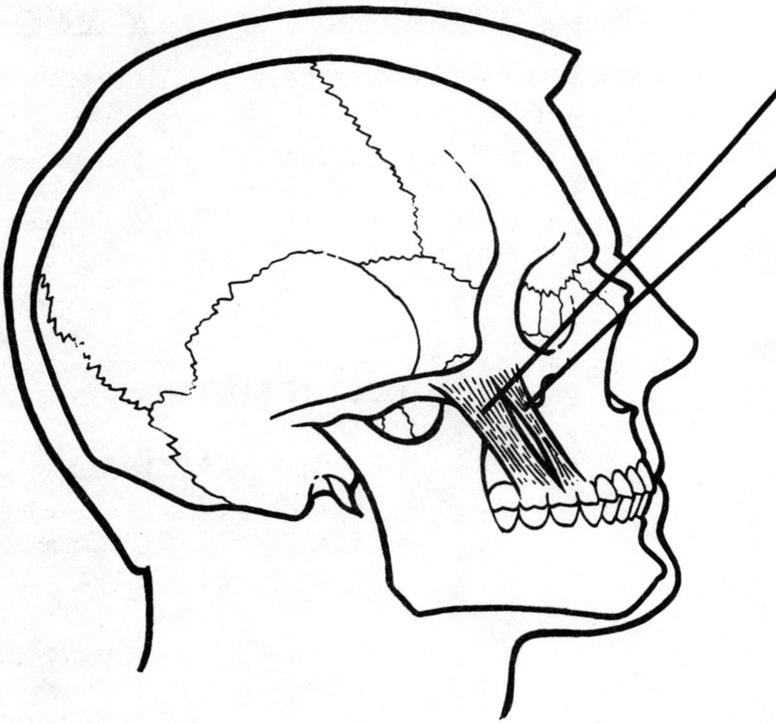

OTHER EXAMPLES:

LONGUS
BREVIS
MAXIMUS
MINIMUS

4. MUSCLES NAMED BY NUMBER (OF ORIGINS)

EXAMPLES:	BICEPS	(BI = 2)
	TRICEPS	(TRI = 3)
	QUADRICEPS	(QUAD = 4)

5. MUSCLES NAMED BY SHAPE

EXAMPLE: TRAPEZIUS (TRAPEZOID)

6. MUSCLES NAMED BY ORIGIN AND INSERTION

EXAMPLE: CARPI ULNARIS

(CARPAL) (ULNA)

LESSON 5 — REVIEW
THE MUSCULAR SYSTEM
HOW MUSCLES ARE NAMED

7. MUSCLES NAMED BY ACTION

WORD	AUDIONYM	VISUAL IMAGE / ASSOCIATION	ACTION
A. flexor	flags	See the **flags decreasing the angle of the joint**!	decreases the angle of a joint
B. extensor	extension cord	See the **extension cord increasing the angle of the joint**!	increases the angle of a joint
C. abductor	Abe duck	See the **Abe duck moving a bone away from the midline of the body**!	moves a bone away from the midline of the body
D. adductor	ad duck	See the **ad duck moving a bone toward the midline of the body**!	moves a bone toward the midline of the body
E. levator	levitate	See someone **levitating** on the mandible **producing an upward movement**!	produces an upward movement
F. depressor	deep presser	See the **deep presser producing a downward movement**!	produces a downward movement
G. supinator	soup	See the **soup** with the **palms** of the hand **up**!	turns palms upward
H. pronator	pro gnat	See the **pro gnat** with the **palm** of a gigantic hand coming **down** on it!	turns the palms downward
I. dorsi flexor	doors of flags	See the **doors of flags** swing open and **turn the toes and ankle upward**!	flexes foot at ankle and turns the toes upward
J. plantar flexor	plant/tar flags	See the **plant** with the **tar flags.** The **foot is extended at the ankle joint and the toes are pointed inferiorly**!	extends the foot at the ankle and points the toes inferiorly
K. invertor	inn, fur door	See the **inn** with the **fur door**. See the gigantic **foot in the roof**!	turns the sole of the foot inward

LESSON 5 — REVIEW
THE MUSCULAR SYSTEM
HOW MUSCLES ARE NAMED

7. MUSCLES NAMED BY ACTION

WORD	AUDIONYM	VISUAL IMAGE / ASSOCIATION	ACTION
L. evertor	elevator	See the **elevator** with the sole of **the foot** sticking **out** of it!	turns the foot outward
M. sphincter	sphinx	See the **sphinx decreasing the size of its opening**!	decreases the size of an opening
N. tensor	tents	See the **tents** with **body parts** being stretched until they are **rigid**!	makes a body part more rigid
O. rotator	rotary	See the **rotary** mower **moving** a **bone around a long ax**!	moves a bone around its longitudinal axis

LESSON 5 — REVIEW
THE MUSCULAR SYSTEM
HOW MUSCLES ARE NAMED

The following examples utilize an illustration of a skeleton in action, since all muscles named according to action refer to their movement of skeletel bones.

7. MUSCLES NAMED BY ACTION

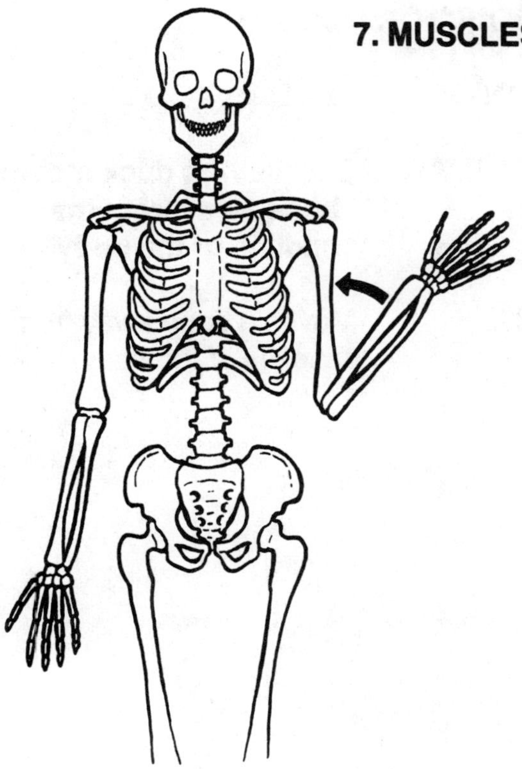

A - FLEXOR MUSCLE

AUDIONYM: Flags

VISUAL IMAGE: See the **flags decreasing the angle of a joint**

ACTION: Decreases the anterior angle of a joint.

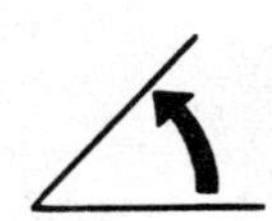

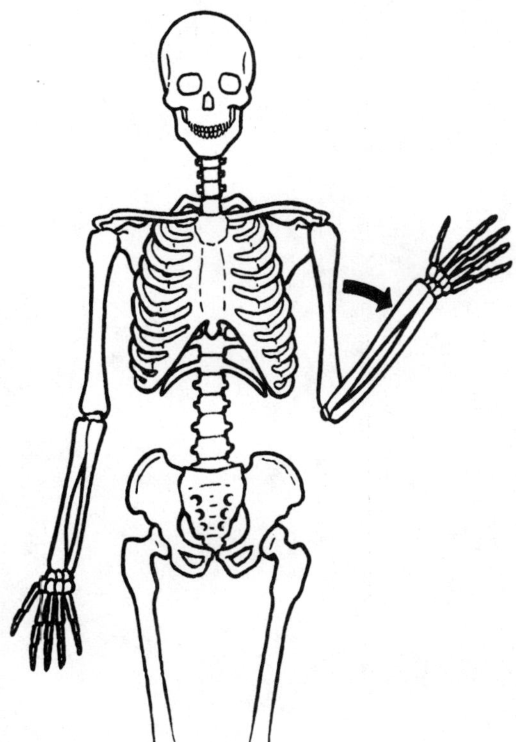

B - EXTENSOR MUSCLE

AUDIONYM: Extension Cord

VISUAL IMAGE: See the **extension cord increasing the angle of a joint**

ACTION: Increases the anterior angle of a joint.

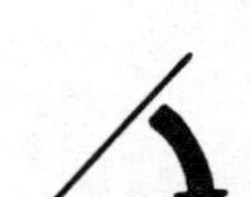

LESSON 5 — REVIEW
THE MUSCULAR SYSTEM
HOW MUSCLES ARE NAMED

7. MUSCLES NAMED BY ACTION (cont.)

C - ABDUCTOR MUSCLE

AUDIONYM: Abe Duck

VISUAL IMAGE: See the **Abe duck moving a bone away from the midline of the body**

ACTION: Moves a bone away from the midline of the body.

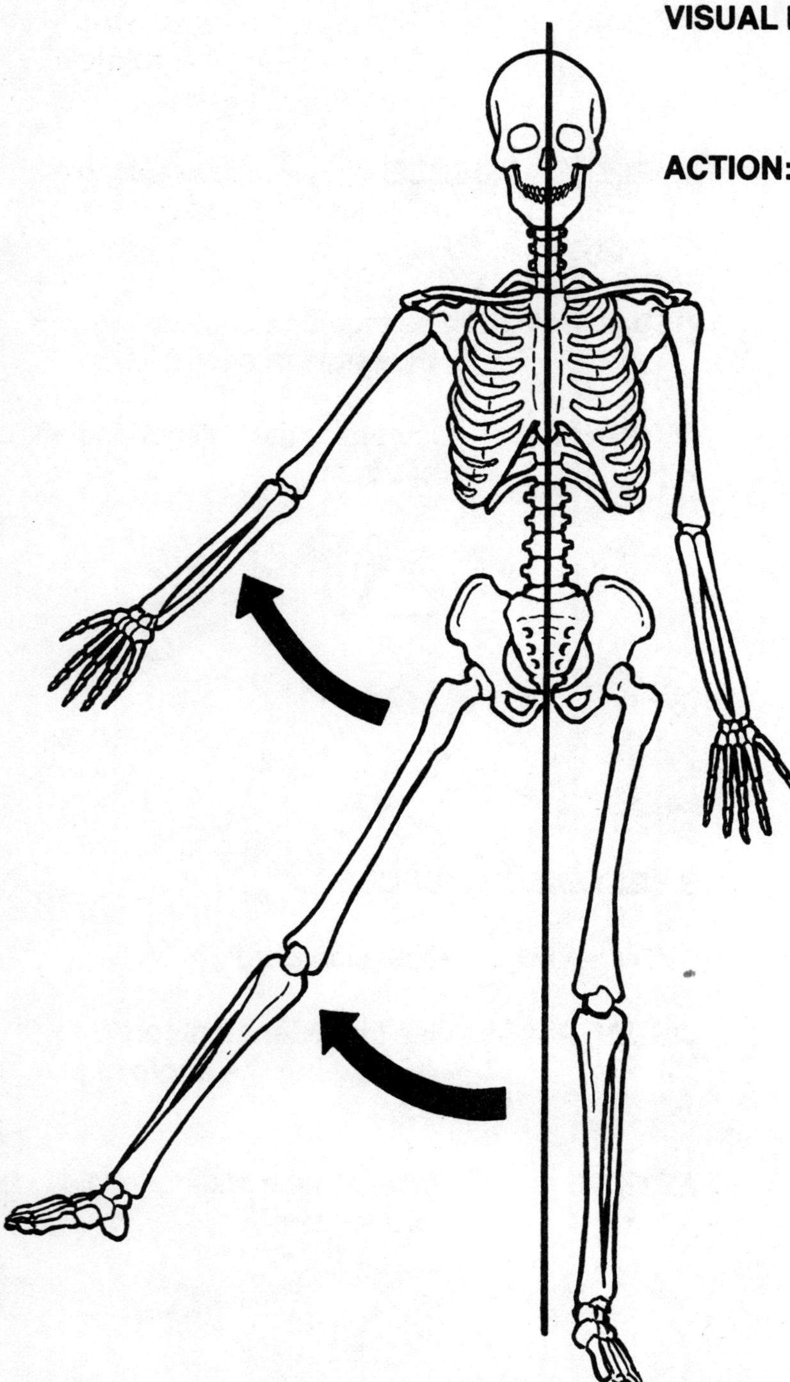

LESSON 5 — REVIEW
THE MUSCULAR SYSTEM
HOW MUSCLES ARE NAMED

7. MUSCLES NAMED BY ACTION (cont.)

D - ADDUCTOR MUSCLE

AUDIONYM: Ad Duck

VISUAL IMAGE: See the **ad duck moving a bone toward the midline of the body**

ACTION: Moves a bone toward the midline of the body.

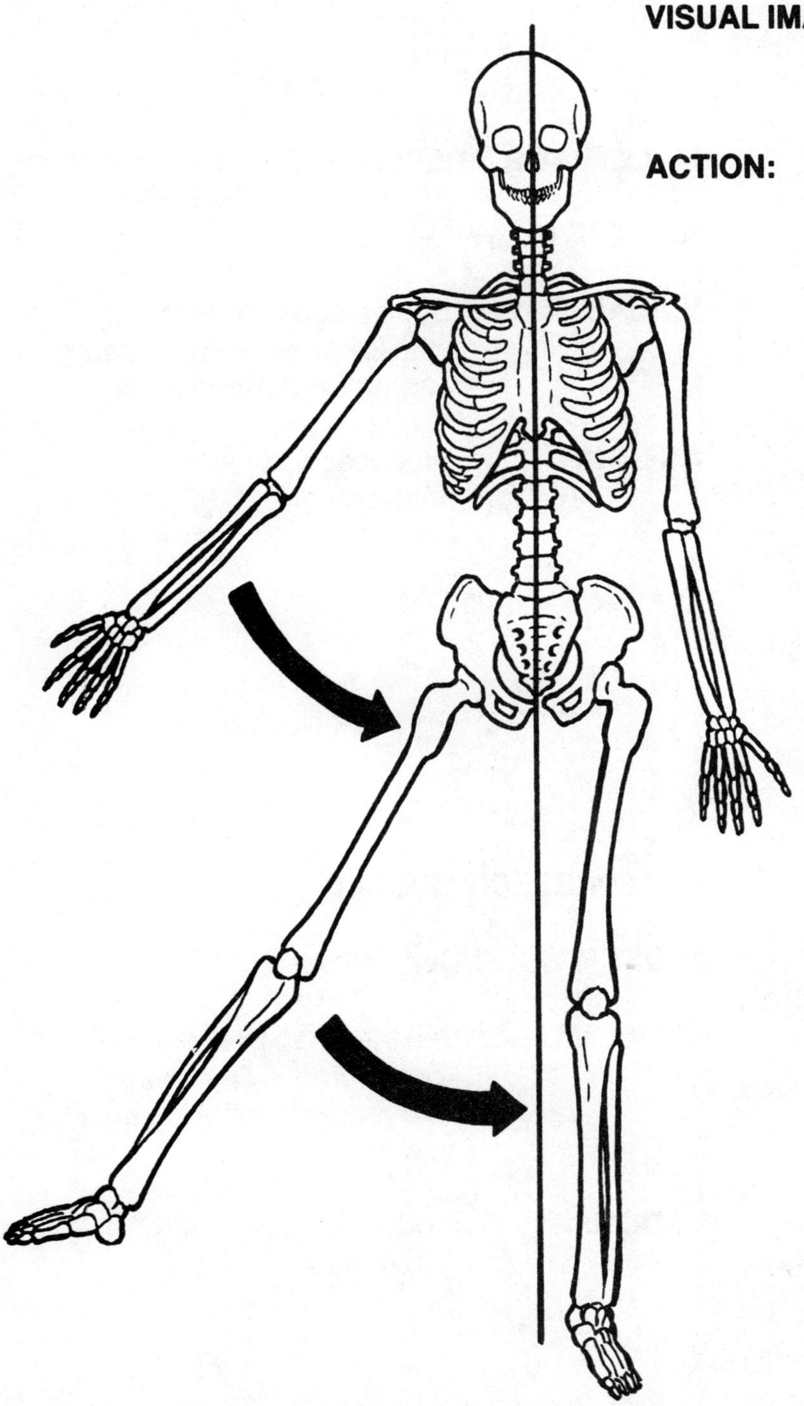

LESSON 5 — REVIEW
THE MUSCULAR SYSTEM
HOW MUSCLES ARE NAMED

7. MUSCLES NAMED BY ACTION (cont.)

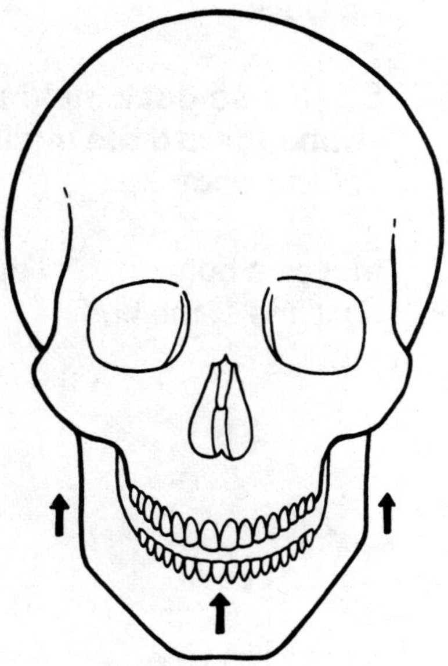

E - LEVATOR MUSCLE

AUDIONYM: Levitate

VISUAL IMAGE: See someone **levitating** on the lower jaw — **producing an upward movement**

ACTION: Produces an upward movement

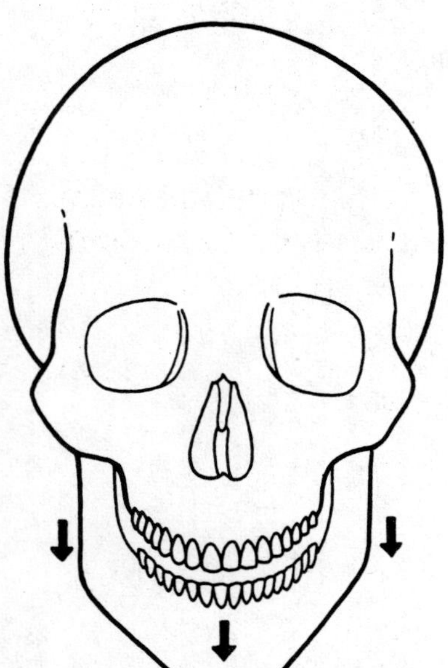

F - DEPRESSOR MUSCLE

AUDIONYM: Deep presser

VISUAL IMAGE: See the **deep presser producing a downward movement** on the lower jaw

ACTION: Produces a downward movement

LESSON 5 — REVIEW
THE MUSCULAR SYSTEM
HOW MUSCLES ARE NAMED

7. MUSCLES NAMED BY ACTION (cont.)

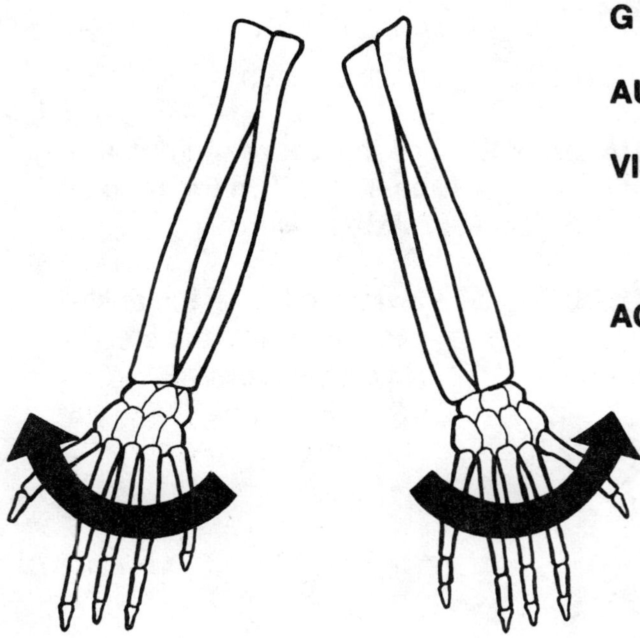

G - SUPINATOR MUSCLE

AUDIONYM: Soup

VISUAL IMAGE: See the **soup** with **palms of hands** sticking out of it! The **palms** are **up**

ACTION: Turns the palms upward or anteriorly

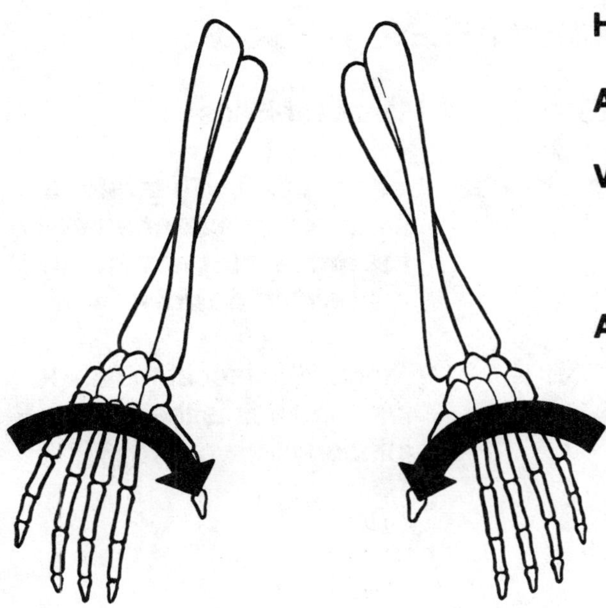

H - PRONATOR MUSCLE

AUDIONYM: Pro Gnat

VISUAL IMAGE: See the **pro gnat** with the **palm** of a **hand** coming **down** on it

ACTION: Turns the palms downward or posteriorly

LESSON 5 — REVIEW
THE MUSCULAR SYSTEM
HOW MUSCLES ARE NAMED

7. MUSCLES NAMED BY ACTION (cont.)

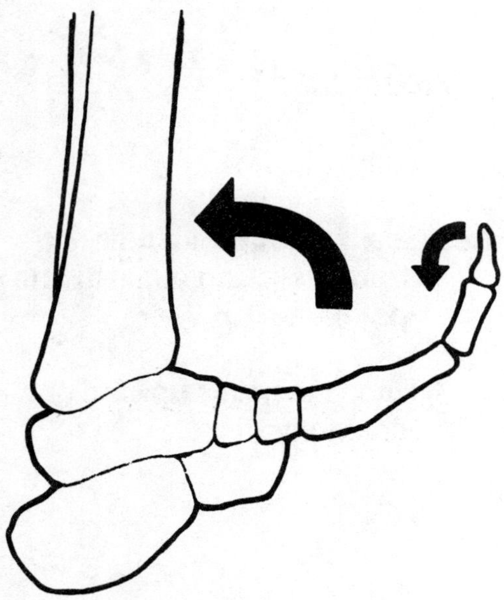

I - DORSIFLEXOR MUSCLE

AUDIONYM: Doors of Flags

VISUAL IMAGE: See the **doors of flags** swing open and **turn the toes and ankle upward**

ACTION: Flexes the foot at the ankle joint and points the toes superiorly (upward)

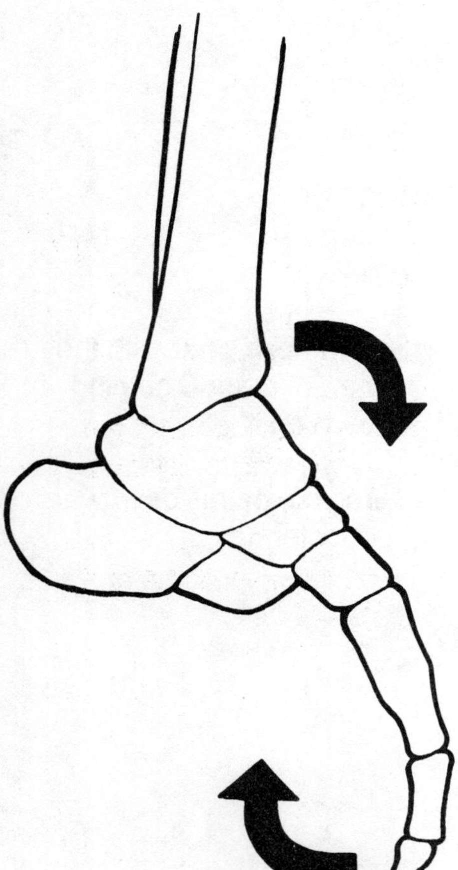

J - PLANTAR FLEXOR MUSCLE

AUDIONYM: Plant / Tar Flags

VISUAL IMAGE: See the **plant** with **tar flags.** It has a **foot extended at the ankle joint** and the **toes** are pointed **downward**

ACTION: Extends the foot at the ankle joint and points the toes inferiorly (downward)

LESSON 5 — REVIEW
THE MUSCULAR SYSTEM
HOW MUSCLES ARE NAMED

7. MUSCLES NAMED BY ACTION (cont.)

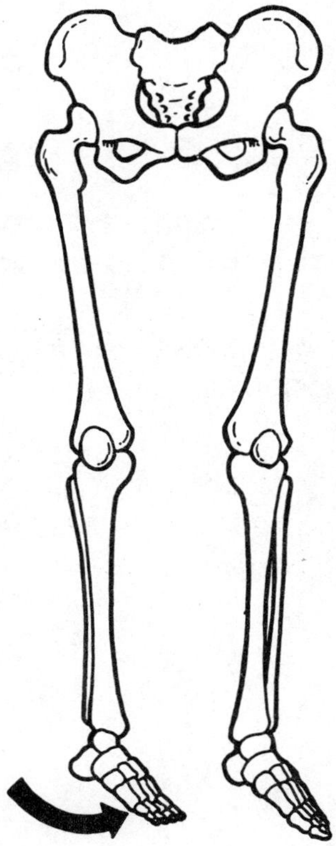

K - INVERTOR MUSCLE

AUDIONYM: Inn/Fur Door

VISUAL IMAGE: See the **inn** with the **fur door**. It has a **foot** down **in** the roof

ACTION: Turns the sole of the foot inward

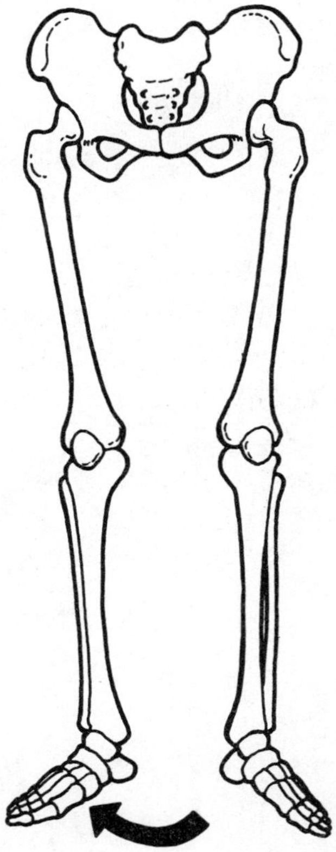

L - EVERTOR MUSCLE

AUDIONYM: Elevator

VISUAL IMAGE: See an **elevator** with the **sole** of a **foot** sticking **out** of it

ACTION: Turns the sole of the foot outward

LESSON 5 — REVIEW
THE MUSCULAR SYSTEM
HOW MUSCLES ARE NAMED

7. MUSCLES NAMED BY ACTION (cont.)

M - SPHINCTER MUSCLE

AUDIONYM: Sphinx

VISUAL IMAGE: See the **sphinx decreasing the size of its opening**

ACTION: Decreases the size of an opening

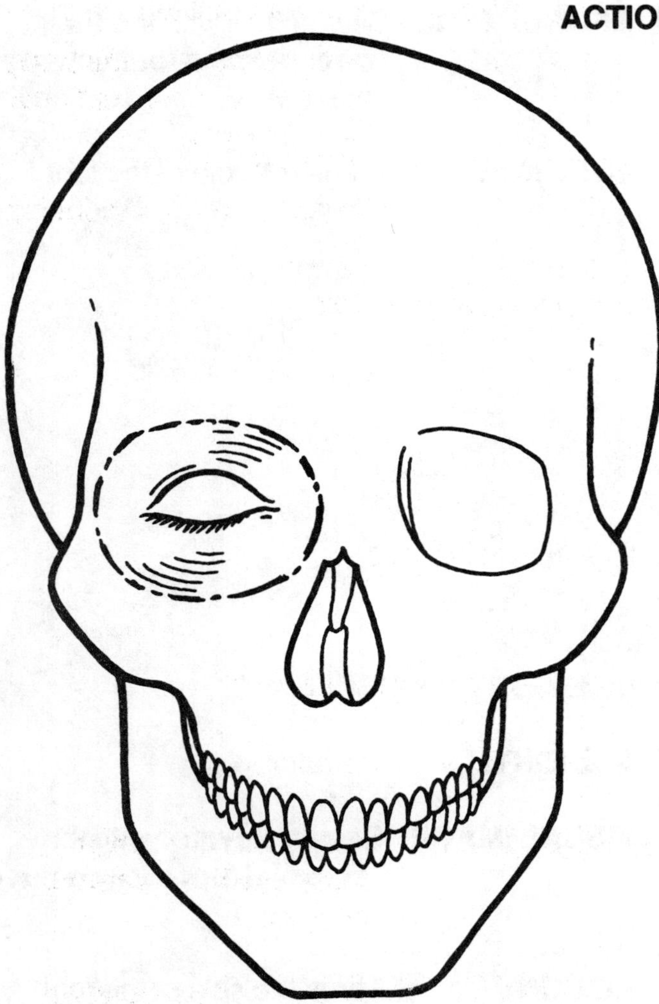

LESSON 5 — REVIEW
THE MUSCULAR SYSTEM
HOW MUSCLES ARE NAMED

7. MUSCLES NAMED BY ACTION (cont.)

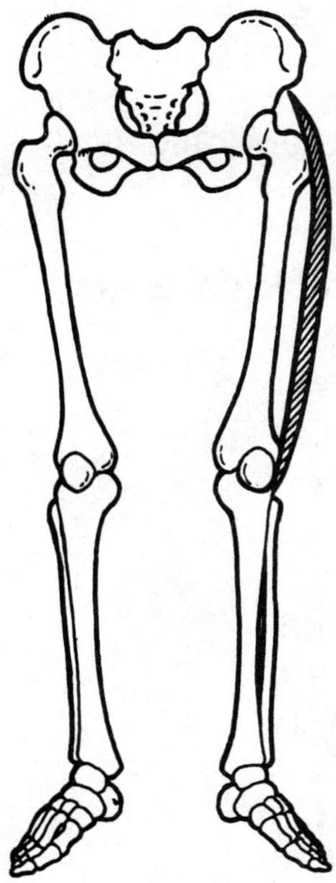

N - TENSOR MUSCLE

AUDIONYM: Tents

VISUAL IMAGE: See the **tents** with the **body parts** being stretched until they are **rigid**

ACTION: Makes a body part more rigid

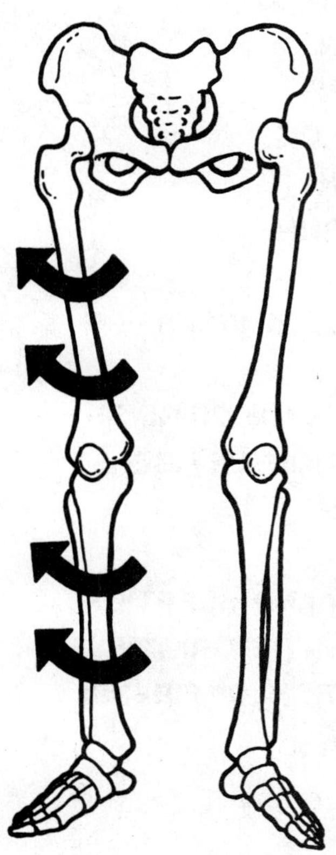

O - ROTATOR MUSCLE

AUDIONYM: Rotary Mower

VISUAL IMAGE: See the **rotary mower moving a bone around a long ax**

ACTION: Moves a bone around its longitudinal axis

LESSON 5 — REVIEW
THE MUSCULAR SYSTEM
HOW MUSCLES ARE NAMED

Following is an example of various types of muscles and how they are named. Review these types of muscles until you can correctly identify how each type is named.

MUSCLE TYPE	NAMED BY:
EXTENSOR	ACTION
TRICEPS	NUMBER (OF ORIGINS)
PRONATOR	ACTION
ADDUCTOR	ACTION
OBLIQUE	DIRECTION (OF FIBERS)
ABDUCTOR	ACTION
EVERTOR	ACTION
LONGUS	SIZE
FLEXOR	ACTION
MAXIMUS	SIZE
DORSIFLEXOR	ACTION
ZYGOMATICUS	LOCATION
ABDOMINIS	LOCATION
FEMORIS	LOCATION
ROTATOR	ACTION
OCCIPITALIS	LOCATION
DEPRESSOR	ACTION
TENSOR	ACTION
INVERTOR	ACTION
LEVATOR	ACTION
TIBIALIS	LOCATION
SPHINCTER	ACTION
TEMPORALIS	LOCATION
MINIMUS	SIZE
CARPI ULNARIS	ORIGIN AND INSERTION
SUPINATOR	ACTION
BICEPS	NUMBER (OF ORIGINS)
TRANSVERSUS	DIRECTION (OF FIBERS)
PLANTAR FLEXOR	ACTION
BREVIS	SIZE
CARPI RADIALIS	ORIGIN AND INSERTION
QUADRICEPS	NUMBER (OF ORIGINS)
RECTUS	DIRECTION (OF FIBERS)
TRAPEZIUS	SHAPE

LESSON 5 — WORKSHEET
THE MUSCULAR SYSTEM
HOW MUSCLES ARE NAMED

40

COMPLETE THE BLANKS:

WORD	AUDIONYM
1. DIRECTION	Book of Directions
2. LOCATION	Locomotive
3. SIZE	S Eyes
4. NUMBER	numbers
5. SHAPE	shake
6. ORIGIN AND INSERTION	orange/ant in short sleeves
7. ACTION	ax

DIRECTION

WORD	AUDIONYM	MEANING
RECTUS	Wreck	straight
TRANS	Trains	Through across
OBLIQUE	(A COMMON TERM)	

ACTION

WORD	AUDIONYM
A. FLEXOR	Flags
B. EXTENSOR	Extension Cord
C. ABDUCTOR	Abe Duck
D. ADDUCTOR	AD Duck
E. LEVATOR	Levitate
F. DEPRESSOR	Deep Presser
G. SUPINATOR	Soup
H. PRONATOR	Procnat
I. DORSIFLEXOR	Doors of Flags
J. PLANTAR FLEXOR	plant Tar Flags
K. INVERTOR	inn Fur door
L. EVERTOR	Elevator
M. SPHINCTER	SpHinX
N. TENSOR	Tents
O. ROTATOR	Rotary

LESSON 5 — WORKSHEET
THE MUSCULAR SYSTEM
HOW MUSCLES ARE NAMED
(THE LINK SYSTEM)

PRINT THE CORRECT LETTER WITHIN THE PARENTHESES

To remember how **muscles are named**, just think of and fill in the audionym for "NAMING OF MUSCLES": muscles are Named by action ?

Then, use the **link system** to recall each audionym in sequence. Under the column marked "AUDIONYM," print the appropriate letter from the audionyms listed below. Under the column marked "MUSCLES ARE NAMED BY," print the appropriate letter from the list below entitled "HOW MUSCLES ARE NAMED."

VISUAL IMAGE	AUDIONYM	MUSCLES ARE NAMED BY:
See (?) with (1)	( )	( )
See (1) with (2)	( )	( )
See (2) with (3)	( )	( )
See (3) with (4)	( )	( )
See (4) with (5)	( )	( )
See (5) with (6)	( )	( )
See (6) with (7)	( )	( )

AUDIONYMS

A. "S" EYES

B. AX

C. NUMBERS

D. ORANGE / ANT IN SHORT SLEEVES

E. (MILK) SHAKE

F. (BOOK OF) DIRECTIONS

G. LOCOMOTIVE

HOW MUSCLES ARE NAMED

A. SIZE

B. NUMBER (OF ORIGINS)

C. ACTION

D. LOCATION

E. SHAPE

F. DIRECTION (OF FIBERS)

G. ORIGIN AND INSERTION

LESSON 5 — WORKSHEET
THE MUSCULAR SYSTEM
HOW MUSCLES ARE NAMED

PRINT THE CORRECT LETTER WITHIN THE PARENTHESES

1. MUSCLES NAMED BY DIRECTION (OF FIBERS)

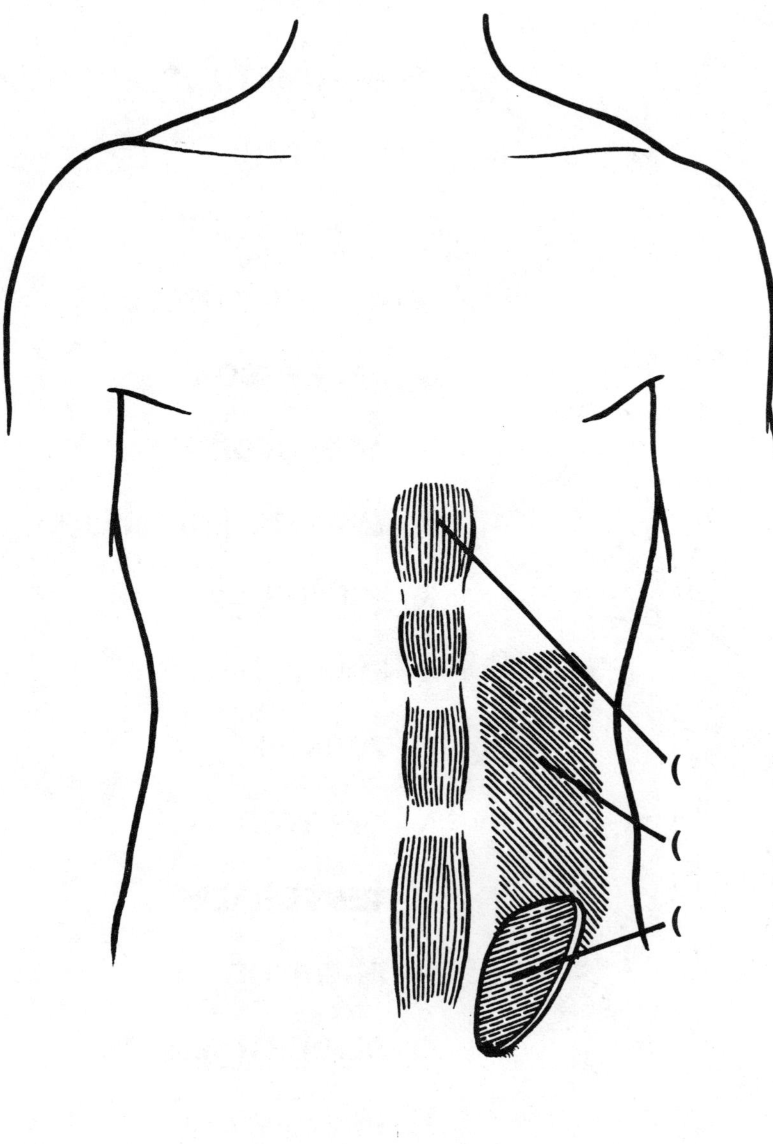

( )
( )
( )

A - OBLIQUE MUSCLE
B - ROTATOR
C - EXTENSOR
D - ZYGOMATICUS MINOR
E - LEVATOR
F - DORSIFLEXOR
G - RECTUS MUSCLE
H - DEPRESSOR
I - ADDUCTOR
J - ZYGOMATICUS MAJOR
K - FLEXOR
L - SPHINCTER
M - TENSOR
N - EVERTOR
O - TEMPORALIS
P - INVERTOR
Q - PLANTAR FLEXOR
R - PRONATOR
S - SUPINATOR
T - ABDUCTOR
U - TRANSVERSE MUSCLE

LESSON 5 — WORKSHEET
THE MUSCULAR SYSTEM
HOW MUSCLES ARE NAMED

PRINT THE CORRECT LETTER WITHIN THE PARENTHESES

2. MUSCLES NAMED BY LOCATION

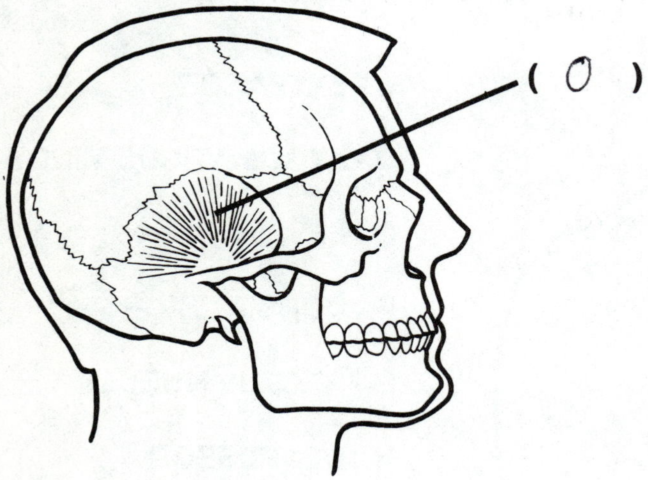

3. MUSCLES NAMED BY SIZE

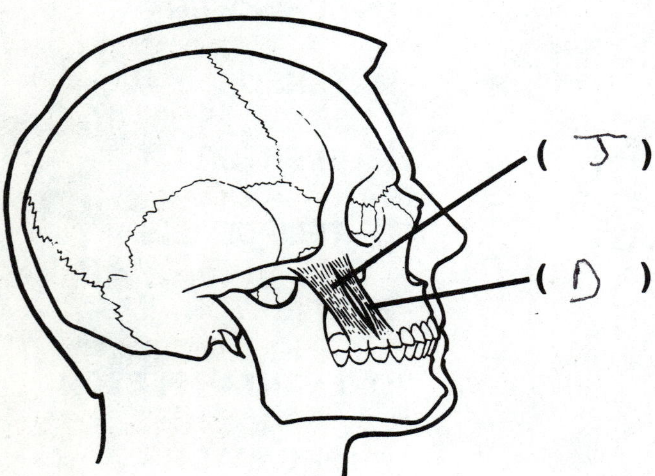

A - OBLIQUE MUSCLE
B - ROTATOR
C - EXTENSOR
D - ZYGOMATICUS MINOR
E - LEVATOR
F - DORSIFLEXOR
G - RECTUS MUSCLE
H - DEPRESSOR
I - ADDUCTOR
J - ZYGOMATICUS MAJOR
K - FLEXOR
L - SPHINCTER
M - TENSOR
N - EVERTOR
O - TEMPORALIS
P - INVERTOR
Q - PLANTAR FLEXOR
R - PRONATOR
S - SUPINATOR
T - ABDUCTOR
U - TRANSVERSE MUSCLE

LESSON 5 — WORKSHEET
THE MUSCULAR SYSTEM
HOW MUSCLES ARE NAMED

PRINT THE CORRECT LETTER WITHIN THE PARENTHESES

4. MUSCLES NAMED BY NUMBER (OF ORIGINS)

From the list below, select **three** types of muscles named by their number of origins.

( ) ( ) ( )

5. MUSCLES NAMED BY SHAPE

From the list below, select **one** muscle named by its shape

( )

6. MUSCLES NAMED BY ORIGIN AND INSERTION

From the list below, select **two** muscles named by their origin and insertion.

( ) ( )

A - OCCIPITALIS
B - DEPRESSOR
C - TENSOR
D - BREVIS
E - CARPI RADIALIS
F - TRICEPS
G - PRONATOR
H - OBLIQUE
I - ABDUCTOR
J - EVERTOR
K - LONGUS
L - RECTUS
M - TRAPEZIUS
N - INVERTOR
O - LEVATOR
P - TIBIALIS
Q - TEMPORALIS
R - MINIMUS
S - CARPI ULNARIS
T - BICEPS
U - TRANSVERSUS
V - MAXIMUS
W - ZYGOMATICUS
X - QUADRICEPS

LESSON 5 — WORKSHEET
THE MUSCULAR SYSTEM
HOW MUSCLES ARE NAMED

PRINT THE CORRECT LETTER WITHIN THE PARENTHESES

7. MUSCLES NAMED BY ACTION

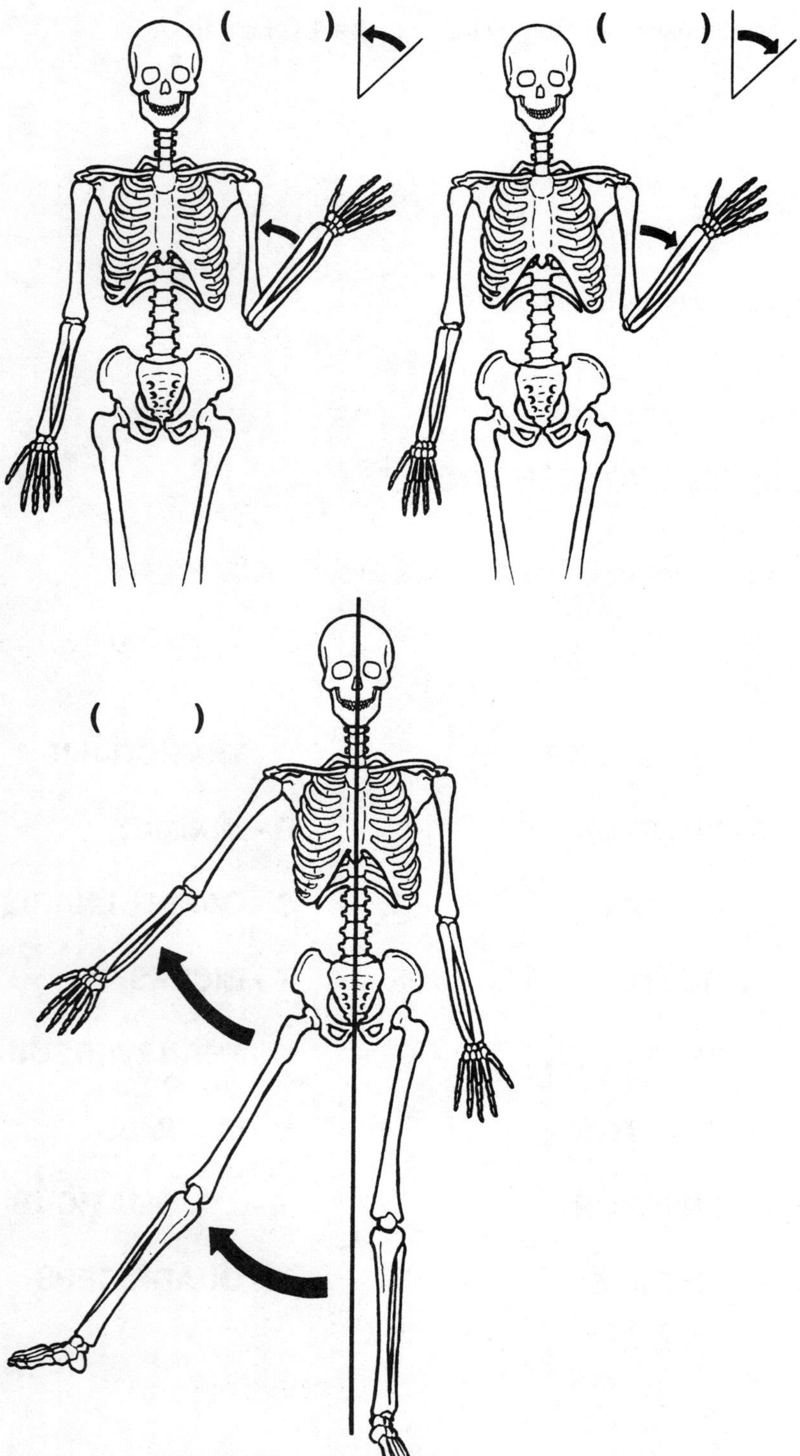

A - OBLIQUE MUSCLE
B - ROTATOR
C - EXTENSOR
D - ZYGOMATICUS MINOR
E - LEVATOR
F - DORSIFLEXOR
G - RECTUS MUSCLE
H - DEPRESSOR
I - ADDUCTOR
J - ZYGOMATICUS MAJOR
K - FLEXOR
L - SPHINCTER
M - TENSOR
N - EVERTOR
O - TEMPORALIS
P - INVERTOR
Q - PLANTAR FLEXOR
R - PRONATOR
S - SUPINATOR
T - ABDUCTOR
U - TRANSVERSE MUSCLE

LESSON 5 — WORKSHEET
THE MUSCULAR SYSTEM
HOW MUSCLES ARE NAMED

PRINT THE CORRECT LETTER WITHIN THE PARENTHESES

7. MUSCLES NAMED BY ACTION (cont.)

( )

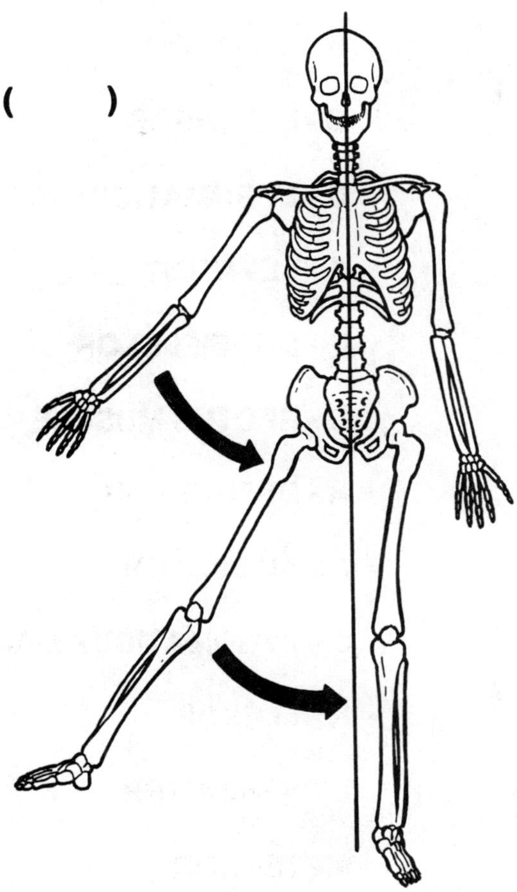

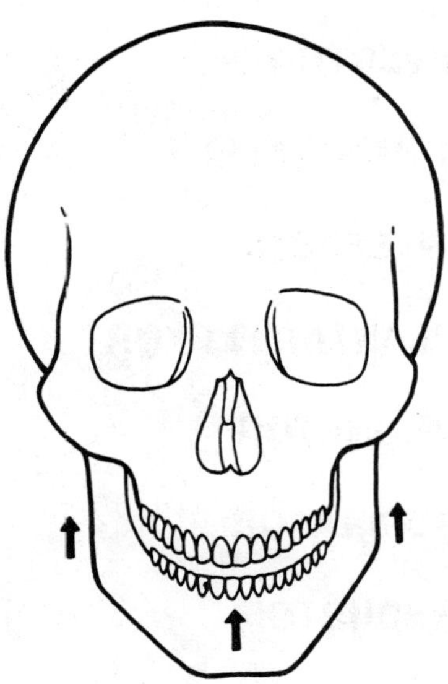

( )

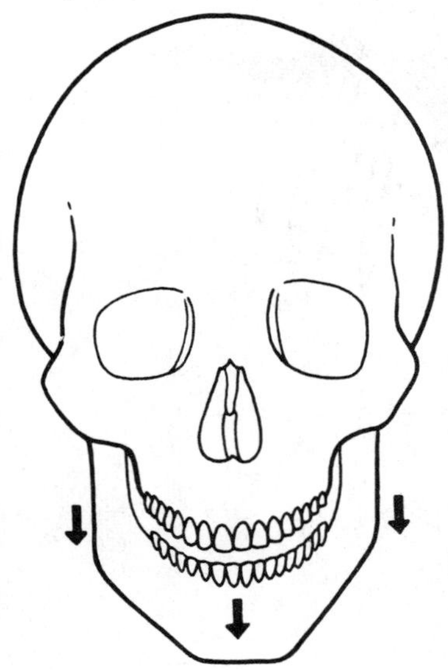

( )

A - OBLIQUE MUSCLE

B - ROTATOR

C - EXTENSOR

D - ZYGOMATICUS MINOR

E - LEVATOR

F - DORSIFLEXOR

G - RECTUS MUSCLE

H - DEPRESSOR

I - ADDUCTOR

J - ZYGOMATICUS MAJOR

K - FLEXOR

L - SPHINCTER

M - TENSOR

N - EVERTOR

O - TEMPORALIS

P - INVERTOR

Q - PLANTAR FLEXOR

R - PRONATOR

S - SUPINATOR

T - ABDUCTOR

U - TRANSVERSE MUSCLE

LESSON 5 — WORKSHEET
THE MUSCULAR SYSTEM
HOW MUSCLES ARE NAMED

PRINT THE CORRECT LETTER WITHIN THE PARENTHESES

7. MUSCLES NAMED BY ACTION (cont.)

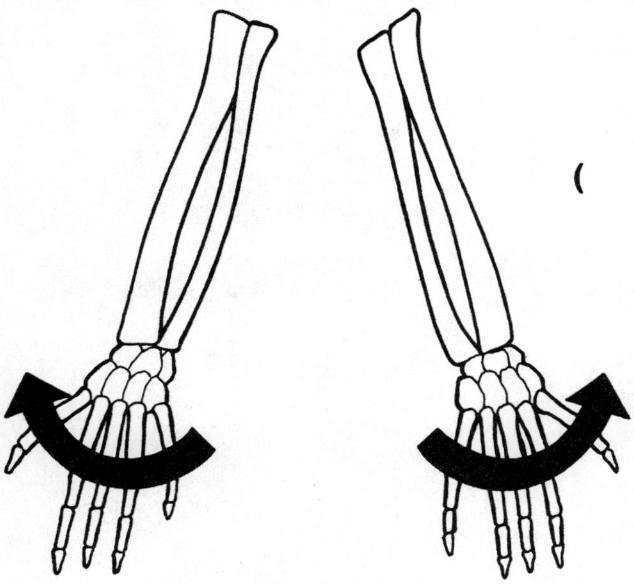

( )

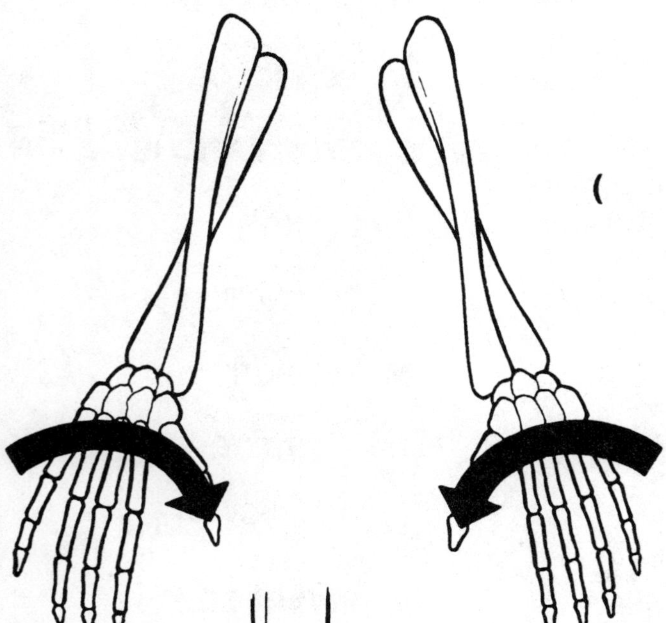

( )

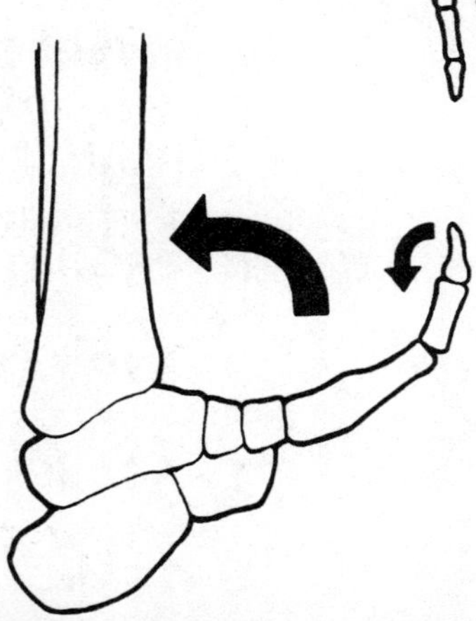

( )

A - OBLIQUE MUSCLE

B - ROTATOR

C - EXTENSOR

D - ZYGOMATICUS MINOR

E - LEVATOR

F - DORSIFLEXOR

G - RECTUS MUSCLE

H - DEPRESSOR

I - ADDUCTOR

J - ZYGOMATICUS MAJOR

K - FLEXOR

L - SPHINCTER

M - TENSOR

N - EVERTOR

O - TEMPORALIS

P - INVERTOR

Q - PLANTAR FLEXOR

R - PRONATOR

S - SUPINATOR

T - ABDUCTOR

U - TRANSVERSE MUSCLE

LESSON 5 — WORKSHEET
THE MUSCULAR SYSTEM
HOW MUSCLES ARE NAMED

PRINT THE CORRECT LETTER WITHIN THE PARENTHESES

7. MUSCLES NAMED BY ACTION (cont.)

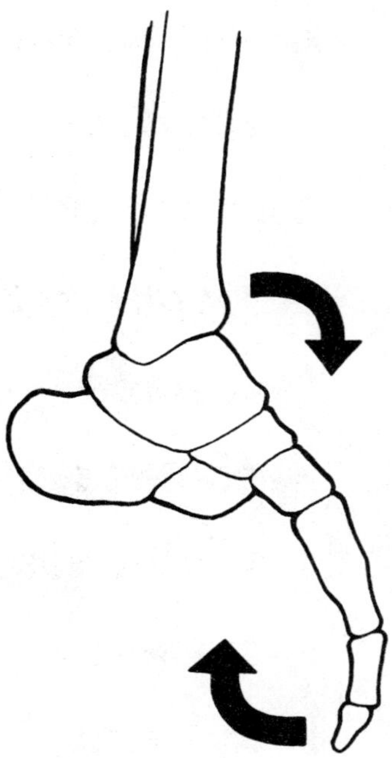

( )

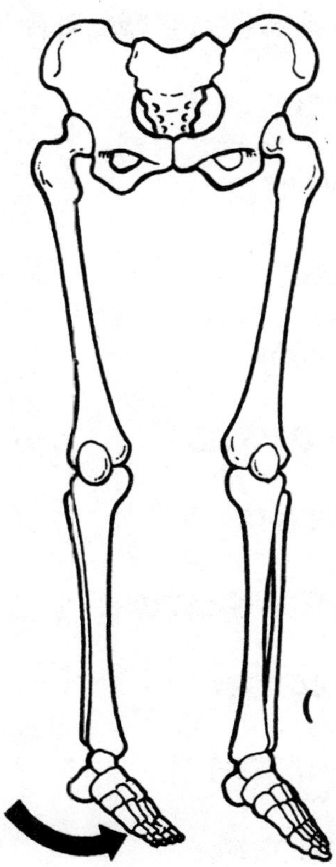

( )

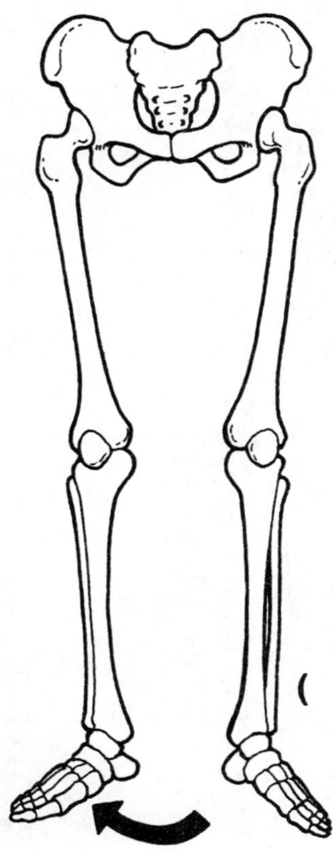

( )

A - OBLIQUE MUSCLE

B - ROTATOR

C - EXTENSOR

D - ZYGOMATICUS MINOR

E - LEVATOR

F - DORSIFLEXOR

G - RECTUS MUSCLE

H - DEPRESSOR

I - ADDUCTOR

J - ZYGOMATICUS MAJOR

K - FLEXOR

L - SPHINCTER

M - TENSOR

N - EVERTOR

O - TEMPORALIS

P - INVERTOR

Q - PLANTAR FLEXOR

R - PRONATOR

S - SUPINATOR

T - ABDUCTOR

U - TRANSVERSE MUSCLE

LESSON 5 — WORKSHEET
THE MUSCULAR SYSTEM
HOW MUSCLES ARE NAMED

PRINT THE CORRECT LETTER WITHIN THE PARENTHESES

7. MUSCLES NAMED BY ACTION (cont.)

( )

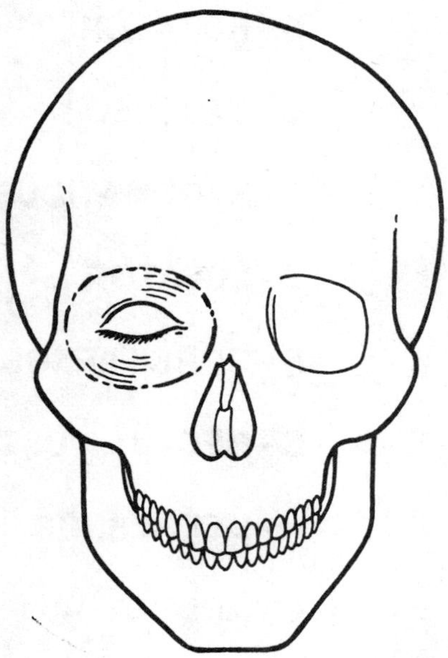

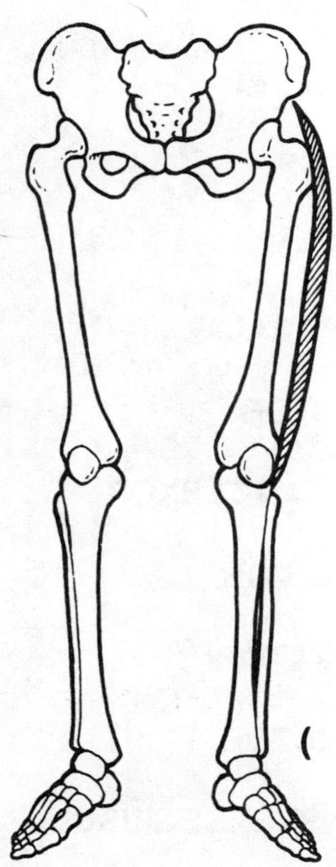

( )

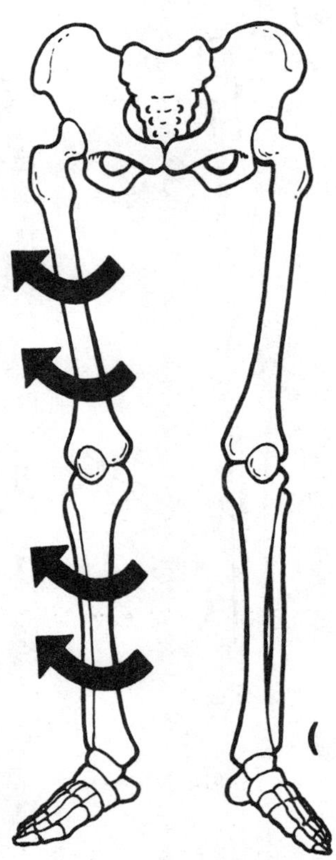

( )

A - OBLIQUE MUSCLE

B - ROTATOR

C - EXTENSOR

D - ZYGOMATICUS MINOR

E - LEVATOR

F - DORSIFLEXOR

G - RECTUS MUSCLE

H - DEPRESSOR

I - ADDUCTOR

J - ZYGOMATICUS MAJOR

K - FLEXOR

L - SPHINCTER

M - TENSOR

N - EVERTOR

O - TEMPORALIS

P - INVERTOR

Q - PLANTAR FLEXOR

R - PRONATOR

S - SUPINATOR

T - ABDUCTOR

U - TRANSVERSE MUSCLE

LESSON 5 — WORKSHEET
THE MUSCULAR SYSTEM
PRINT THE CORRECT LETTER WITHIN THE PARENTHESES

HOW MUSCLES ARE NAMED

From the list marked "HOW MUSCLES ARE NAMED," select the letter which most closely describes how each of the following types of muscles are named. Mark the letter in the parentheses:

MUSCLE	NAMED BY:
OCCIPITALIS	(E)
DEPRESSOR	(D)
EXTENSOR	(D)
TENSOR	(D)
BREVIS	(B)
ADDUCTOR	(D)
CARPI RADIALIS	(G)
TRICEPS	(F)
PRONATOR	(D)
OBLIQUE	(A)
FLEXOR	(D)
ABDUCTOR	(D)
EVERTOR	(D)
LONGUS	(B)
RECTUS	(A)
DORSI FLEXOR	(D)
TRAPEZIUS	(C)
INVERTOR	(D)
LEVATOR	(D)
ROTATOR	(D)
TIBIALIS	(E)
TEMPORALIS	(E)
MINIMUS	(B)
SPHINCTER	(D)
CARPI ULNARIS	(G)
BICEPS	(F)
TRANSVERSUS	(A)
SUPINATOR	(D)
MAXIMUS	(B)
ZYGOMATICUS	(E)
PLANTAR FLEXOR	(D)
ABDOMINIS	(E)
FEMORIS	(E)
QUADRICEPS	(F)

HOW MUSCLES ARE NAMED

A - DIRECTION (OF FIBERS)
B - SIZE
C - SHAPE
D - ACTION
E - LOCATION
F - NUMBER (OF ORIGINS)
G - ORIGIN AND INSERTION

LESSON 6

THE INTEGUMENTARY SYSTEM

THE SKIN AND ITS DERIVATIVES

- CUTIS (SKIN)
- HAIR
- GLANDS
- NAILS

REMEMBER!

1st ***Pronounce*** *the name of the body part or term*
2nd ***Recall*** *and* ***pronounce*** *the audionym*
3rd ***For body parts: visualize*** *the audionym in place*
For terms: visualize *the association*
4th ***Pronounce*** *the name of the body part or term again.*

LESSON 6 — REVIEW
THE INTEGUMENTARY SYSTEM
THE SKIN AND ITS DERIVATIVES

AUDIONYMS

WORD	AUDIONYM
EPIDERMIS	A PEA/DORMATS
DERMIS	DOORMATS
SUBCUTANEOUS TISSUE	SUB/CUESTICK/TISSUE
HAIR SHAFT	HAIR SHIFT (GEAR SHIFT)
ROOT	ROOT
NAIL	NAIL
NAIL BODY	NAIL/BODY
FREE EDGE	FREEZER HEDGE
NAIL ROOT	NAIL/ROOT
NAIL BED	NAIL/BED

ASSOCIATIONS

WORD	AUDIONYM	VISUAL IMAGE / ASSOCIATION	MEANING
cutis	cuestick	See the **cuesticks** covering the **skin**!	skin
sebaceous (gland)	sea base	See a **sea base** with an **oil** rig on it!	oil (gland)
sudoriferous (gland)	suit of furs	See someone wearing a **suit of furs.** He is **sweating**!	sweat (gland)

LESSON 6 — REVIEW
THE INTEGUMENTARY SYSTEM

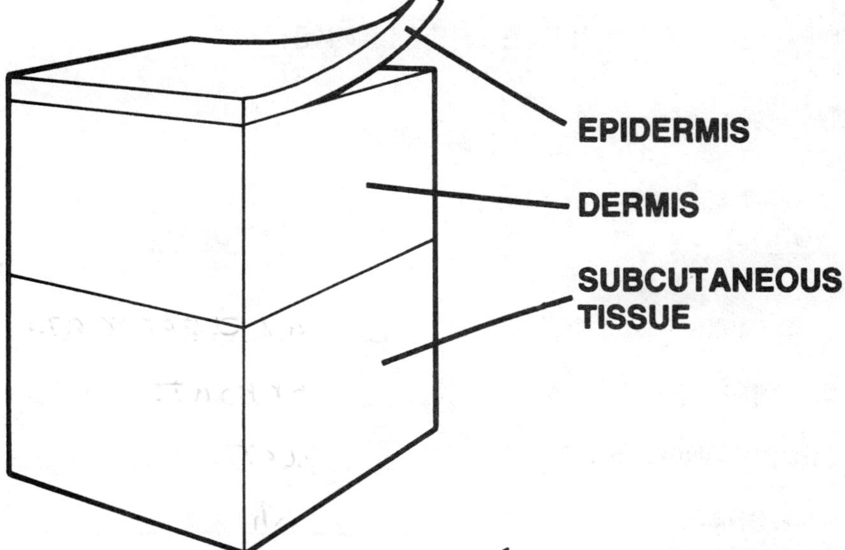

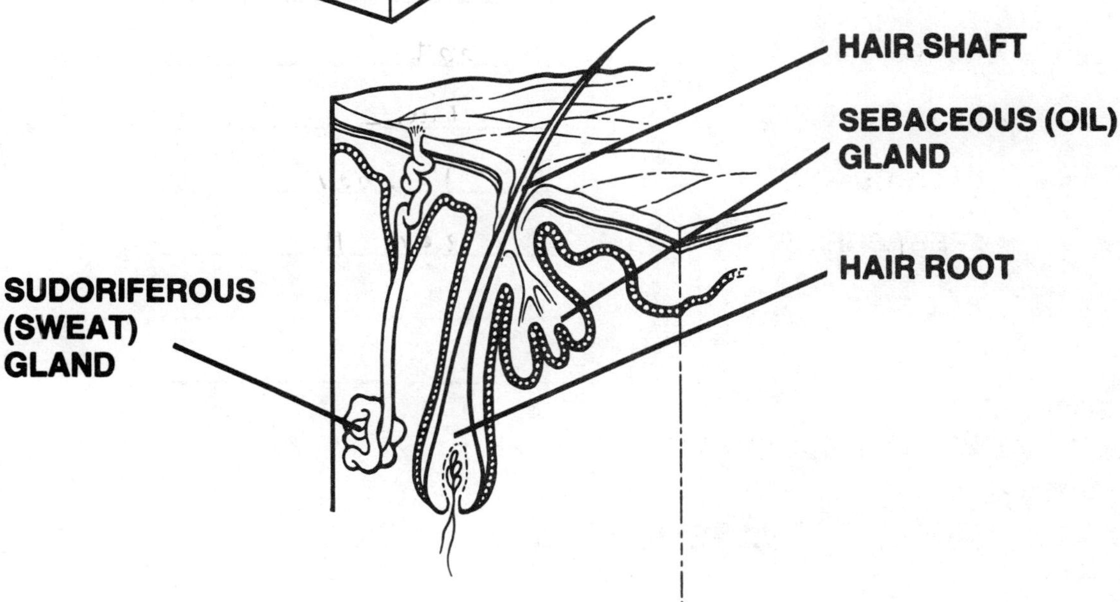

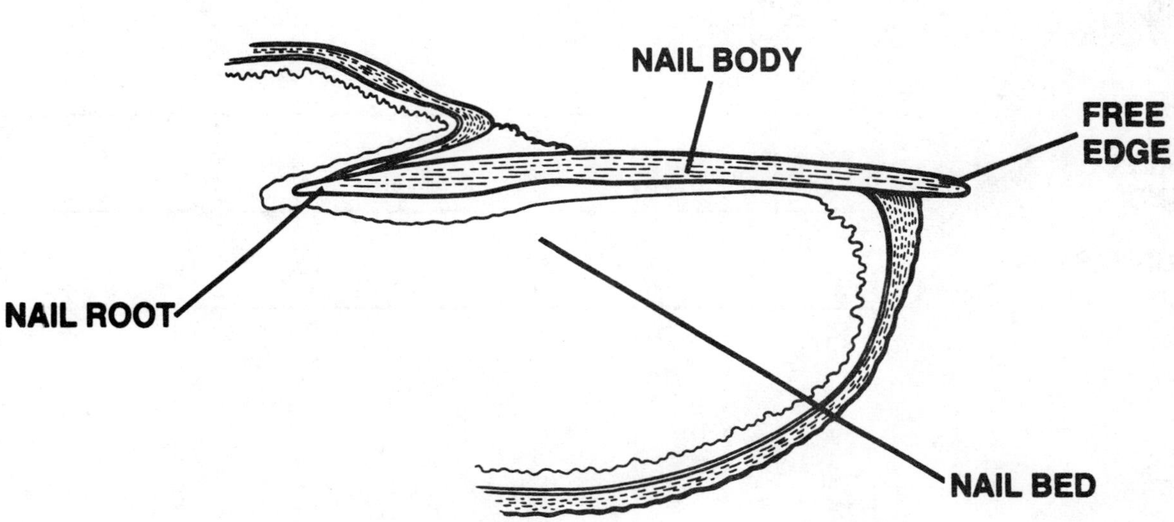

LESSON 6 — WORKSHEET
THE INTEGUMENTARY SYSTEM

COMPLETE THE BLANKS:

AUDIONYMS

WORD	AUDIONYM
EPIDERMIS	a Pea/doormats
DERMIS	Doormats
SUBCUTANEOUS TISSUE	Sub/cuestick/Tissue
HAIR SHAFT	Hair Shift (Gear shift)
ROOT	Root
NAIL	nail
NAIL BODY	Nail/body
FREE EDGE	Freezer Hedge
NAIL ROOT	Nail Root
NAIL BED	Nail Bed

ASSOCIATIONS

WORD	AUDIONYM	MEANING
CUTIS	Cuestick	skin
SEBACEOUS (GLAND)	Sea base	oil (Glands)
SUDORIFEROUS (GLAND)	Suit of furs	Sweat (Glands)

LESSON 6 — WORKSHEET
THE INTEGUMENTARY SYSTEM

PRINT THE CORRECT LETTER WITHIN THE PARENTHESES

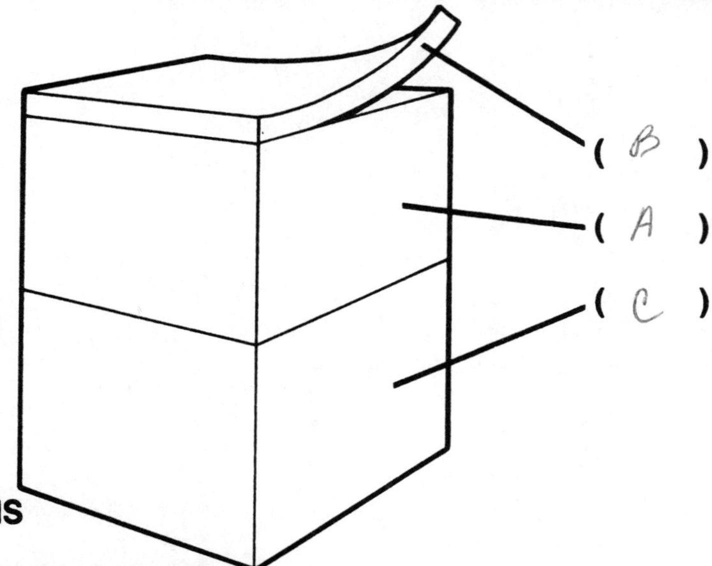

A - DERMIS

B - EPIDERMIS

C - SUBCUTANEOUS TISSUE

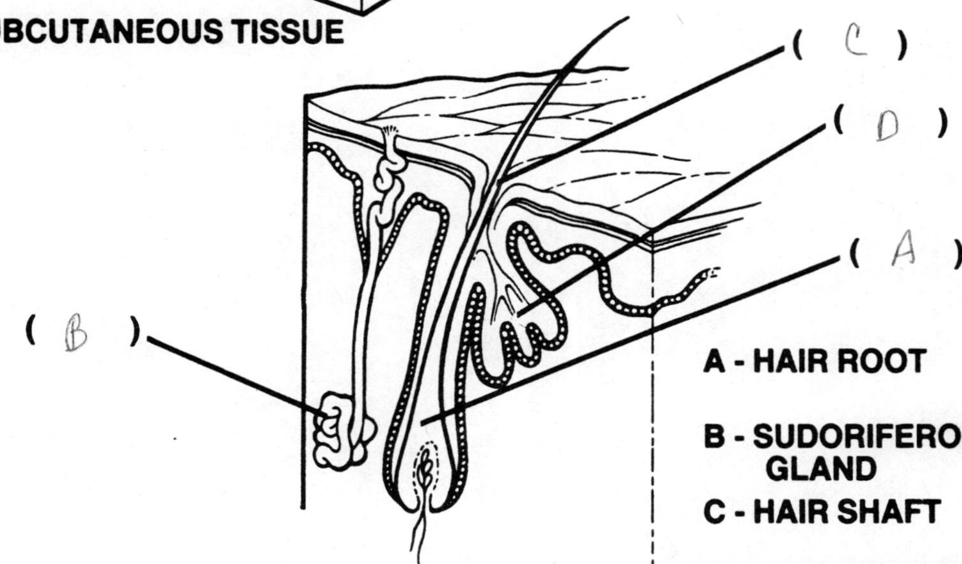

A - HAIR ROOT

B - SUDORIFEROUS (SWEAT) GLAND

C - HAIR SHAFT

D - SEBACEOUS (OIL) GLAND

A - NAIL BED

B - NAIL ROOT

C - FREE EDGE

D - NAIL BODY

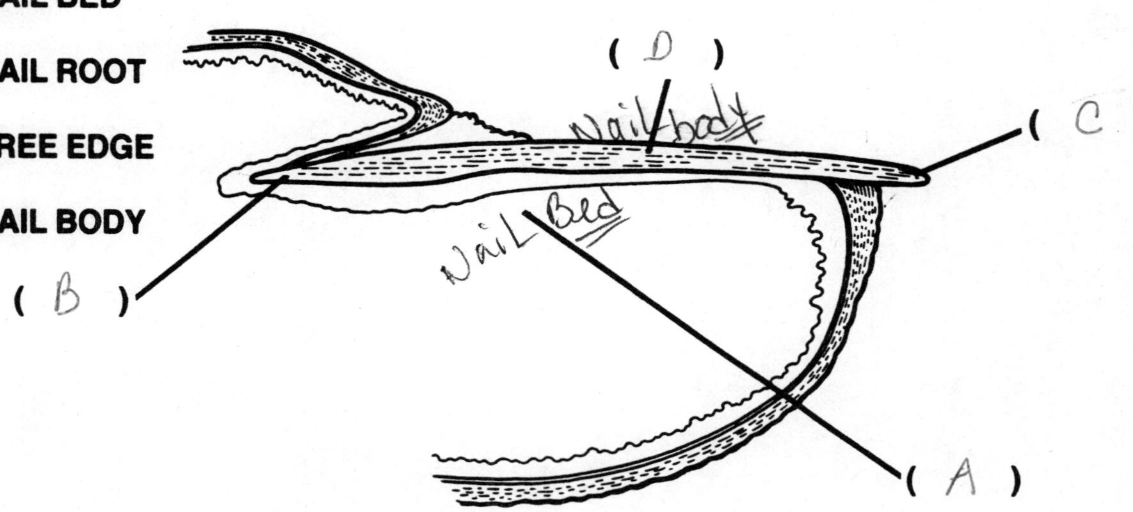

LESSON 7

THE RESPIRATORY SYSTEM

	NUMBER
● NASAL CAVITY	2
● PHARYNX	1
● LARYNX	1
● TRACHEA	1
● BRONCHUS	2
● LUNG	2

REMEMBER!

1st ***Pronounce*** *the name of the body part or term*
2nd ***Recall*** *and* ***pronounce*** *the audionym*
3rd ***For body parts: visualize*** *the audionym in place*
For terms: visualize *the association*
4th ***Pronounce*** *the name of the body part or term again.*

LESSON 7 — REVIEW
THE RESPIRATORY SYSTEM

AUDIONYMS

WORD	AUDIONYM
NASAL CAVITY	NASAL SPRAY
PHARYNX	FIRE RINGS
LARYNX	LAYER INKS
TRACHEA	TRAY KEY
BRONCHUS	BRONCO
LUNG	LUNG

LESSON 7 — REVIEW
THE RESPIRATORY SYSTEM

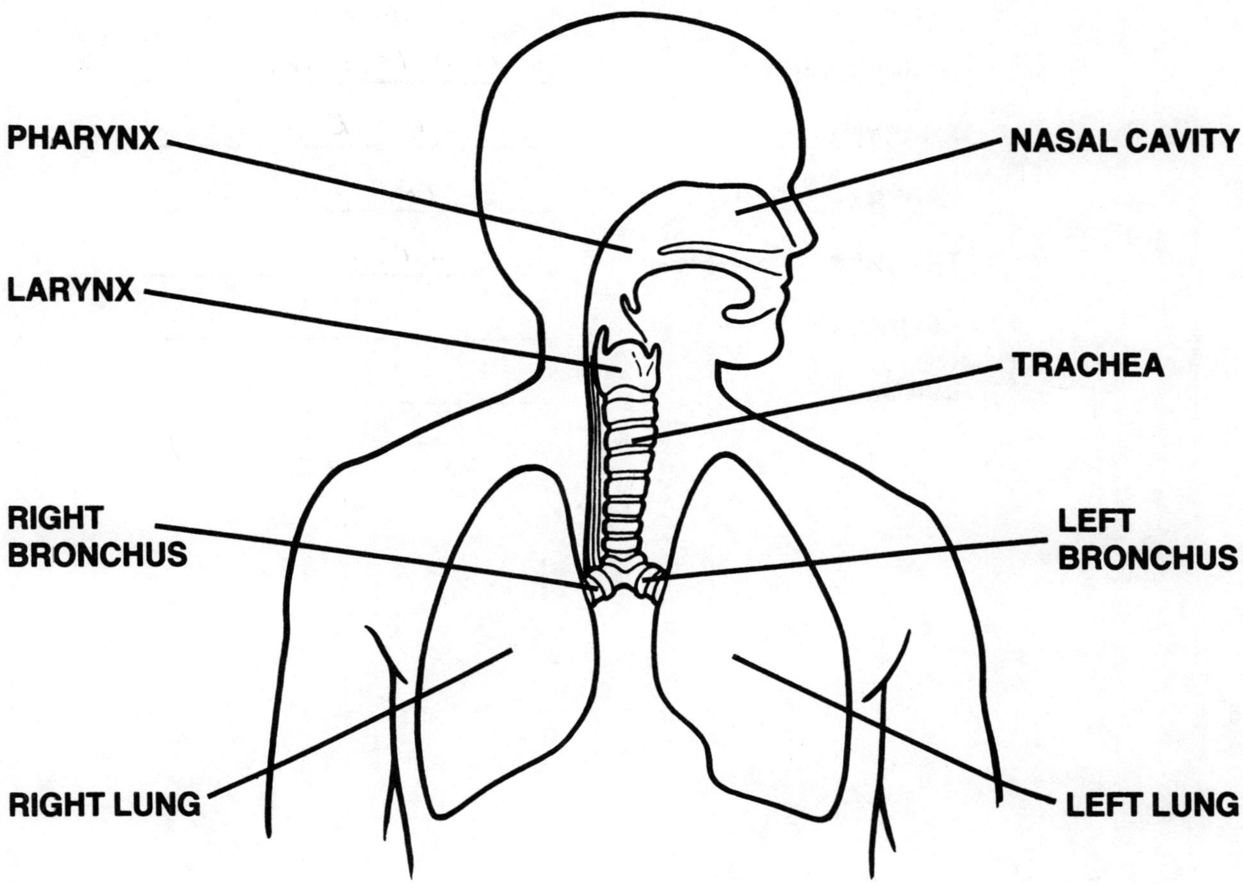

LESSON 7 — WORKSHEET
THE RESPIRATORY SYSTEM

COMPLETE THE BLANKS:

AUDIONYMS

WORD	AUDIONYM
NASAL CAVITY	Nasal spray
PHARYNX	Fire Rings
LARYNX	Layer inks
TRACHEA	Thay Key
BRONCHUS	Broncho
LUNG	Lung

LESSON 7 — WORKSHEET
THE RESPIRATORY SYSTEM

PRINT THE CORRECT LETTER WITHIN THE PARENTHESES

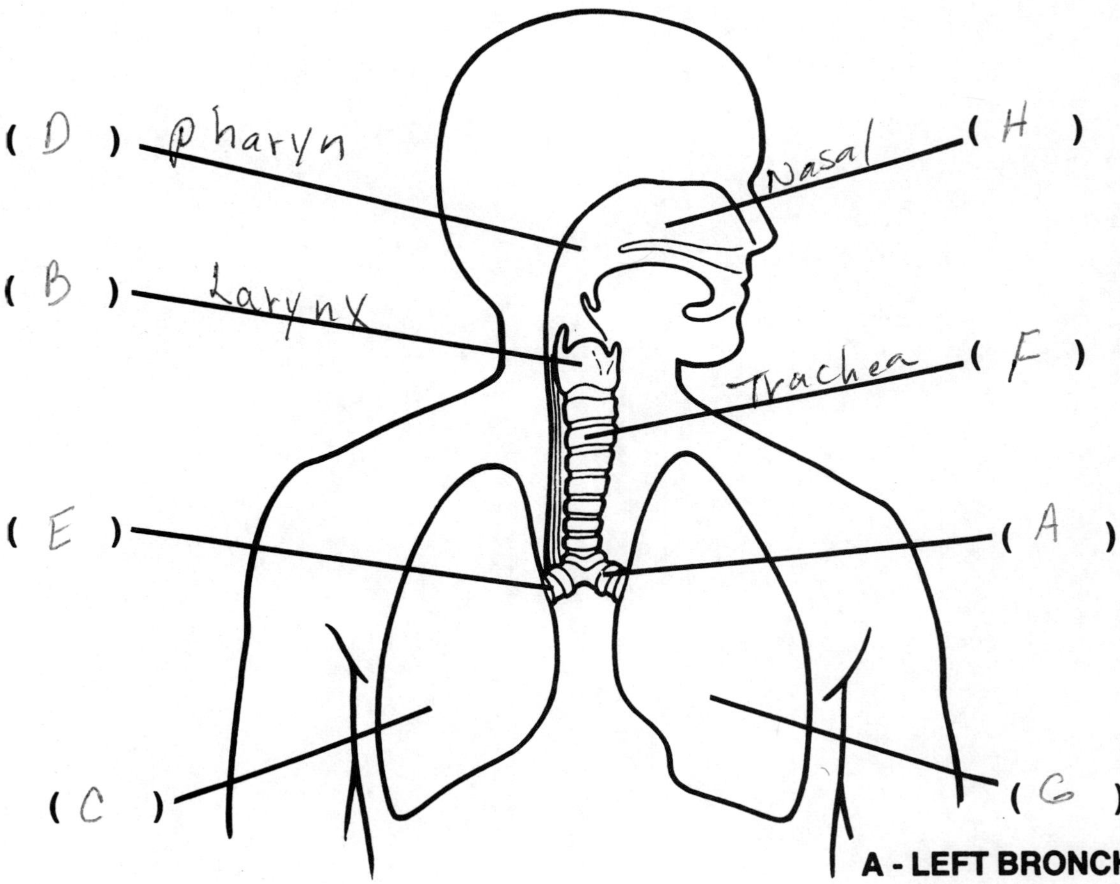

A - LEFT BRONCHUS

B - LARYNX

C - RIGHT LUNG

D - PHARYNX

E - RIGHT BRONCHUS

F - TRACHEA

G - LEFT LUNG

H - NASAL CAVITY

LESSON 8

THE NERVOUS SYSTEM

PART A

THE CENTRAL NERVOUS SYTEM

- PRINCIPAL PARTS OF THE BRAIN
- PRINCIPAL PARTS OF THE SPINAL CORD

REMEMBER!

1st *Pronounce the name of the body part or term*
2nd ***Recall** and **pronounce** the audionym*
3rd ***For body parts: visualize** the audionym in place*
***For terms: visualize** the association*
4th ***Pronounce** the name of the body part or term again.*

LESSON 8 — REVIEW
THE NERVOUS SYSTEM
PART A
THE CENTRAL NERVOUS SYSTEM

AUDIONYMS

WORD	AUDIONYM
CENTRAL (NERVOUS SYSTEM)	CENT
PERIPHERAL (NERVOUS SYSTEM)	PEAR HALF

PRINCIPAL PARTS OF THE BRAIN

WORD	AUDIONYM
CEREBELLUM	CELERY/BELL
CEREBRUM	CELERY/BROOM
THALAMUS	TALL MOOSE
HYPOTHALAMUS	HIPPO/TALL MOOSE
MIDBRAIN	MEAT/BRAIN
PONS	POND
MEDULLA	MEDAL

PRINCIPAL PARTS OF THE SPINAL CORD

WORD	AUDIONYM
WHITE MATTER	WHITE MAT
GRAY MATTER	GRAY MAT
CENTRAL CANAL	CENT/CAN

LESSON 8 — REVIEW
THE NERVOUS SYSTEM
PART A
THE CENTRAL NERVOUS SYSTEM

PRINCIPAL PARTS OF THE BRAIN

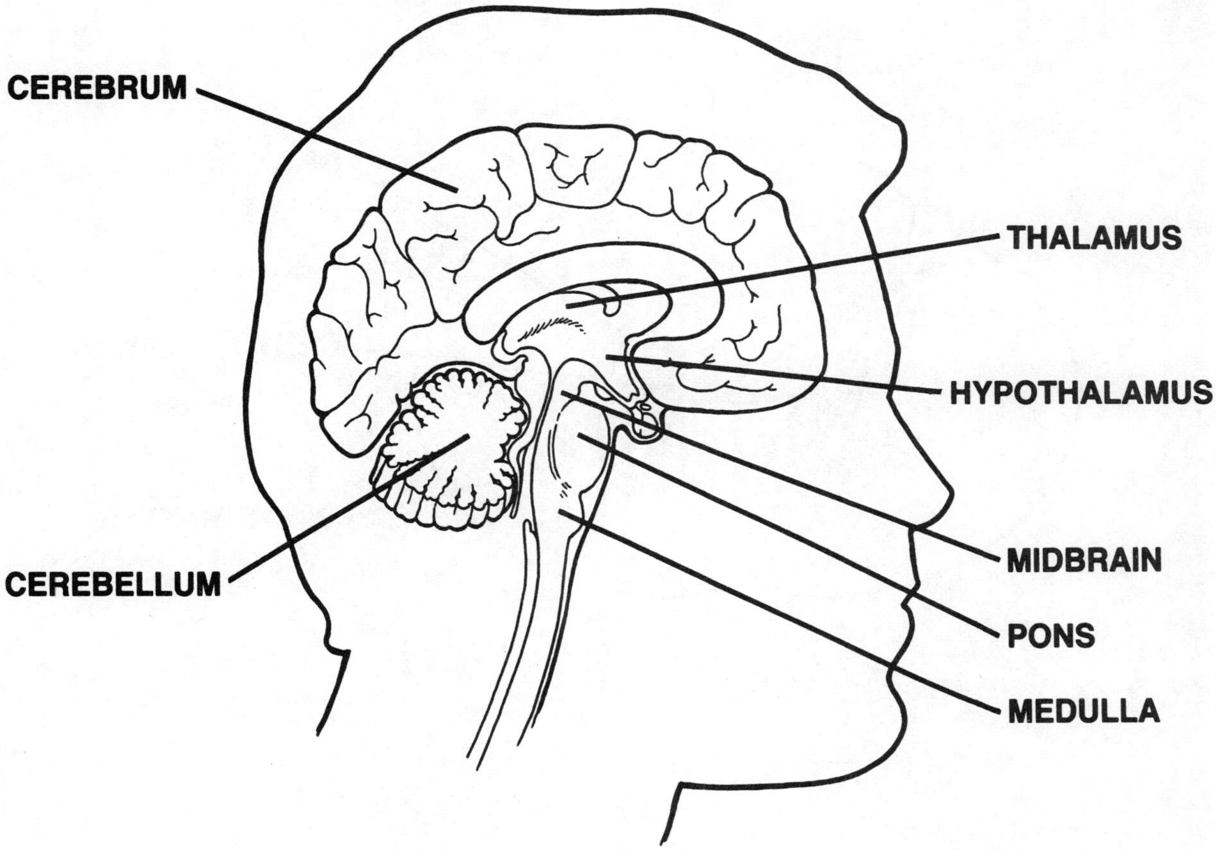

LESSON 8 — REVIEW
THE NERVOUS SYSTEM
PART A
THE CENTRAL NERVOUS SYSTEM

PRINCIPAL PARTS OF THE SPINAL CORD

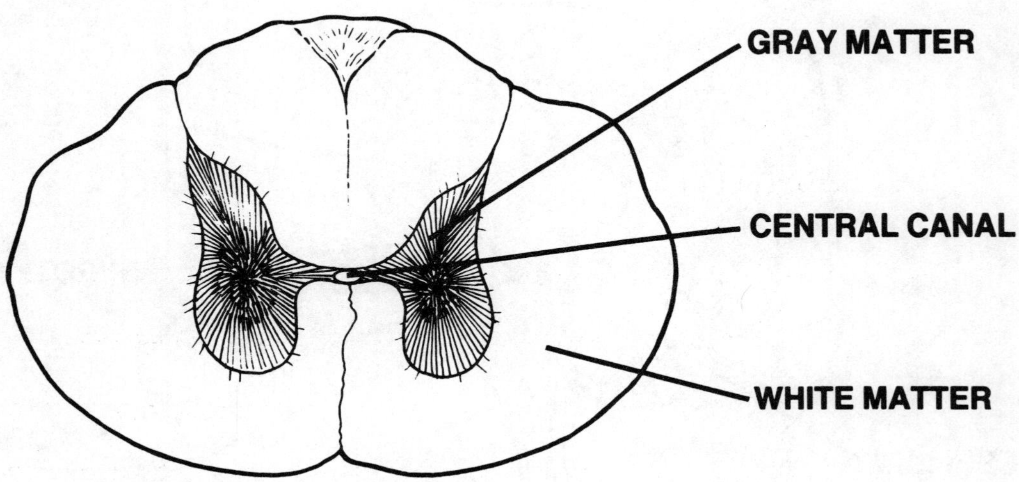

LESSON 8 — WORKSHEET
THE NERVOUS SYSTEM
PART A
THE CENTRAL NERVOUS SYSTEM

COMPLETE THE BLANKS:

AUDIONYMS

WORD	AUDIONYM
CENTRAL (Nervous System)	Cent
PERIPHERAL (Nervous System)	Pear Half

PRINCIPAL PARTS OF THE BRAIN

WORD	AUDIONYM
CEREBELLUM	Celery Bell
CEREBRUM	Celery Broom
THALAMUS	Tall moose
HYPOTHALAMUS	Hipp TAll moose
MIDBRAIN	meat Brain
PONS	Pond
MEDULLA	Medal

PRINCIPAL PARTS OF THE SPINAL CORD

WORD	AUDIONYM
WHITE MATTER	white mat
GRAY MATTER	Gray mat
CENTRAL CANAL	cent/can

LESSON 8 — WORKSHEET
THE NERVOUS SYSTEM

PRINT THE CORRECT LETTER WITHIN THE PARENTHESES

PRINCIPAL PARTS OF THE BRAIN

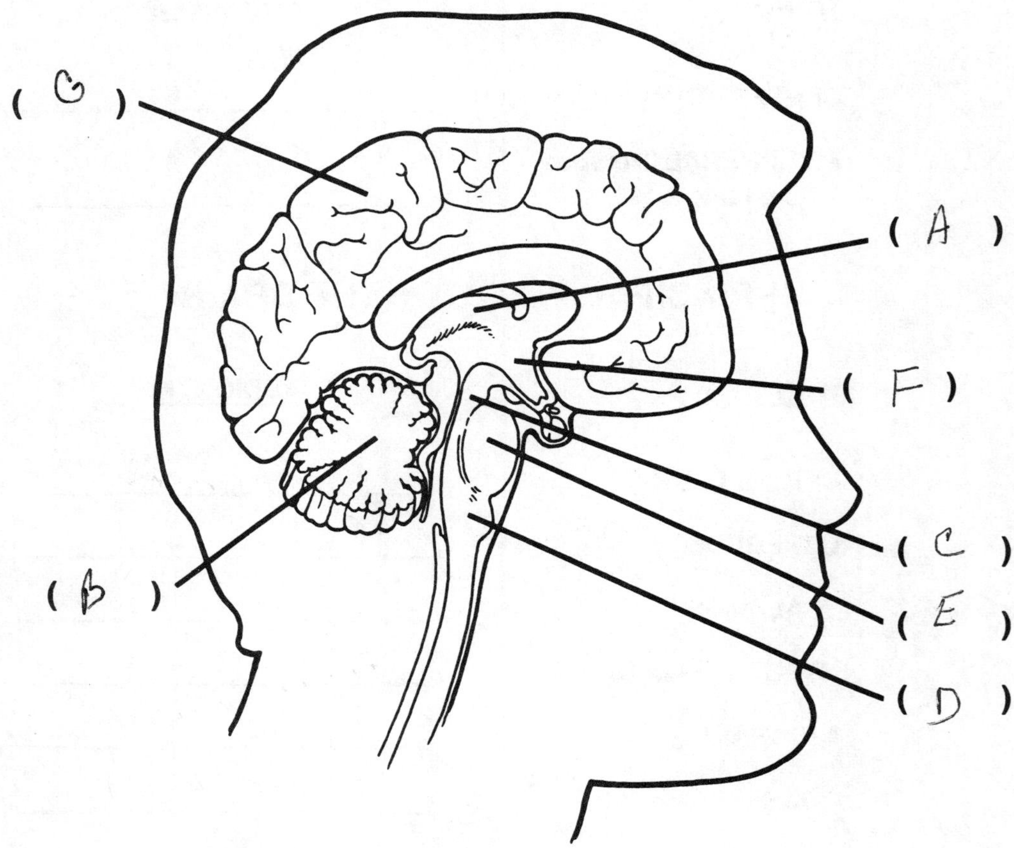

A - THALAMUS

B - CEREBELLUM

C - MIDBRAIN

D - MEDULLA

E - PONS

F - HYPOTHALAMUS

G - CEREBRUM

LESSON 8 — WORKSHEET
THE NERVOUS SYSTEM

PRINT THE CORRECT LETTER WITHIN THE PARENTHESES

PRINCIPAL PARTS OF THE SPINAL CORD

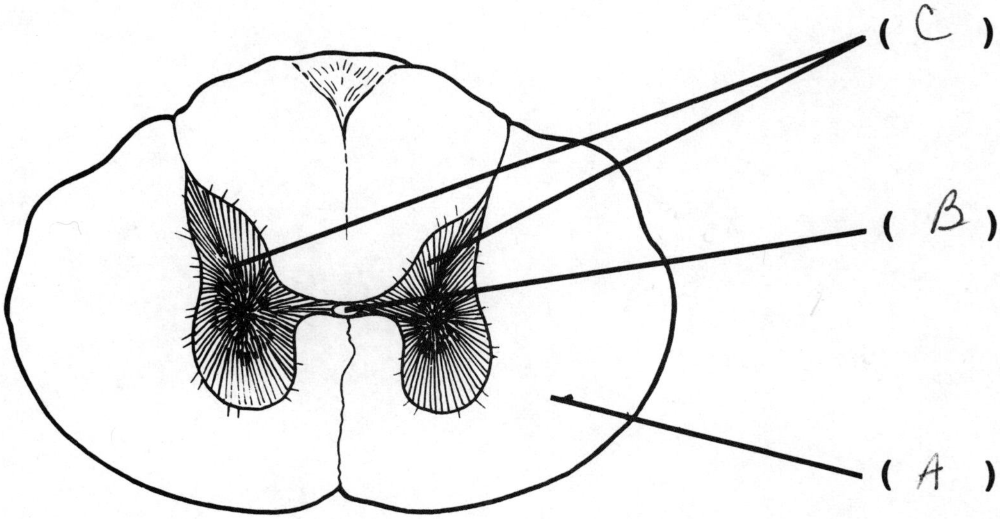

A - WHITE MATTER

B - CENTRAL CANAL

C - GRAY MATTER

LESSON 8

THE NERVOUS SYSTEM

PART B

THE PERIPHERAL NERVOUS SYSTEM

- CRANIAL NERVES (12 PAIRS)
- SPINAL NERVES (31 PAIRS)
- PRINCIPAL PLEXUSES
- TERMS
- SYMPATHETIC NERVES
- PARASYMPATHETIC NERVES

REMEMBER!

1st ***Pronounce*** *the name of the body part or term*
2nd ***Recall*** *and* ***pronounce*** *the audionym*
3rd ***For body parts: visualize*** *the audionym in place*
For terms: visualize *the association*
4th ***Pronounce*** *the name of the body part or term again.*

LESSON 8 — REVIEW
THE NERVOUS SYSTEM
PART B
THE PERIPHERAL NERVOUS SYSTEM

WORD	AUDIONYM	VISUAL IMAGE / ASSOCIATION	MEANING
plexus	plaques	See the **plaques** covered with **nets** of **spinal nerves**!	networks of spinal nerves
afferent	a fur ant	See **a fur ant carrying sand/cereal (messages) to the central nervous system**!	carries (sensory) messages to the central nervous system
efferent	evergreen	See the **evergreen** with the **motor** carrying **messages from the central nervous system to all parts of the body**!	carries (motor) impulses (messages) to all parts of the body
sympathetic	symphony	See the **symphony** playing **emergency** vehicles (in the thoracolumbar region of the spinal cord)!	acts in cases of emergency
para sympathetic	parrot symphony	See the **parrot symphony** playing **body organs** (in the craniosacral regions of the spinal cord)!	regulates the function of body organs
somatic nervous system	sombrero attic	See the **sombrero attic**,it has **skeleton with muscles in it**!	serves the skeletal (or voluntary) muscles
sciatic nerve	ice attic	See the **ice attic** in place!	largest and longest nerve in the body

THE CRANIAL NERVES

WORD	AUDIONYM
OLFACTORY	OIL FACTORY
OPTIC	OPAL
OCULOMOTOR	OCTOPUS/MOTOR
TROCHLEAR	TRUCK/LURE
TRIGEMINAL	TREE/GEM
ABDUCENS	ABE/TWO CENTS
FACIAL	FACE
VESTIBULOCOCHLEAR	VEST/BULL/COCOA
GLOSSOPHARYNGEAL	GLASS OF FIRE RINGS
VAGUS	VEGAS
ACCESSORY	AX
HYPOGLOSSAL	HIPPO/GLASSES

LESSON 8 — REVIEW
THE NERVOUS SYSTEM
PART B
THE PERIPHERAL NERVOUS SYSTEM
THE CRANIAL NERVES

HOW TO REMEMBER THE 12 PAIRS OF CRANIAL NERVES IN SEQUENCE
(From the AUDIOVISUAL PROGRAM)

To remember the names of the 12 pairs of cranial nerves, just recall the audionym for "cranial nerves" — **crane/nerves** (A **crane** with **nerves** all over it).

Then, use the LINK SYSTEM to recall each audionym in sequence:

ROMAN NUMERAL	VISUAL IMAGE / ASSOCIATION	NERVE
I	See the **crane/nerves** with an **oil factory** bursting out of it!	olfactory
II	See the **oil factory** with **opals** floating out of its smoke stacks!	optic
III	See the **opal** with an **octopus/motor** bursting out of it!	oculomotor
IV	See the **octopus/motor** holding a **truck/ lure**!	trochlear
V	See the **truck/lure** with a **tree/gem (a tree with gems)** growing out of it!	trigeminal
VI	See the **tree/gem** with **Abe/two cents** bursting out of it!	abducens
VII	See **Abe/two cents** with a **face** bursting out of it!	facial
VIII	See the **face** with a **vest/bull/cocoa** coming out of it!	vestibulocochlear
IX	See the **vest/bull/cocoa** with a **glass of fire rings** coming out of it!	glossopharyngeal
X	See the **glass of fire rings** with a **vegas** sign rising out of it!	vagus
XI	See the **vegas** sign with an **ax** smashing it!	accessory
XII	See the **ax** with a **hippo/glasses** standing on it!	hypoglossal

LESSON 8 — REVIEW
THE NERVOUS SYSTEM
PART B
THE PERIPHERAL NERVOUS SYSTEM

THE CRANIAL NERVES
(12 PAIRS)

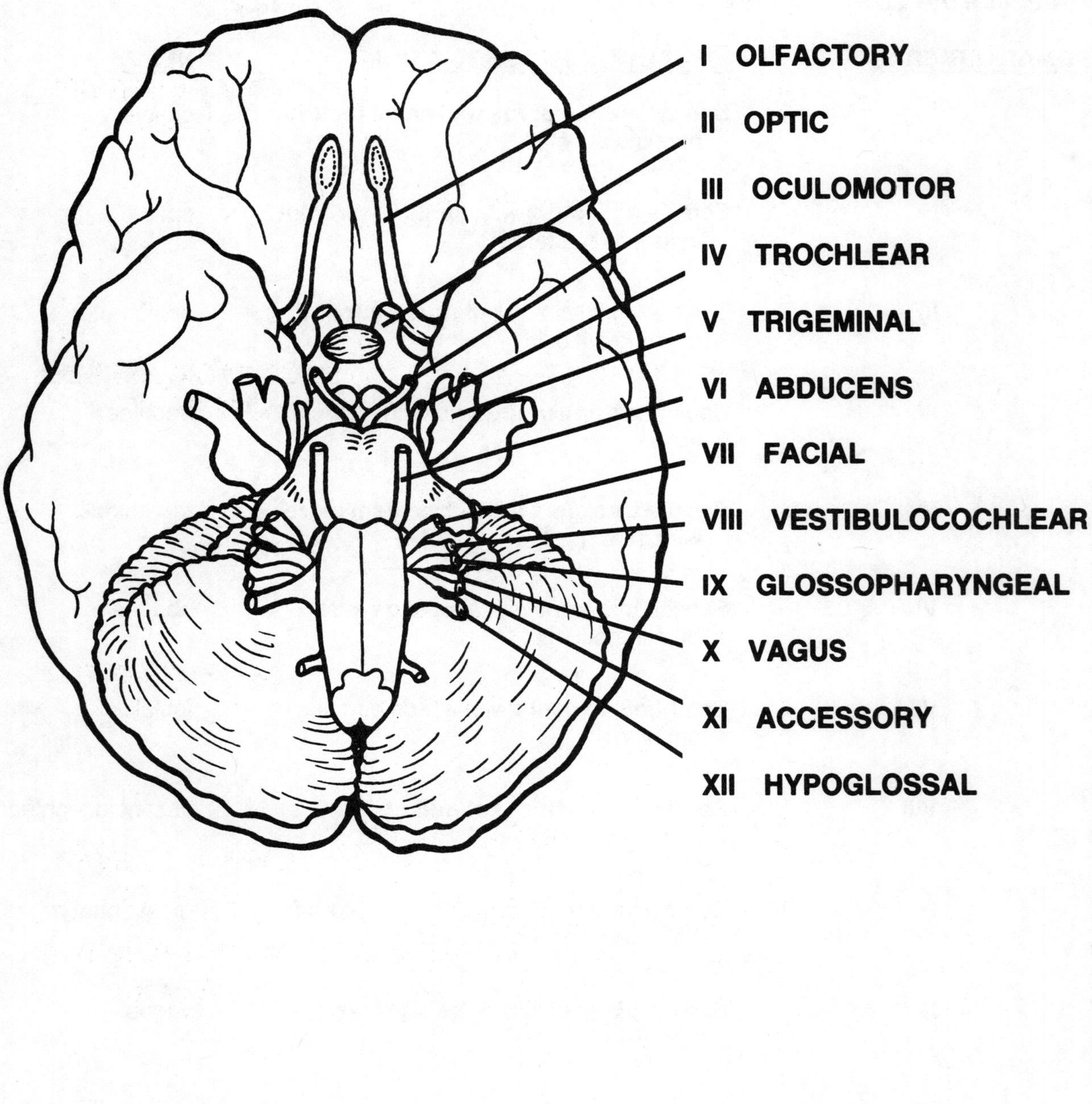

LESSON 8 — REVIEW
THE NERVOUS SYSTEM
SPINAL NERVES
(31 PAIRS)

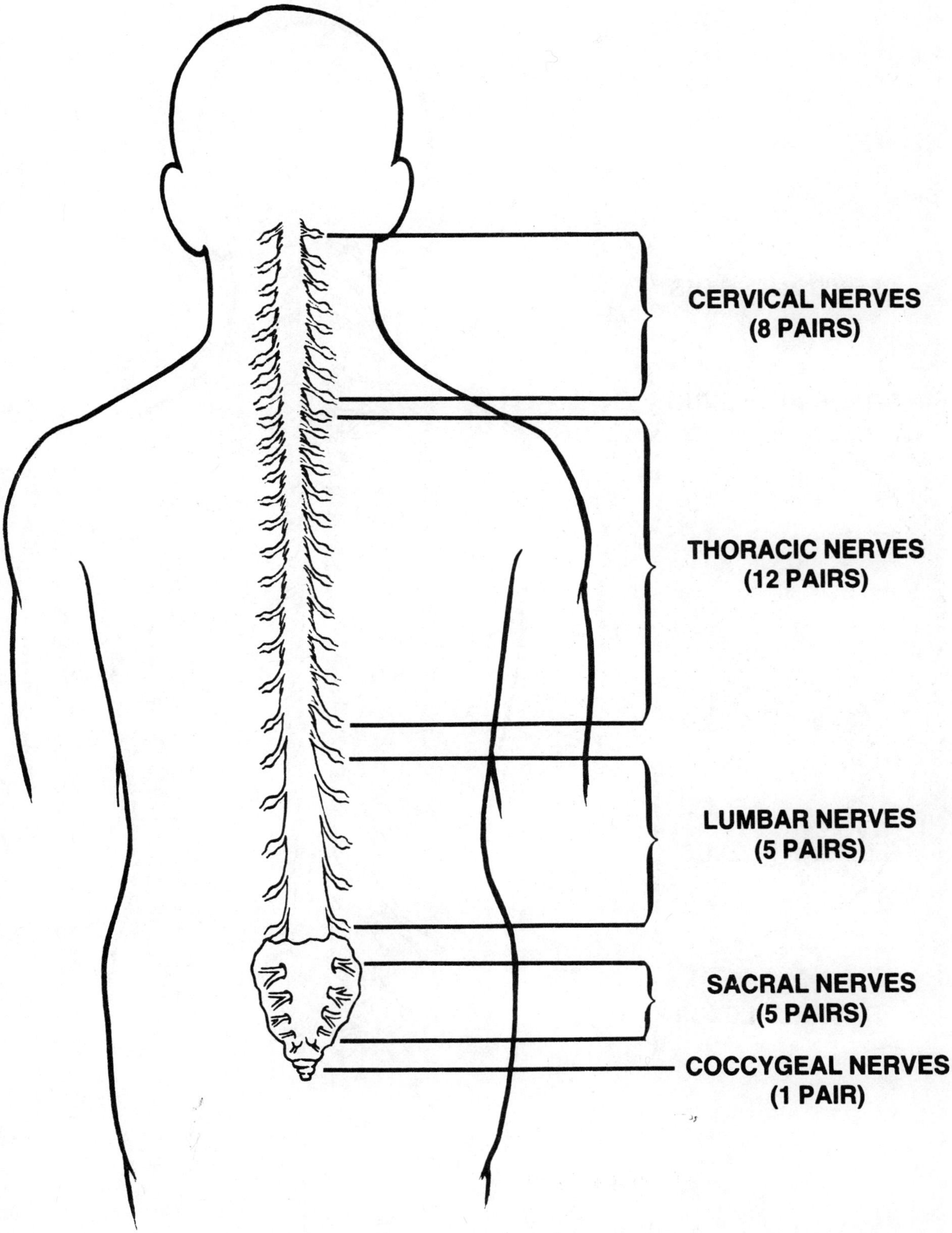

POSTERIOR VIEW

LESSON 8 — REVIEW
THE NERVOUS SYSTEM
PLEXUSES

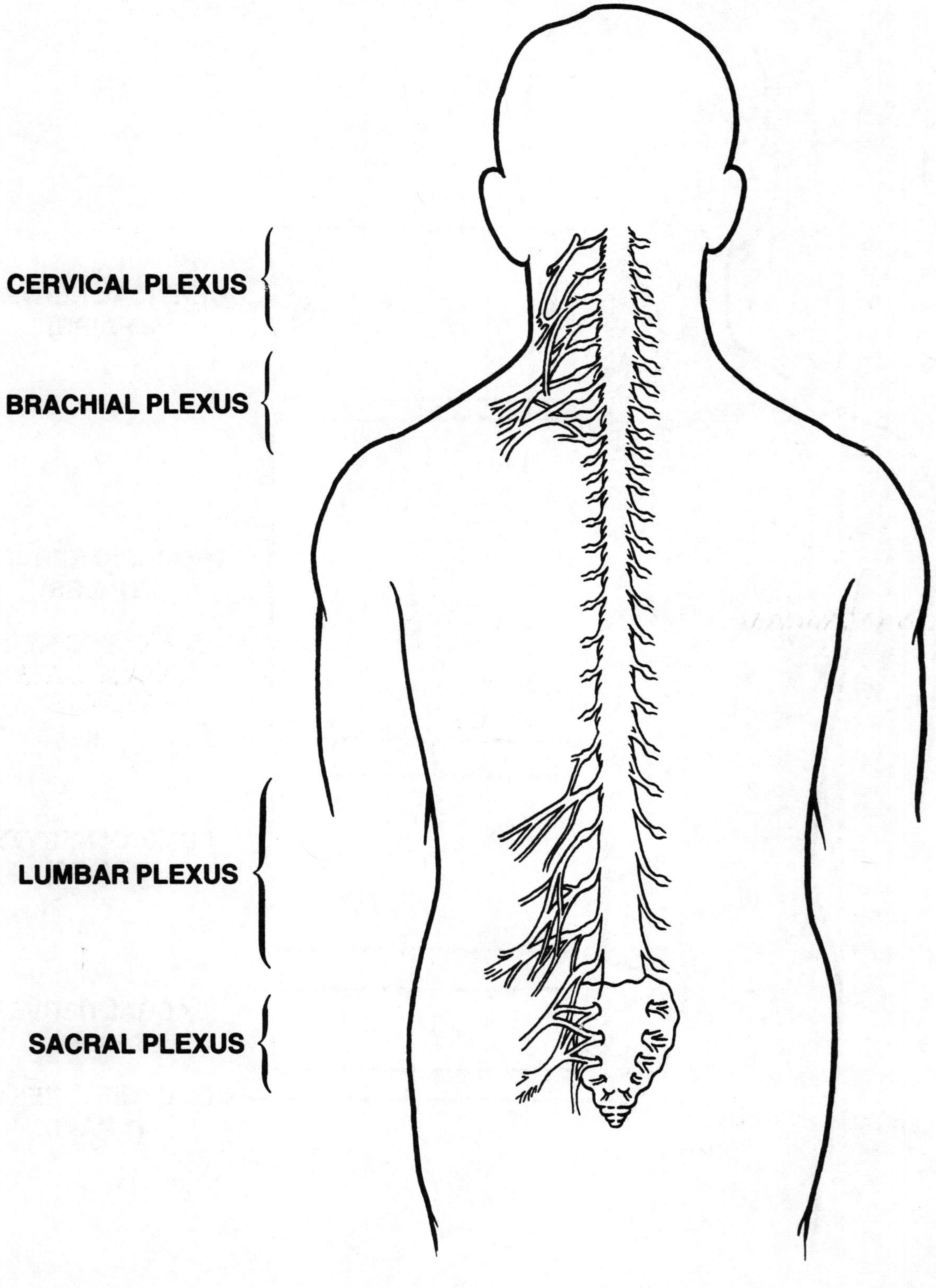

LESSON 8 — REVIEW
THE NERVOUS SYSTEM
PART B
THE PERIPHERAL NERVOUS SYSTEM

SYMPATHETIC AND PARASYMPATHETIC NERVES

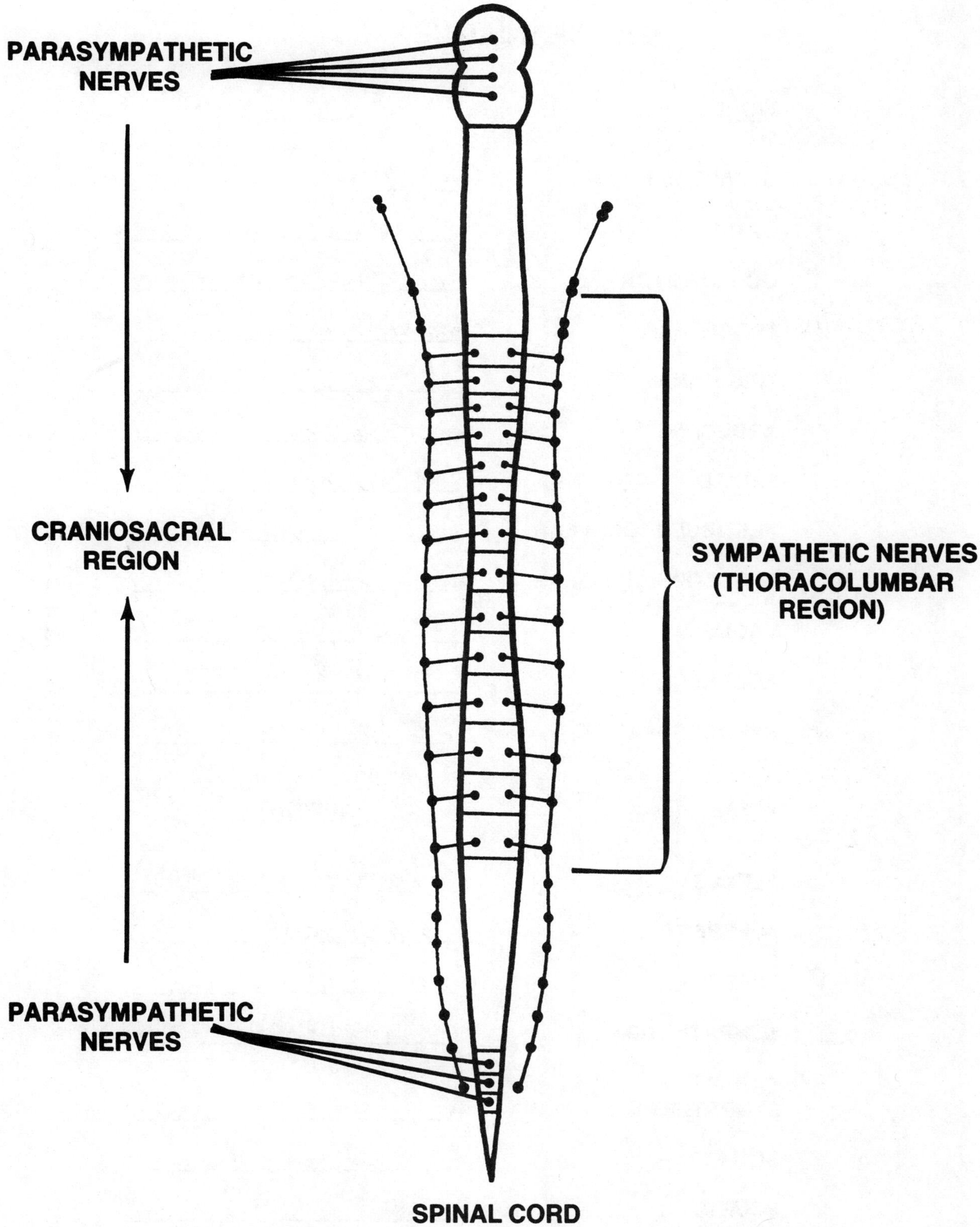

LESSON 8 — WORKSHEET
THE NERVOUS SYSTEM
PART B
THE PERIPHERAL NERVOUS SYSTEM

COMPLETE THE BLANKS:

THE CRANIAL NERVES

	WORD	AUDIONYM
I	OLFACTORY	Crane/nerves c oil Factory bursting out of it
II	OPTIC	oil factory c opals Floating out of its smoke stack
III	OCULOMOTOR	opal c octopus/motor bursting out of it
IV	TROCHLEAR	octopus/motor Holding a Truck Lure
V	TRIGEMINAL	Truck Lure c a Tree Gem
VI	ABDUCENS	Tree Gem c abe/2 cents
VII	FACIAL	abe 2/cents c a Face
VIII	VESTIBULOCOCHLEAR	Face c a vest/bull/cocoa
IX	GLOSSOPHARYNGEAL	vest/bull, cocoa c a glass of Fire rings
X	VAGUS	Glass of Fire rings c Vegas sign
XI	ACCESSORY	vegas sign c ax smashing it
XII	HYPOGLOSSAL	ax c hippo Glasses standing on it

WORD	AUDIONYM
PLEXUS	Plaques
AFFERENT	a Fur ant
EFFERENT	ever green
SYMPATHETIC	Symphony
PARA SYMPATHETIC	parrot Symphony
SOMATIC	Sombrera attic
SCIATIC	Ice attic

LESSON 8 — WORKSHEET
THE NERVOUS SYSTEM
PART B
THE PERIPHERAL NERVOUS SYSTEM

PRINT THE CORRECT LETTER WITHIN THE PARENTHESES

SCIATIC NERVE	(E)	
PLEXUS	(G)	
EFFERENT NERVES	(D)	
AFFERENT NERVES	(B)	
SYMPATHETIC NERVES	(H)	( )
PARASYMPATHETIC NERVES	(A)	( )
SOMATIC NERVOUS SYSTEM (VOLUNTARY)	(F)	

A - REGULATE THE FUNCTION OF BODY ORGANS

B - CARRY (SENSORY) MESSAGES TO THE CENTRAL NERVOUS SYSTEM

C - ORIGINATE IN CRANIOSACRAL REGION OF SPINAL CORD

D - CARRY (MOTOR) IMPULSES (MESSAGES) TO ALL PARTS OF THE BODY

E - THE LARGEST AND LONGEST NERVE IN THE BODY

F - SERVES THE SKELETAL MUSCLES

G - NETWORK OF SPINAL NERVES

H - ACT IN CASES OF EMERGENCY

I - ORIGINATE IN THORACOLUMBAR REGION OF SPINAL CORD

LESSON 8 — WORKSHEET
THE NERVOUS SYSTEM

PRINT THE CORRECT LETTER WITHIN THE PARENTHESES

CRANIAL NERVES

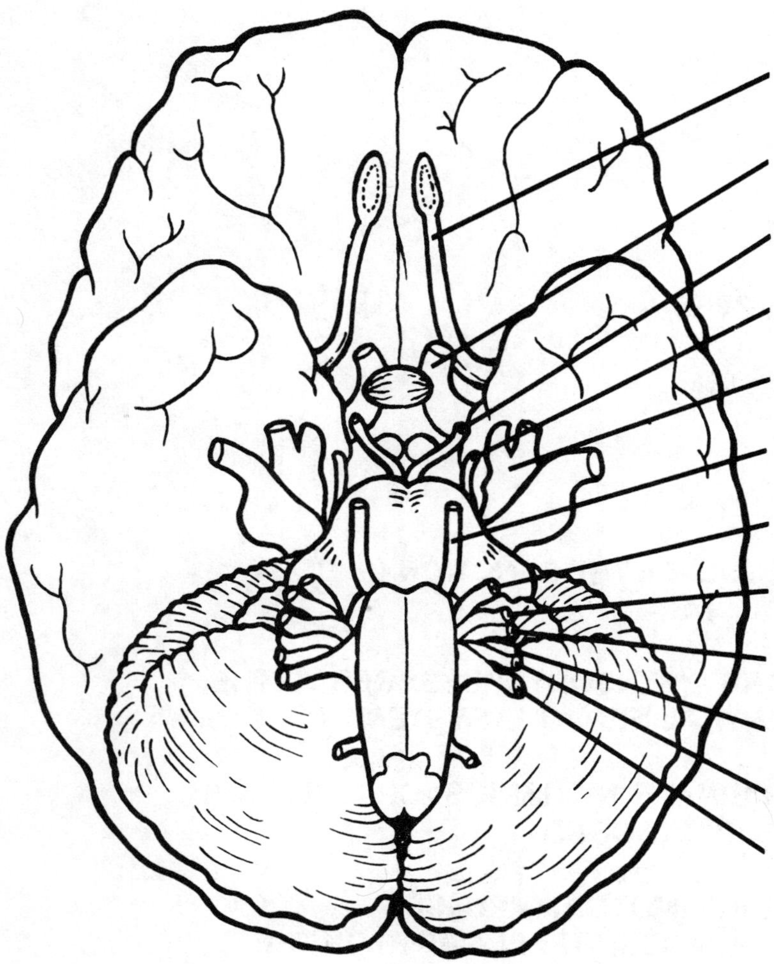

(E) I
(C) II
(A) III
(F) IV
(D) V
(L) VI
(G) VII
(V) VIII
(H) IX
(J) X
(I) XI
(B) XII

A - OCULOMOTOR

B - HYPOGLOSSAL

C - OPTIC

D - TRIGEMINAL

E - OLFACTORY

F - TROCHLEAR

G - FACIAL

H - GLOSSOPHARYNGEAL

I - ACCESSORY

J - VAGUS

K - VESTIBULOCOCHLEAR

L - ABDUCENS

LESSON 8 — WORKSHEET
THE NERVOUS SYSTEM
SPINAL NERVES

PRINT THE CORRECT LETTER WITHIN THE PARENTHESES

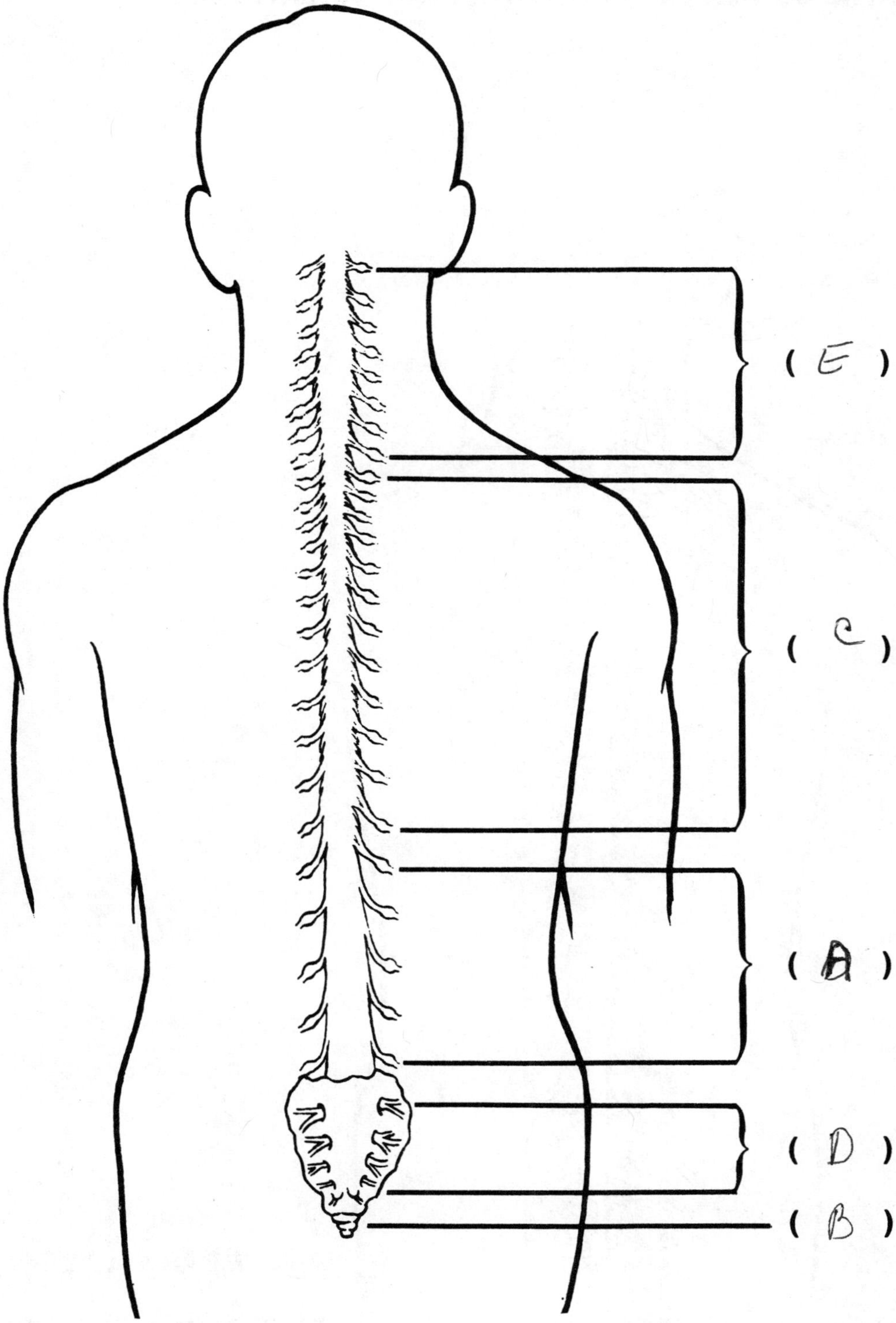

A - LUMBAR NERVES
B - COCCYGEAL NERVES
C - THORACIC NERVES
D - SACRAL NERVES
E - CERVICAL NERVES

POSTERIOR VIEW

LESSON 8 — WORKSHEET
THE NERVOUS SYSTEM
PLEXUSES

PRINT THE CORRECT LETTER WITHIN THE PARENTHESES

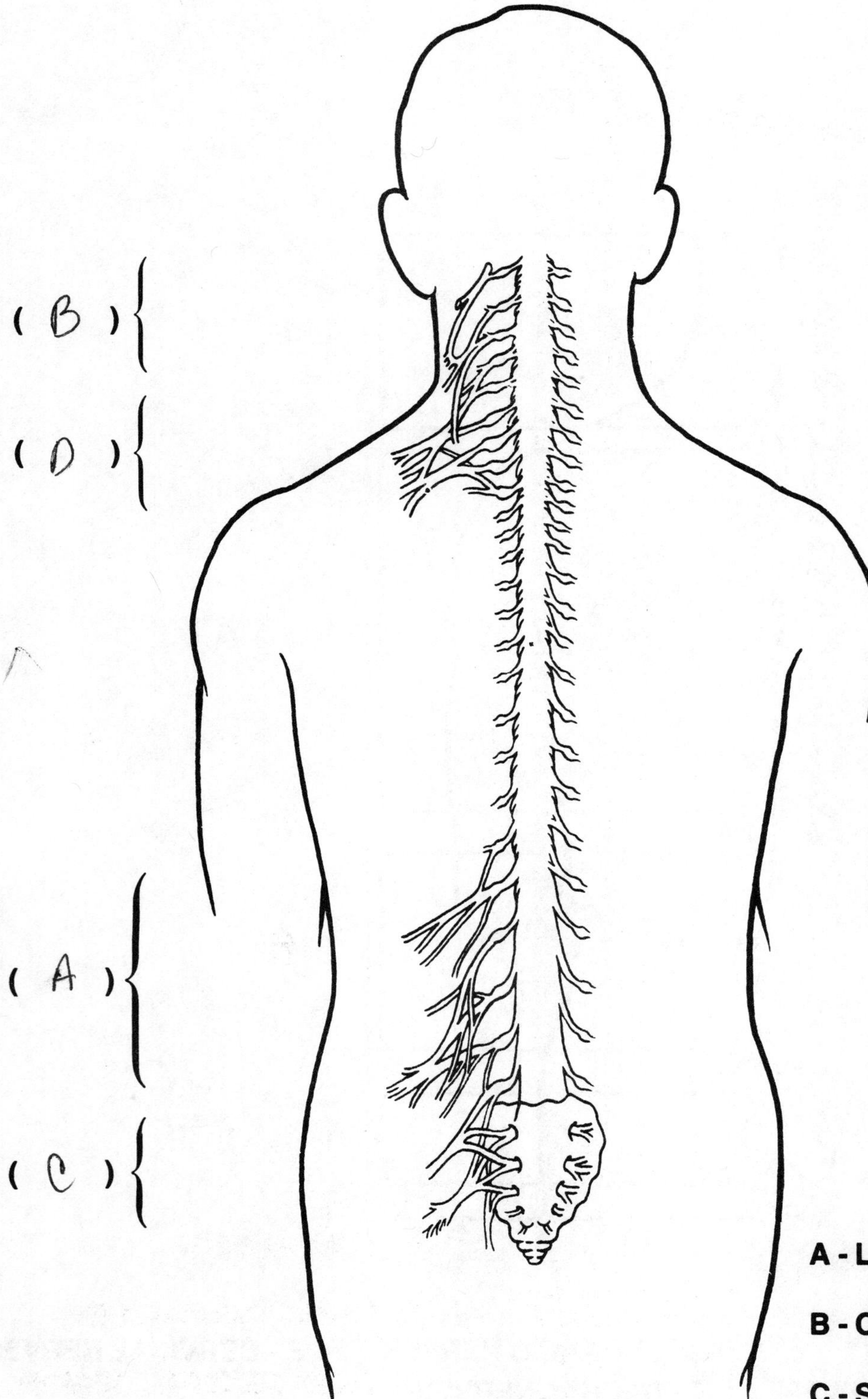

A - LUMBAR PLEXUS

B - CERVICAL PLEXUS

C - SACRAL PLEXUS

D - BRACHIAL PLEXUS

LESSON 8 — WORKSHEET
THE NERVOUS SYSTEM
PART B
THE PERIPHERAL NERVOUS SYSTEM

PRINT THE CORRECT LETTER WITHIN THE PARENTHESES

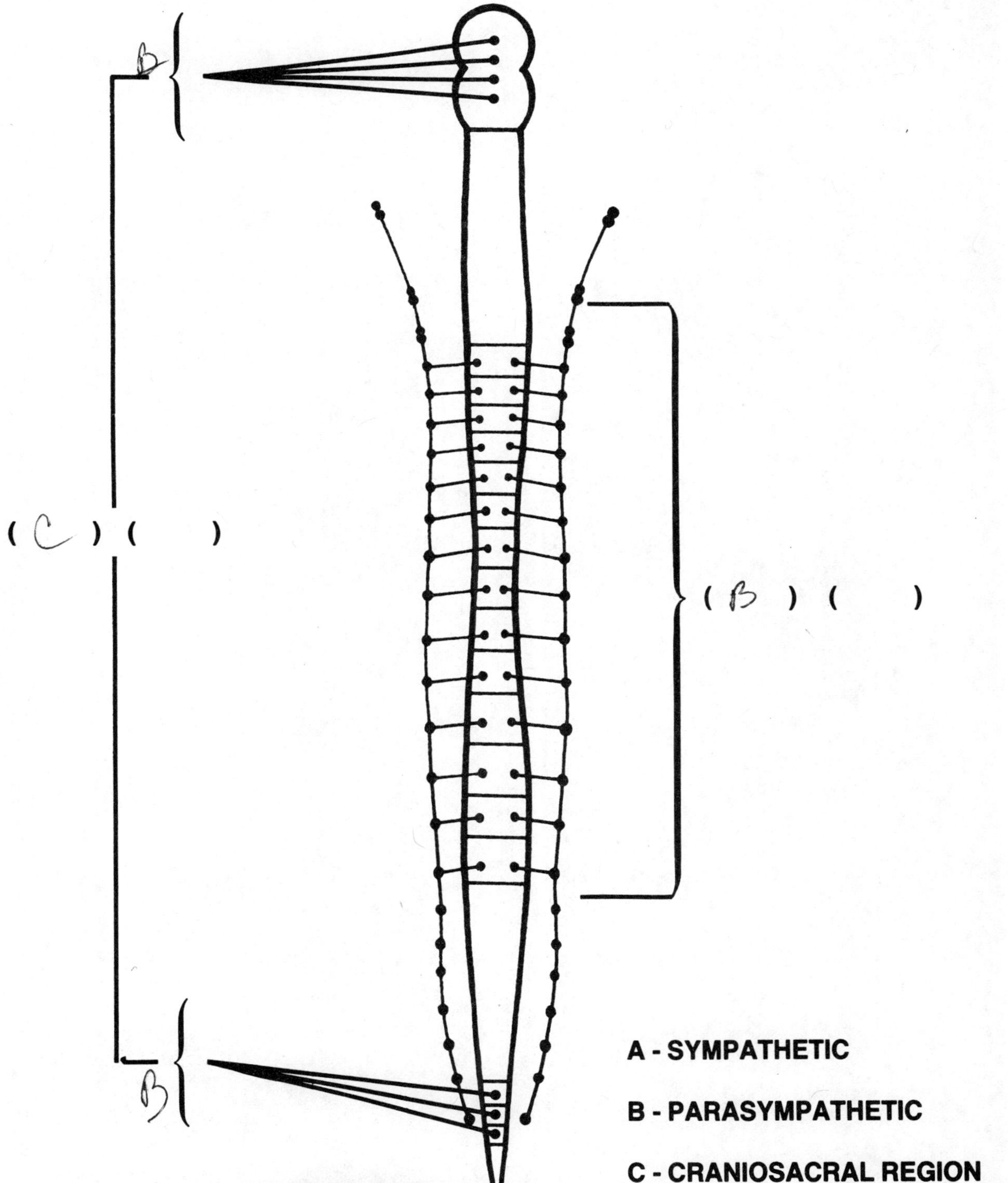

LESSON 9

SENSORY ORGAN

THE EYE

- PRINCIPAL PARTS OF THE EYEBALL

REMEMBER!

1st **Pronounce** *the name of the body part or term*
2nd **Recall** *and* **pronounce** *the audionym*
3rd **For body parts: visualize** *the audionym in place*
For terms: visualize *the association*
4th **Pronounce** *the name of the body part or term again.*

LESSON 9 — REVIEW
SENSORY ORGAN
THE EYE

AUDIONYMS

WORD	AUDIONYM
IRIS	ICE
LENS	LENS
PUPIL	PURPLE PILL
CORNEA	CORN
SCLERA	SCHOLAR
SUSPENSORY LIGAMENT	SUSPENDERS/LICORICE
CONJUNCTIVA	CONE/JUNK
RETINA	RED TUNA
CHOROID	CORE
CILIARY BODY	CELERY/BODY
ANTERIOR CAVITY	ANT/CALF
AQUEOUS HUMOR	AQUA HAMMER
POSTERIOR CAVITY	POSTER/CALF
VITREOUS HUMOR	"V" TREE/HAMMER
OPTIC NERVE	OPAL/NURSE

LESSON 9 — REVIEW
SENSORY ORGAN
THE EYE
PRINCIPAL PARTS OF THE EYEBALL

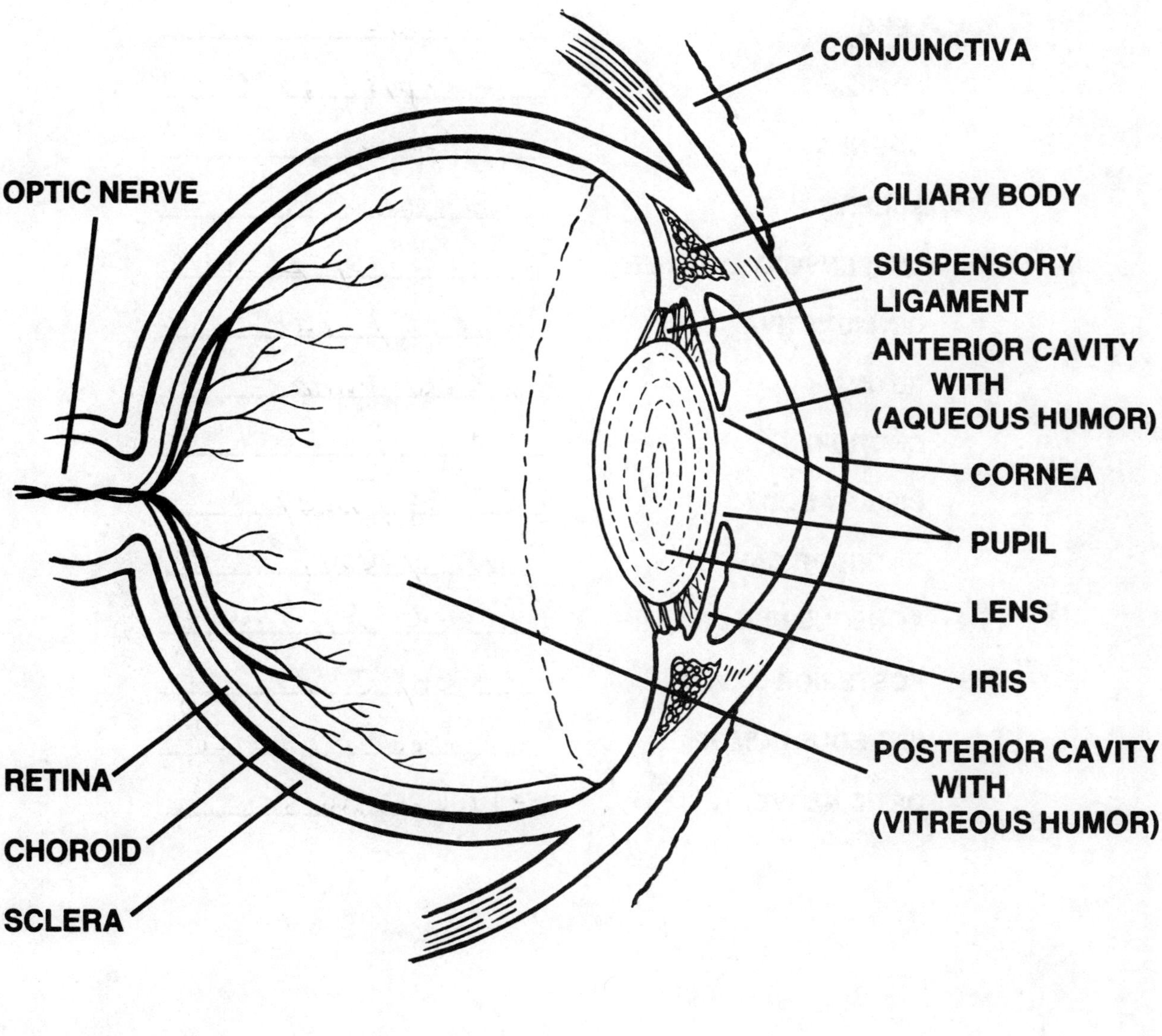

LESSON 9 — WORKSHEET
SENSORY ORGAN
THE EYE

COMPLETE THE BLANKS:

WORD	AUDIONYM
IRIS	Ice
LENS	Lens
PUPIL	Purple Pill
CORNEA	Corn
SCLERA	Scholar
SUSPENSORY LIGAMENT	Suspenders/ Licorice
CONJUNCTIVA	Cone / Junk
RETINA	Red Tuna
CHOROID	Core
CILIARY BODY	Celery / body
ANTERIOR CAVITY	Ant / Calf
AQUEOUS HUMOR	Aqua Hammer
POSTERIOR CAVITY	Poster / Calf
VITREOUS HUMOR	"V" Tree Hammer
OPTIC NERVE	Opal Nurse

LESSON 9 — WORKSHEET
SENSORY ORGAN
THE EYE
PRINCIPAL PARTS OF THE EYEBALL

PRINT THE CORRECT LETTER WITHIN THE PARENTHESES

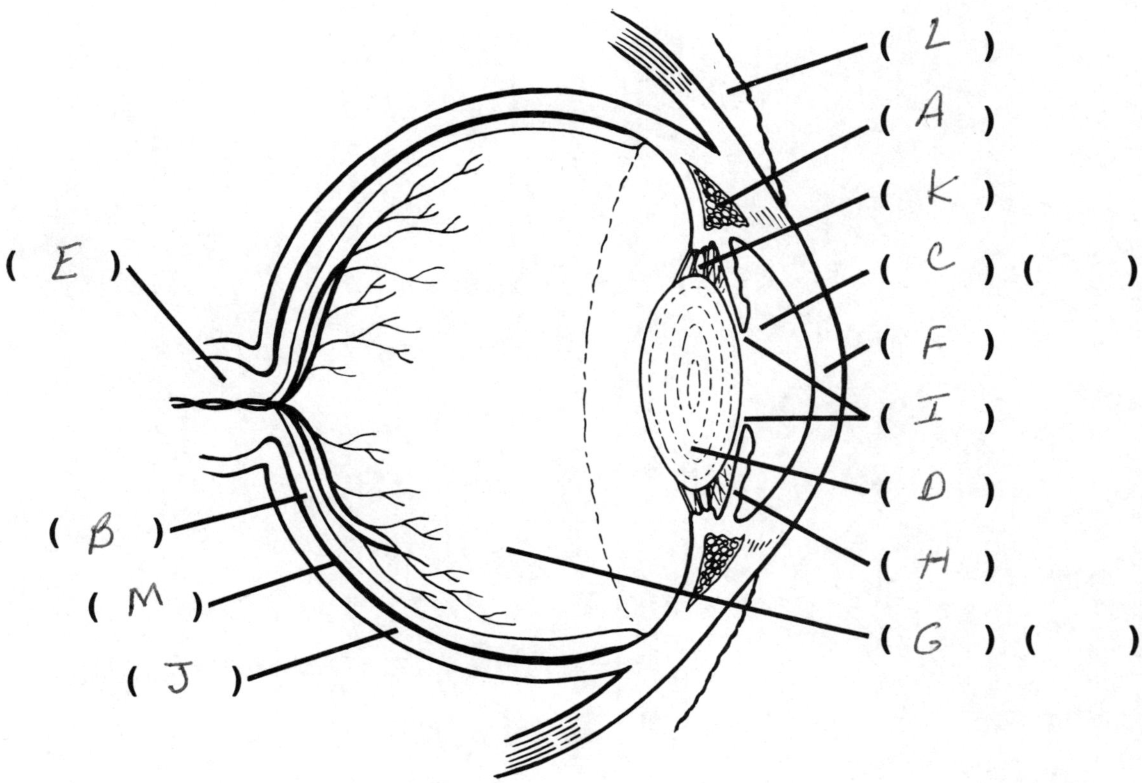

A - CILIARY BODY
B - RETINA
C - ANTERIOR CAVITY
D - LENS
E - OPTIC NERVE
F - CORNEA
G - POSTERIOR CAVITY
H - IRIS
I - PUPIL
J - SCLERA
K - SUSPENSORY LIGAMENT
L - CONJUNCTIVA
M - CHOROID
N - VITREOUS HUMOR
O - AQUEOUS HUMOR

LESSON 10

SENSORY ORGAN

THE EAR

- PRINCIPAL PARTS OF THE EAR

REMEMBER!

1st ***Pronounce*** *the name of the body part or term*
2nd ***Recall*** *and* ***pronounce*** *the audionym*
3rd ***For body parts: visualize*** *the audionym in place*
For terms: visualize *the association*
4th ***Pronounce*** *the name of the body part or term again.*

LESSON 10 — REVIEW
SENSORY ORGAN
THE EAR

AUDIONYMS

WORD	AUDIONYM
PINNA	PINA COLADA
AUDITORY CANAL	AUDITORIUM
TYMPANIC MEMBRANE	TYMPANI
MALLEUS (HAMMER)	MOLASSES
INCUS (ANVIL)	INKS
STAPES (STIRRUP)	STAPLES
VESTIBULE	VEST/BULL
COCHLEA	COCKLESHELL
SEMI-CIRCULAR CANAL	SEMI-CIRCLE/CAN

LESSON 10 — REVIEW
SENSORY ORGAN
THE EAR

PRINCIPAL PARTS OF THE EAR

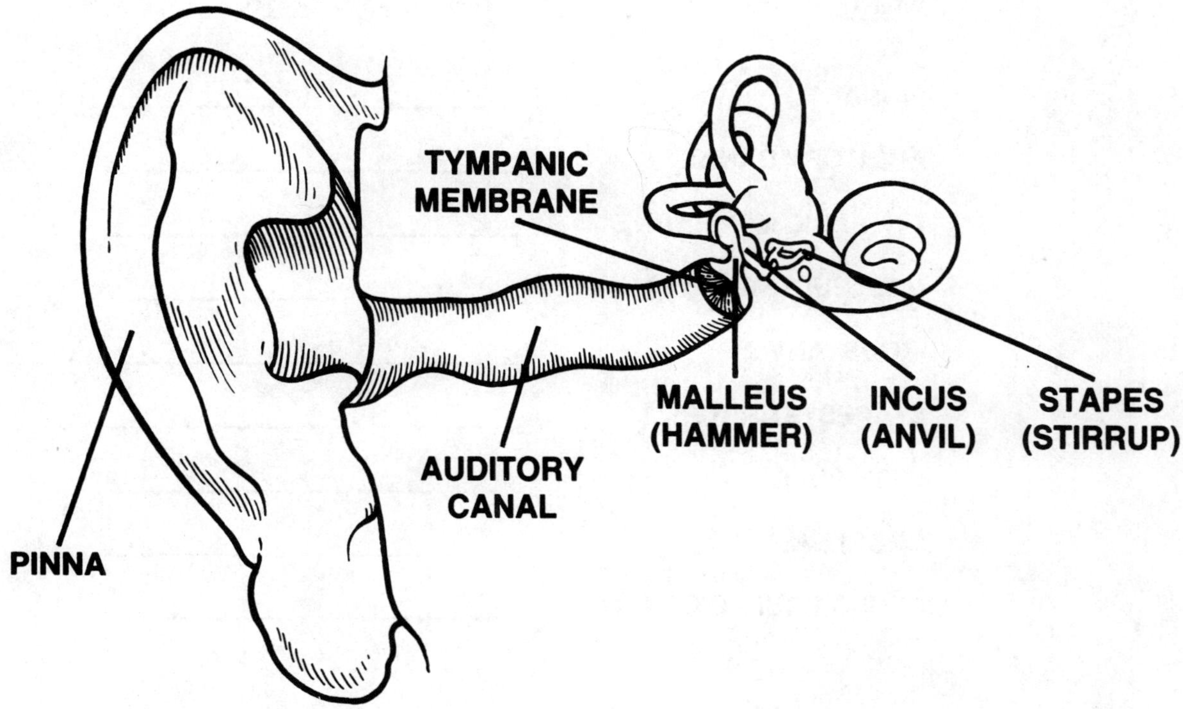

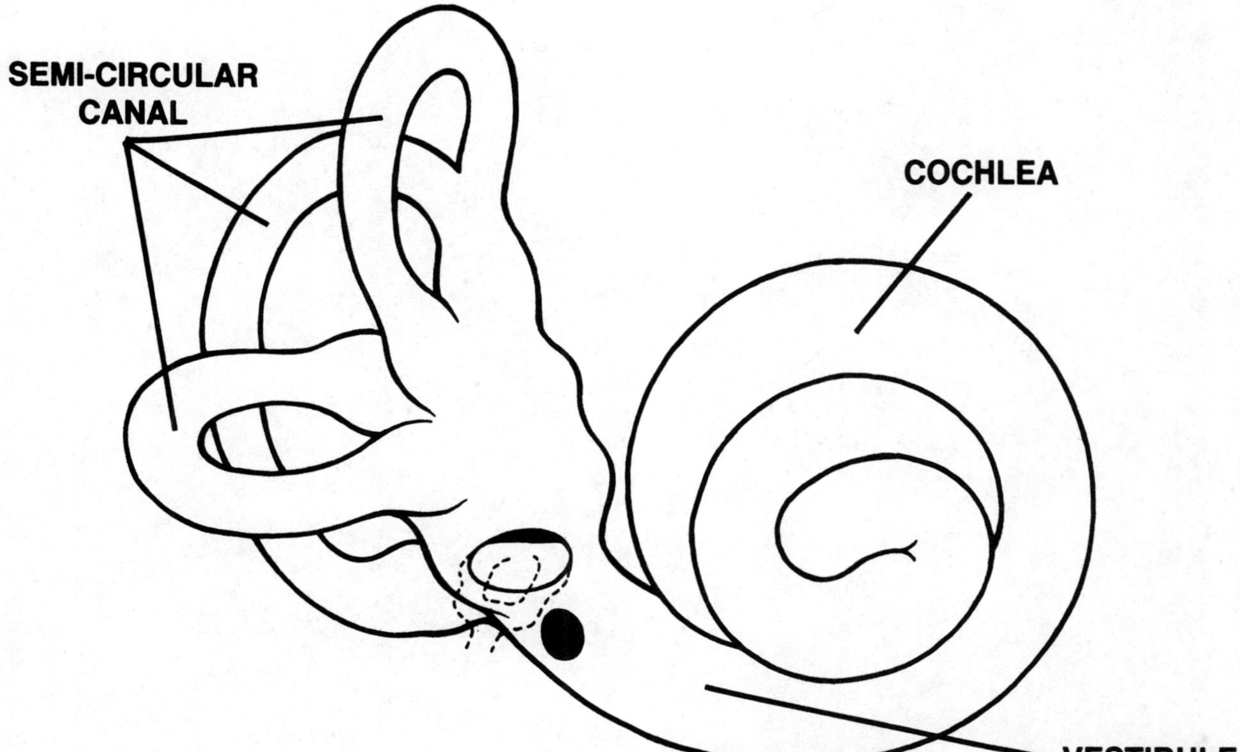

LESSON 10 — WORKSHEET
SENSORY ORGAN
THE EAR

COMPLETE THE BLANKS:

WORD	AUDIONYM
PINNA	Pina Colada
AUDITORY CANAL	Audiotorium
TYMPANIC MEMBRANE	Tympani
MALLEUS (HAMMER)	Molasses
INCUS (ANVIL)	inks
STAPES (STIRRUP)	Staples
VESTIBULE	Vest / Bull
COCHLEA	Cockle shell
SEMI-CIRCULAR CANAL	semi-circle / can

LESSON 10 — WORKSHEET
SENSORY ORGAN
THE EAR
PRINCIPAL PARTS OF THE EAR

PRINT THE CORRECT LETTER WITHIN THE PARENTHESES

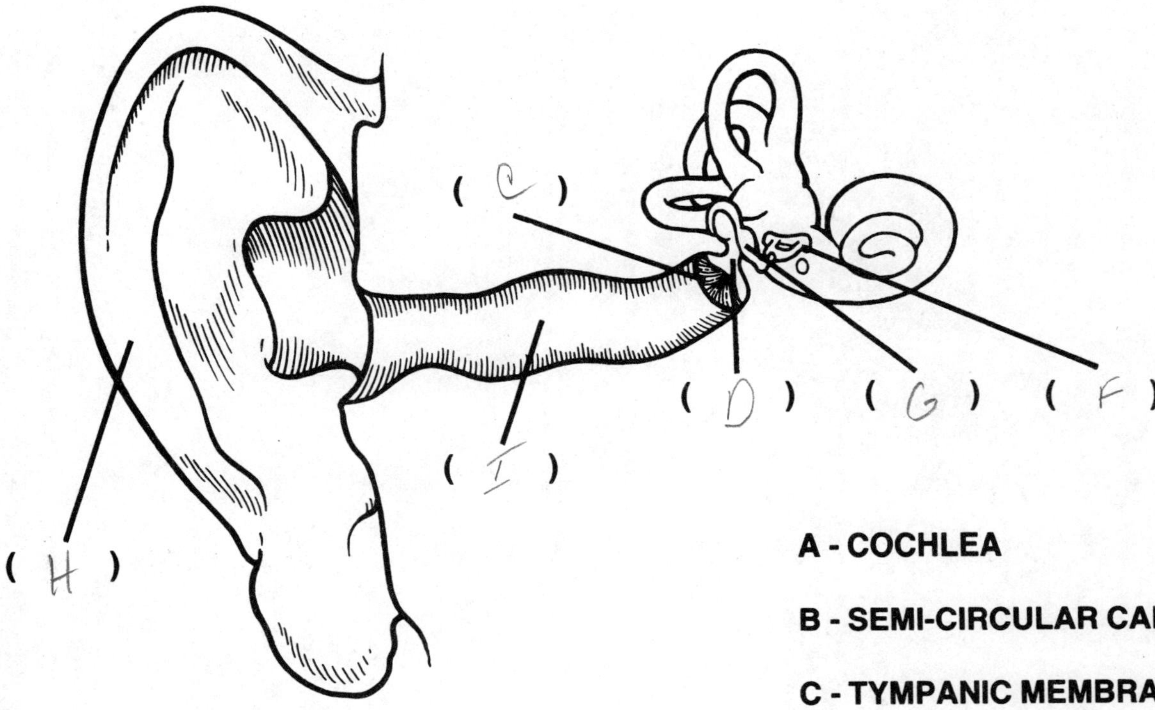

A - COCHLEA

B - SEMI-CIRCULAR CANALS

C - TYMPANIC MEMBRANE

D - MALLEUS (HAMMER)

E - VESTIBULE

F - STAPES (STIRRUP)

G - INCUS (ANVIL)

H - PINNA

I - AUDITORY CANAL

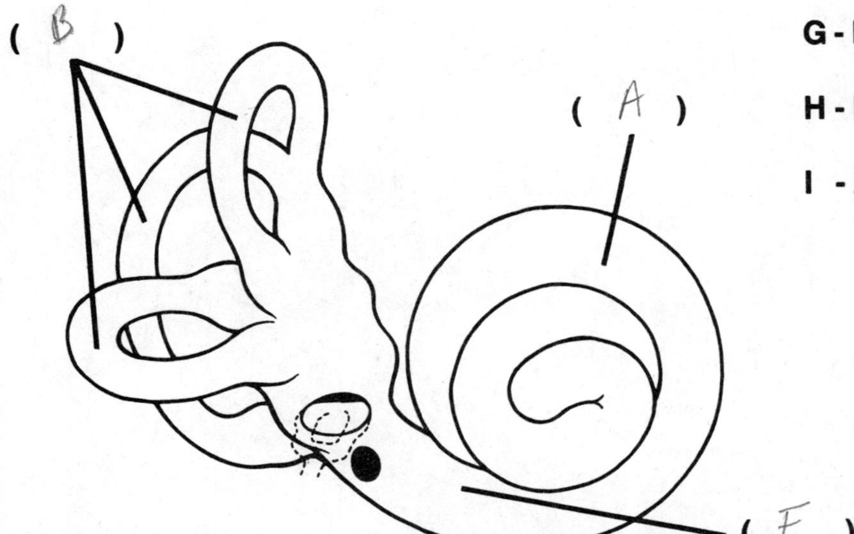

LESSON 11

THE CARDIOVASCULAR SYSTEM

- NAMES AND LOCATIONS OF ARTERIES
- NAMES AND LOCATIONS OF VEINS
- STRUCTURAL RELATIONSHIP OF VESSELS
- PRINCIPAL PARTS OF THE HEART

REMEMBER!

1st ***Pronounce** the name of the body part or term*
2nd ***Recall** and **pronounce** the audionym*
3rd ***For body parts: visualize** the audionym in place*
***For terms: visualize** the association*
4th ***Pronounce** the name of the body part or term again.*

LESSON 11 — REVIEW
THE CARDIOVASCULAR SYSTEM

AUDIONYMS

WORD	AUDIONYM
ATRIUM	ATRIUM
VENTRICLE	VENT
BICUSPID	BICYCLE/CUSTARD
TRICUSPID	TRICYCLE/CUSTARD
AORTA	HAY/OAR
ARTERY	ARTWORK
ARTERIOLE	ARTWORK/OWL
CAPILLARY	CAP
VENULE	VANILLA
VEIN	(WEATHER) VANE
VENA CAVA	"V" NECK/CUFF
CORONARY	CANARY
CAROTID	CARROT
JUGULAR	JUG
SAPHENOUS	SAPPHIRE

LESSON 11 — REVIEW
THE CARDIOVASCULAR SYSTEM
PRINCIPAL ARTERIES OF NECK AND HEAD

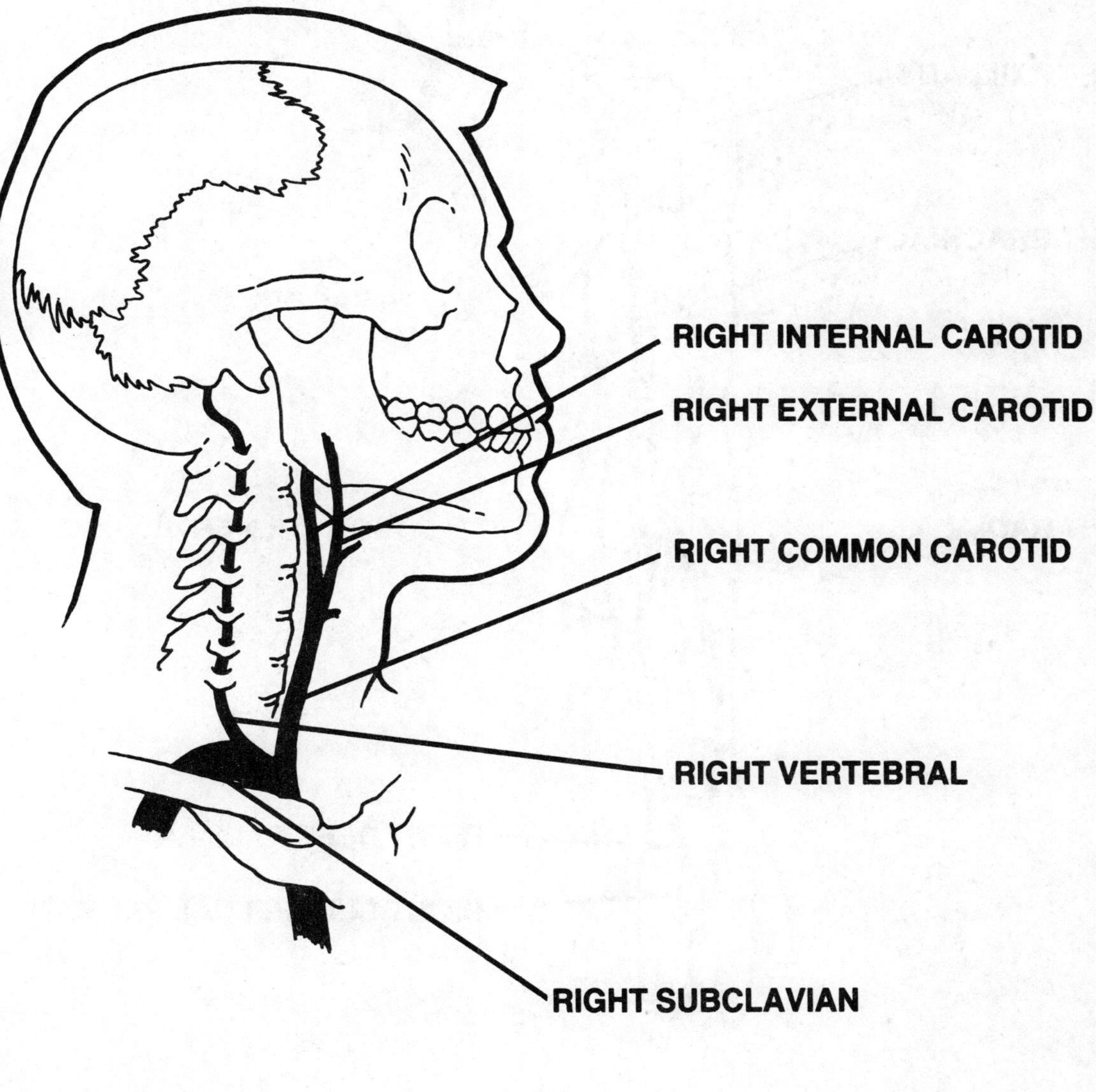

RIGHT LATERAL VIEW

LESSON 11 — REVIEW
THE CARDIOVASCULAR SYSTEM
PRINCIPAL ARTERIES OF RIGHT UPPER EXTREMITY

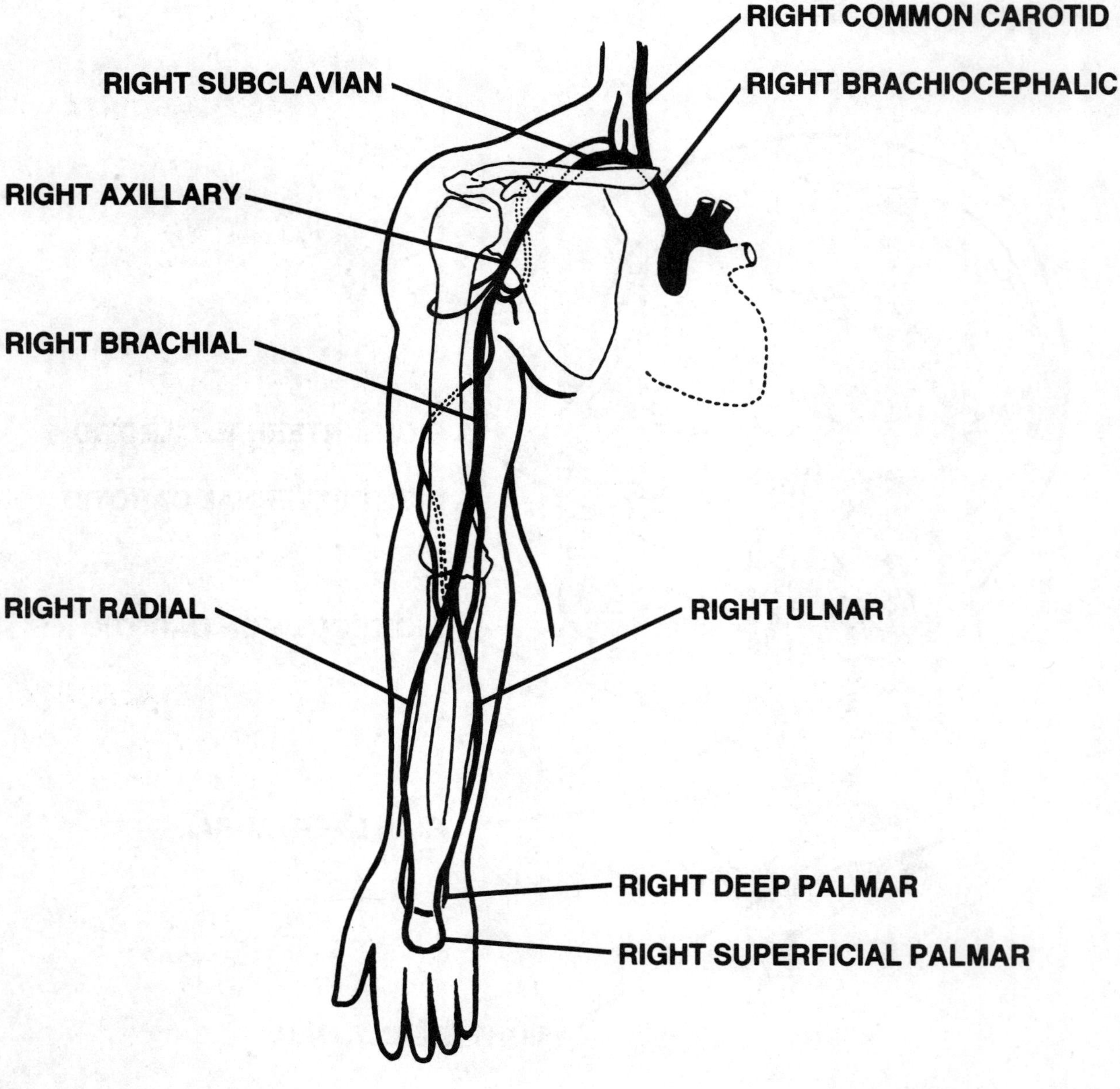

ANTERIOR VIEW

LESSON 11 — REVIEW
THE CARDIOVASCULAR SYSTEM
PRINCIPAL DIVISIONS OF AORTA

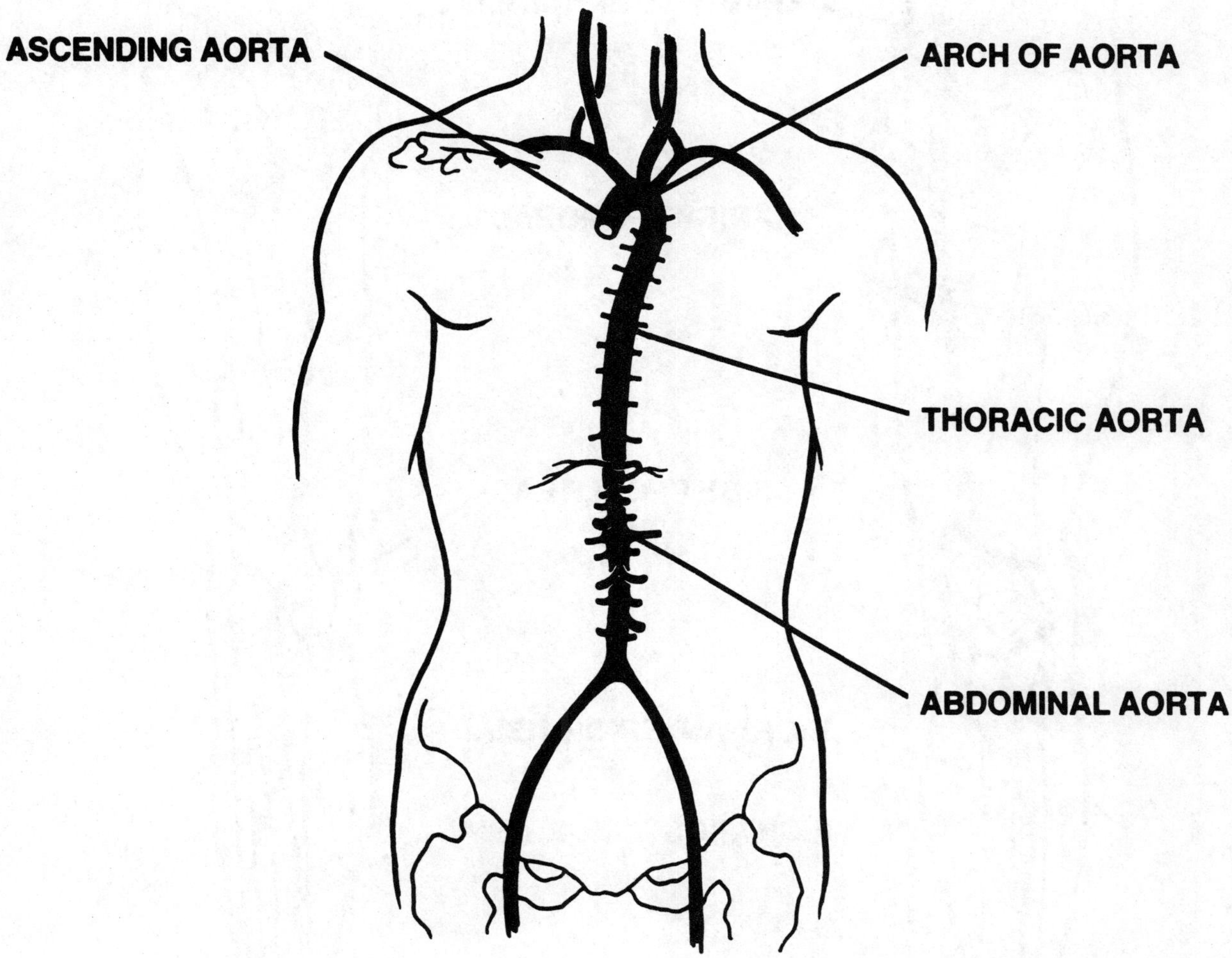

LESSON 11 — REVIEW
THE CARDIOVASCULAR SYSTEM
PRINCIPAL ARTERIES OF THE PELVIS AND RIGHT LOWER EXTREMITY

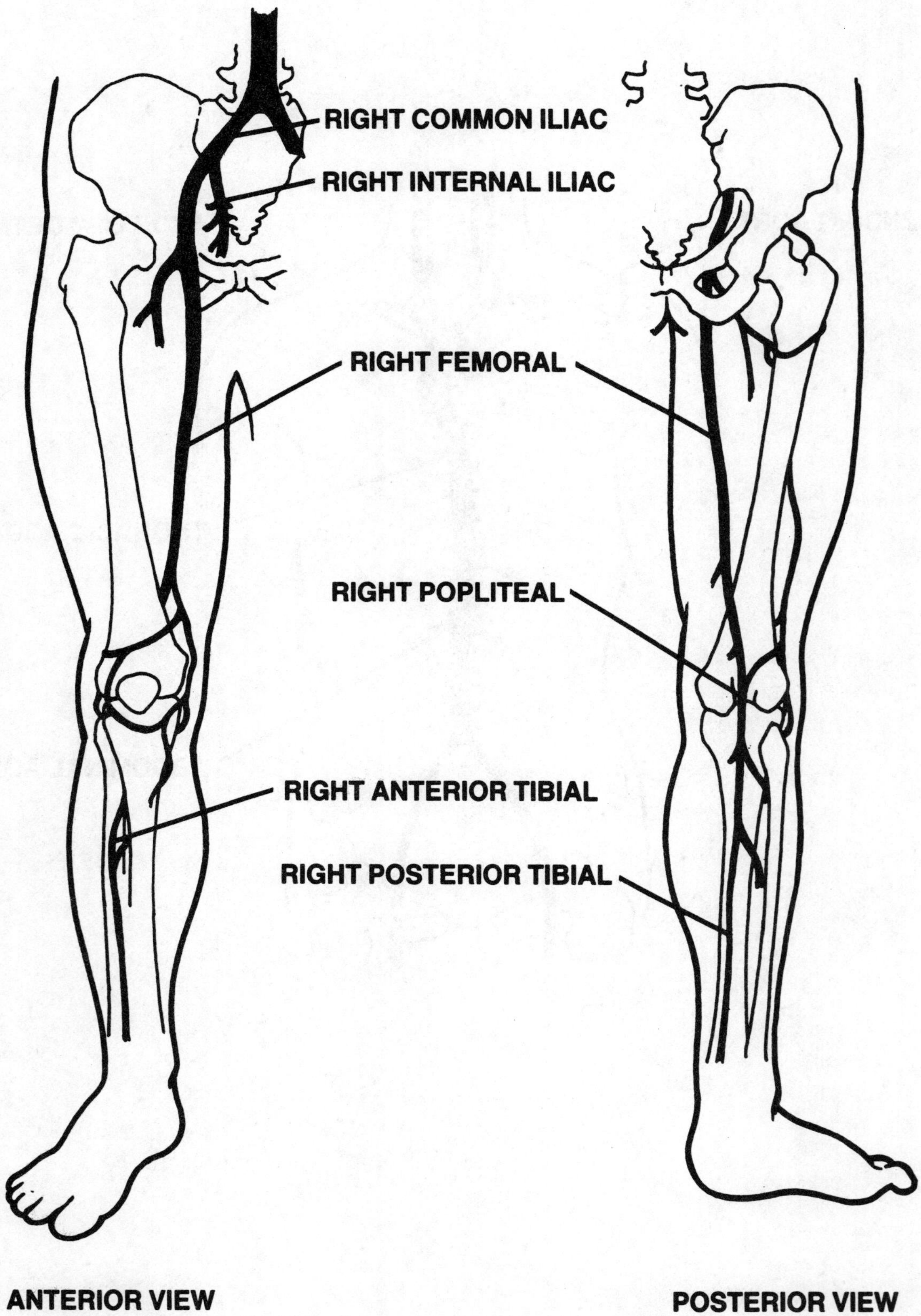

LESSON 11 — REVIEW
THE CARDIOVASCULAR SYSTEM
PRINCIPAL VEINS OF THE HEAD AND NECK

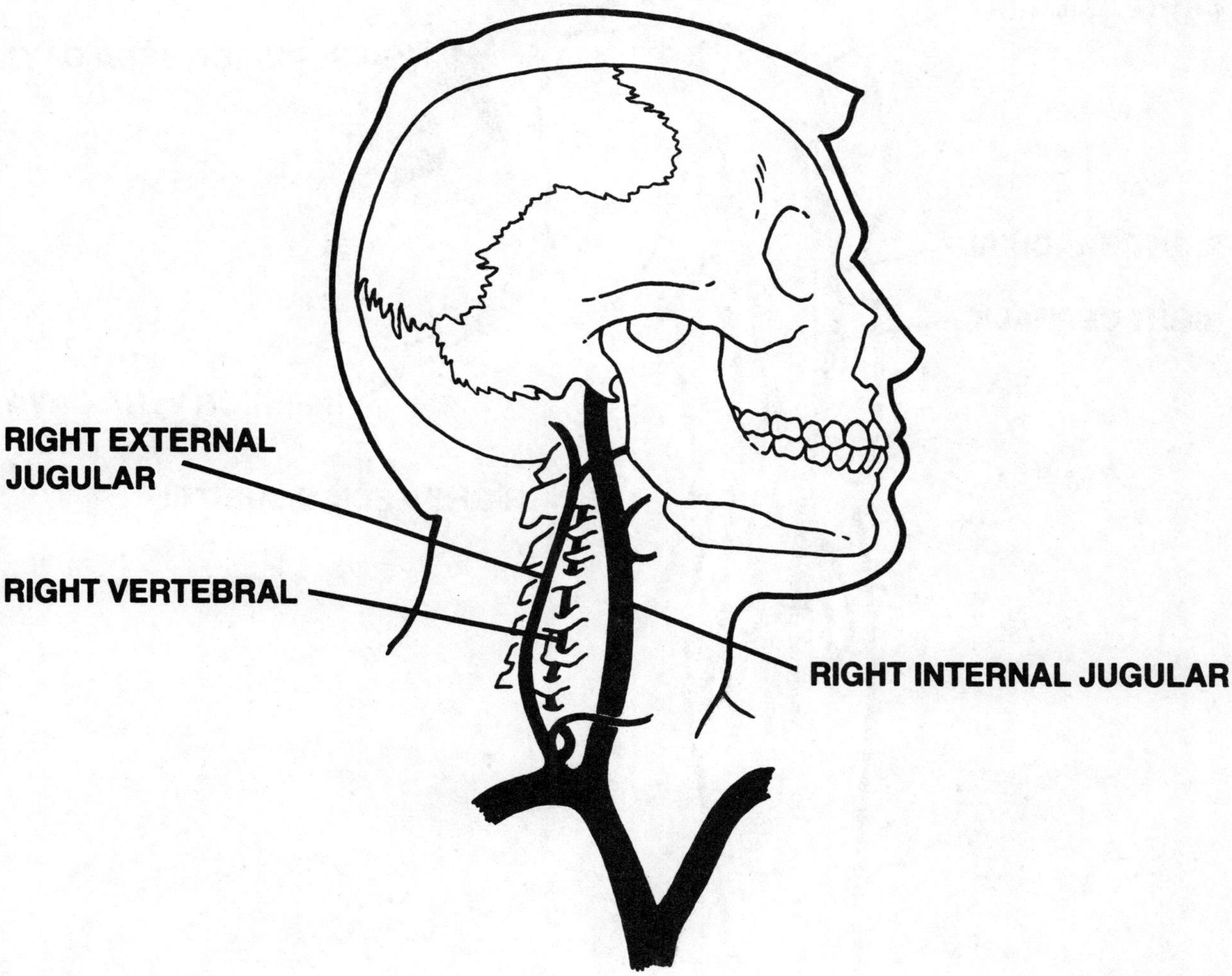

RIGHT LATERAL VIEW

LESSON 11 — REVIEW
THE CARDIOVASCULAR SYSTEM
PRINCIPAL VEINS OF THE RIGHT UPPER EXTREMITY

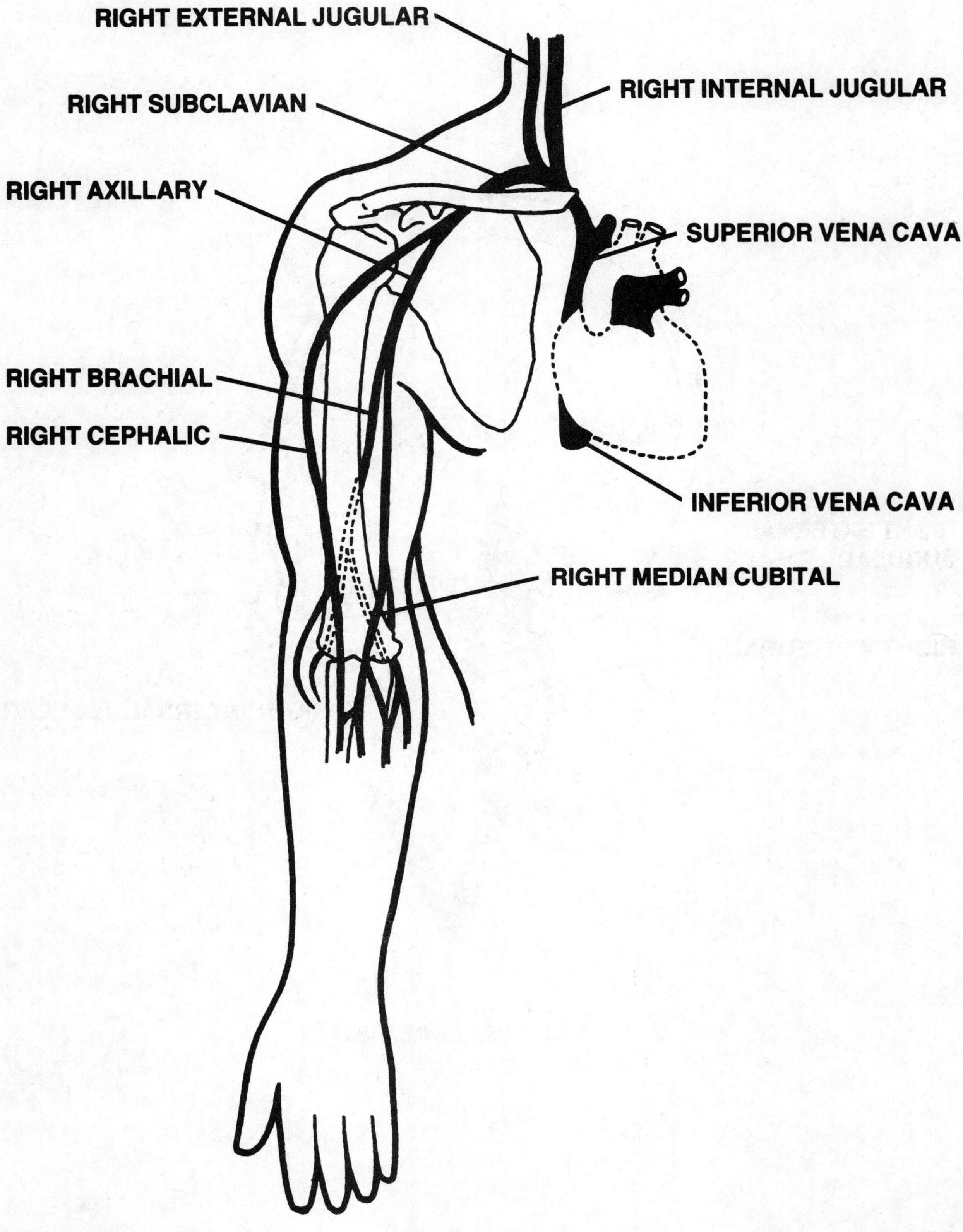

ANTERIOR VIEW

LESSON 11 — REVIEW
THE CARDIOVASCULAR SYSTEM
PRINCIPAL VEINS OF THE THORAX, ABDOMEN, AND PELVIS

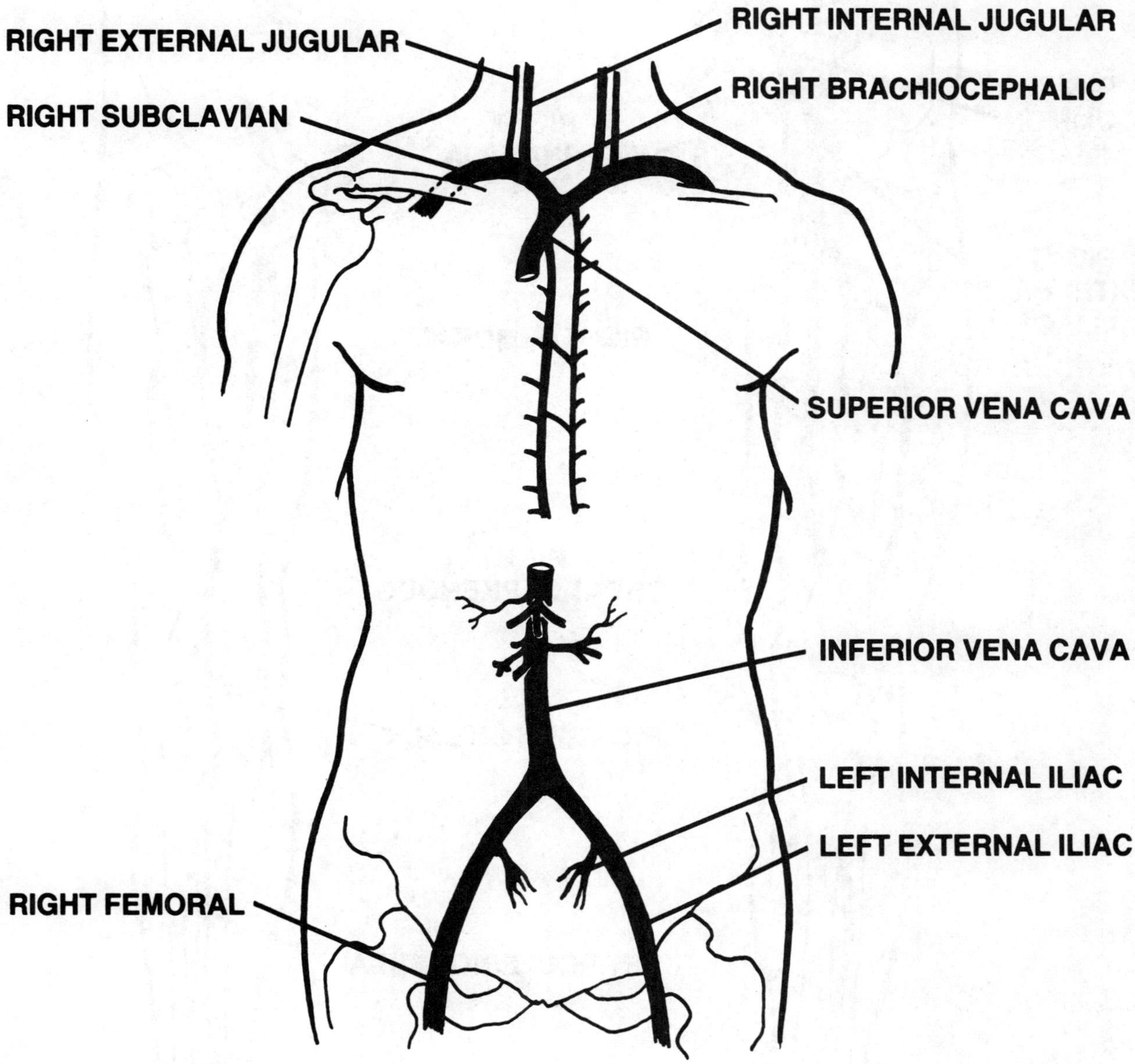

ANTERIOR VIEW

LESSON 11 — REVIEW
THE CARDIOVASCULAR SYSTEM
PRINCIPAL VEINS OF THE PELVIS AND RIGHT LOWER EXTREMITY

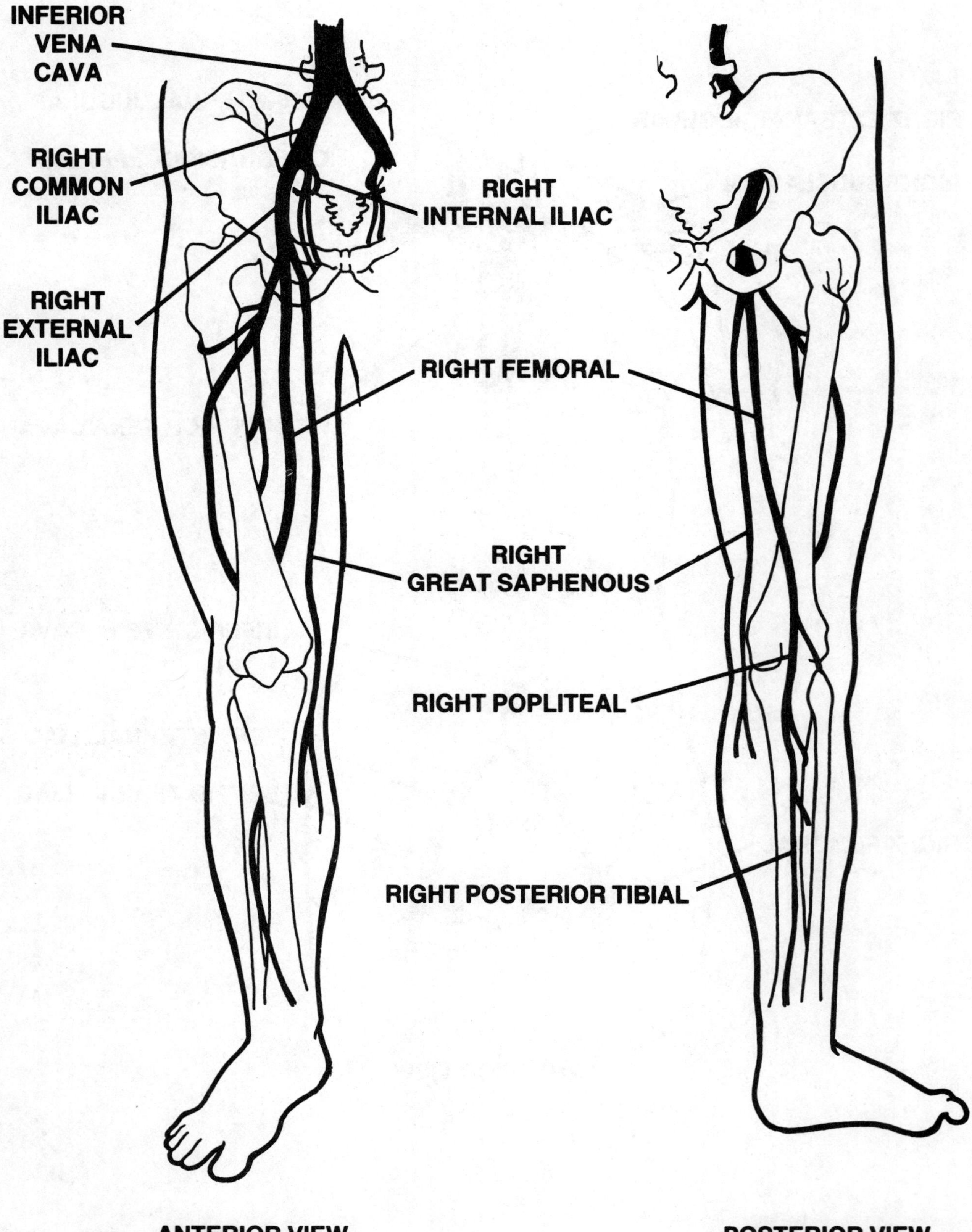

LESSON 11 — REVIEW
THE CARDIOVASCULAR SYSTEM
STRUCTURAL RELATIONSHIP OF VESSELS

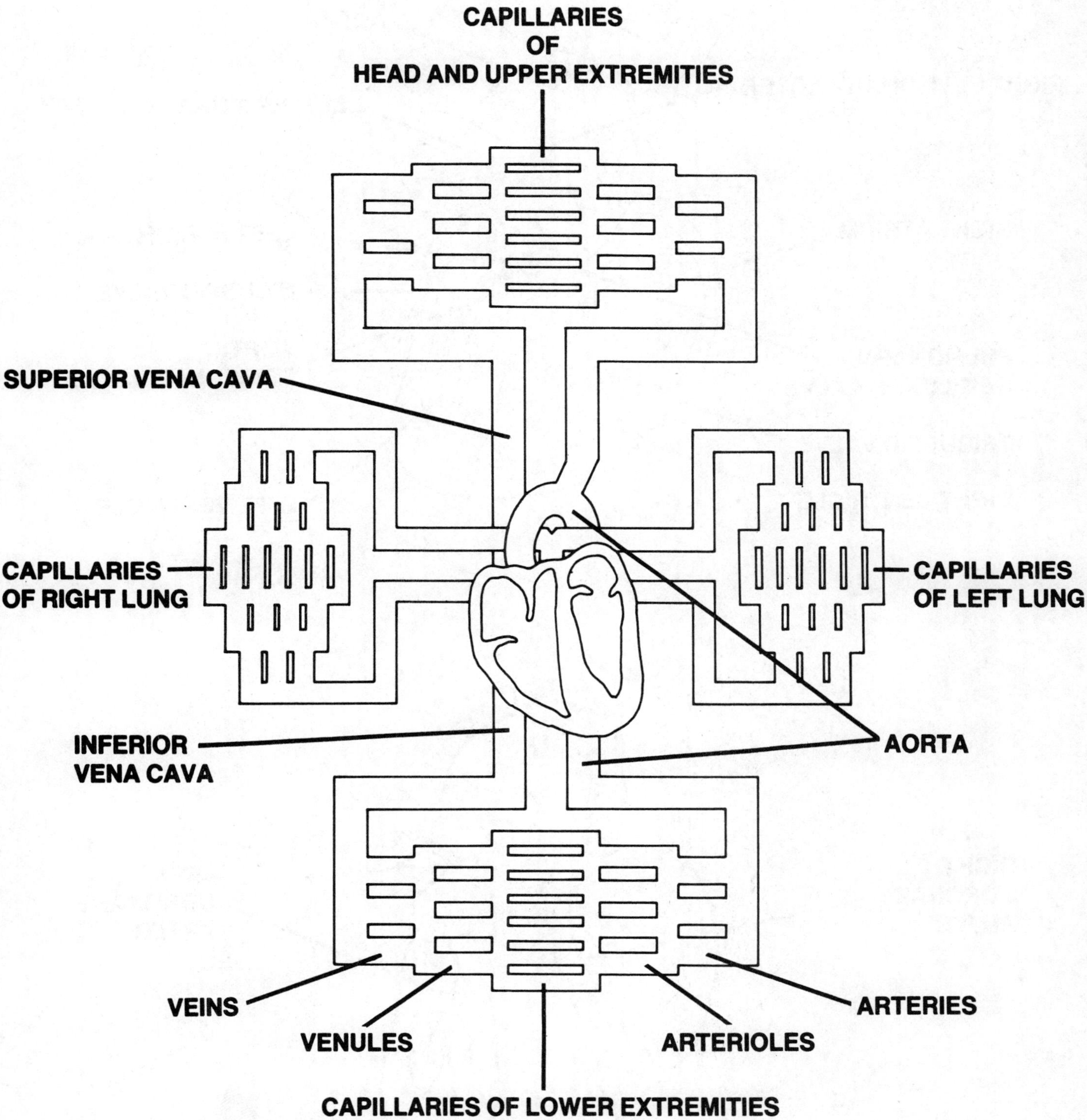

LESSON 11 — REVIEW
THE CARDIOVASCULAR SYSTEM
THE HEART

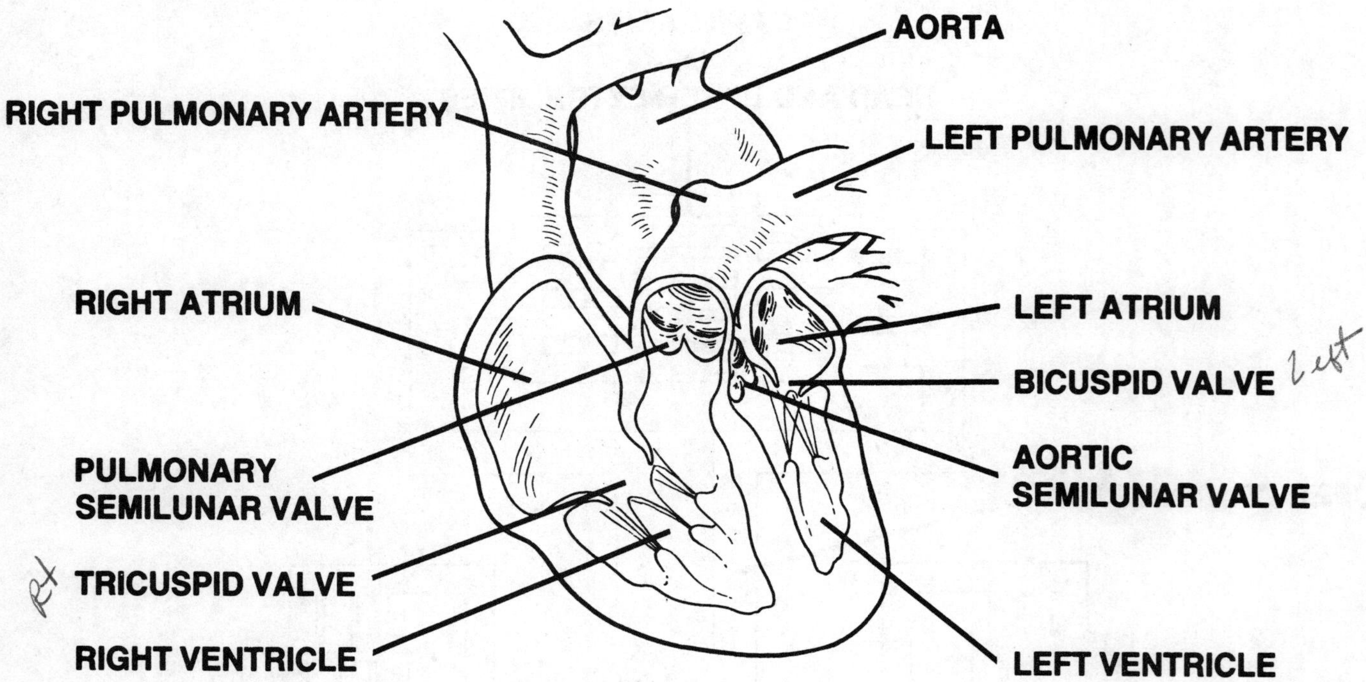

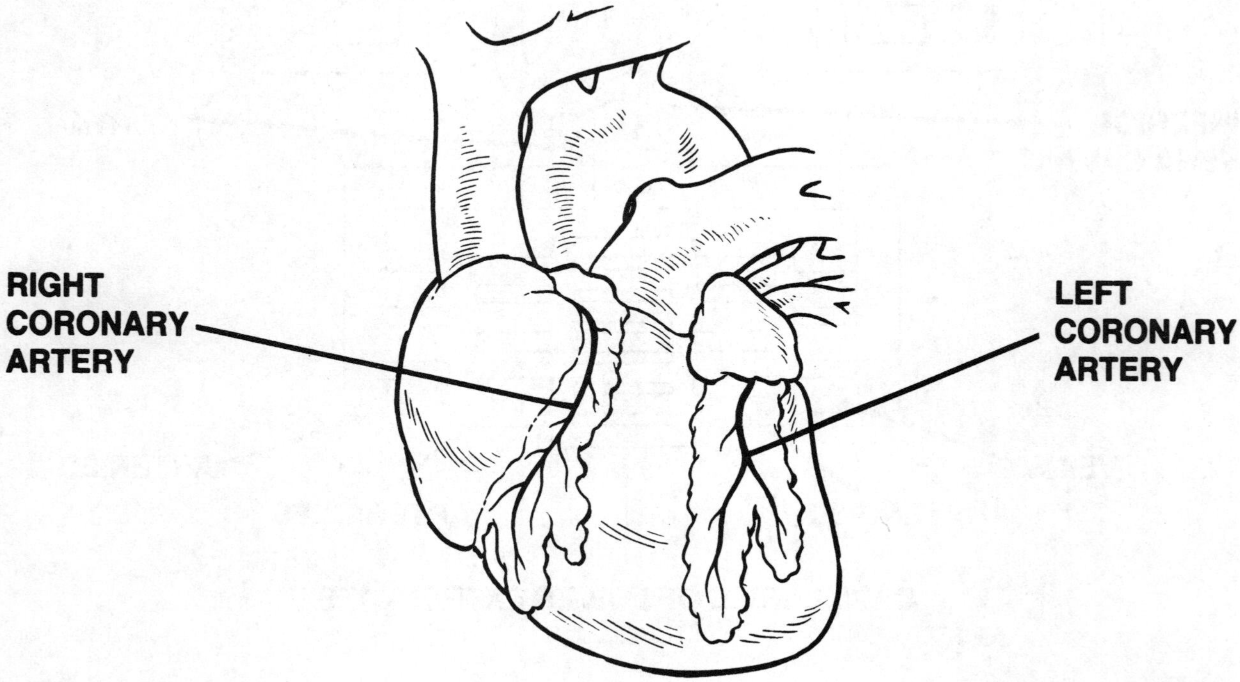

LESSON 11 — WORKSHEET
THE CARDIOVASCULAR SYSTEM

COMPLETE THE BLANKS:

AUDIONYMS

WORD		AUDIONYM
ATRIUM		Atrium
VENTRICLE		Vent
BICUSPID	Left	Bicycle / custard
TRICUSPID	Rt	Tricycle / custard
AORTA		Hay / oar
ARTERY		Artwork
ARTERIOLE		Artwork / owl
CAPILLARY		cap
VENULE		Vanilla
VEIN		weather / vane
VENA CAVA		"V" neck / cuff
CORONARY		Canary
CAROTID		Carrot
JUGULAR		Jug
SAPHENOUS		sapphire

LESSON 11 — WORKSHEET
THE CARDIOVASCULAR SYSTEM
PRINCIPAL ARTERIES OF NECK AND HEAD

PRINT THE CORRECT LETTER WITHIN THE PARENTHESES

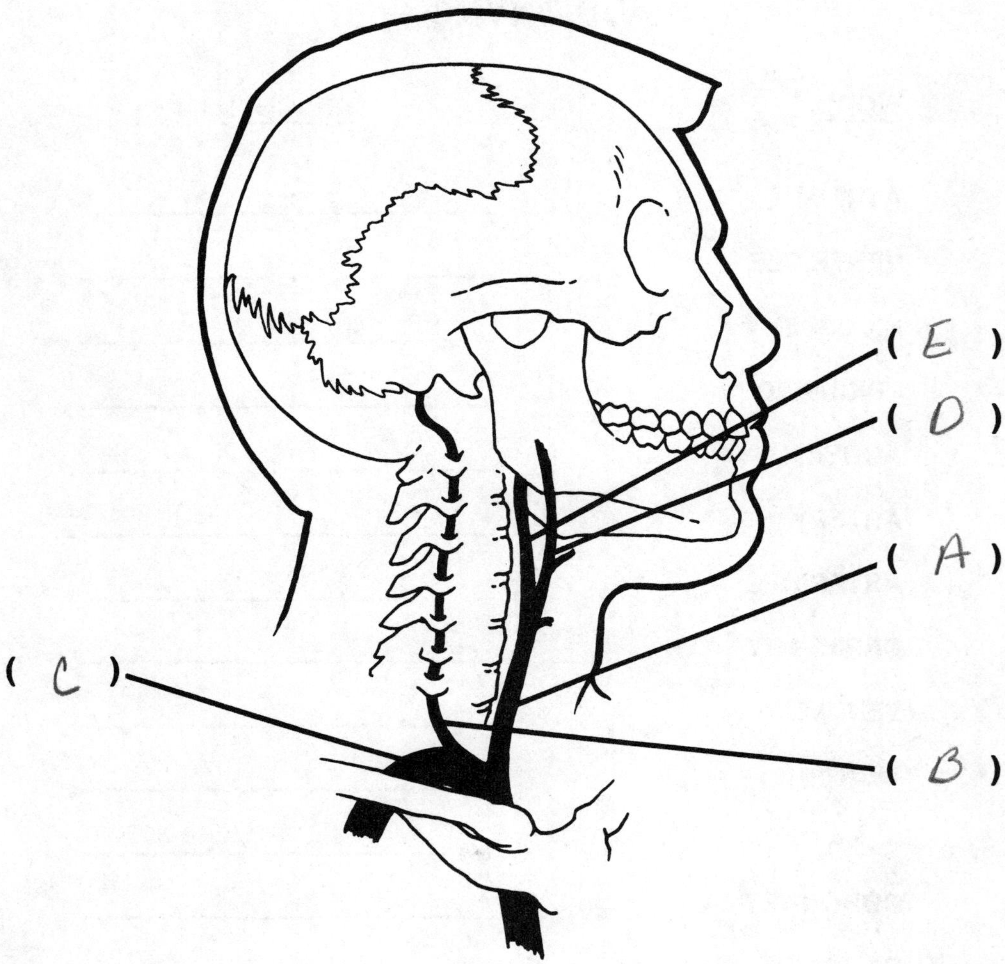

RIGHT LATERAL VIEW

A - RIGHT COMMON CAROTID

B - RIGHT VERTEBRAL

C - RIGHT SUBCLAVIAN

D - RIGHT EXTERNAL CAROTID

E - RIGHT INTERNAL CAROTID

LESSON 11 — WORKSHEET
THE CARDIOVASCULAR SYSTEM
PRINCIPAL ARTERIES OF THE RIGHT UPPER EXTREMITY

PRINT THE CORRECT LETTER WITHIN THE PARENTHESES

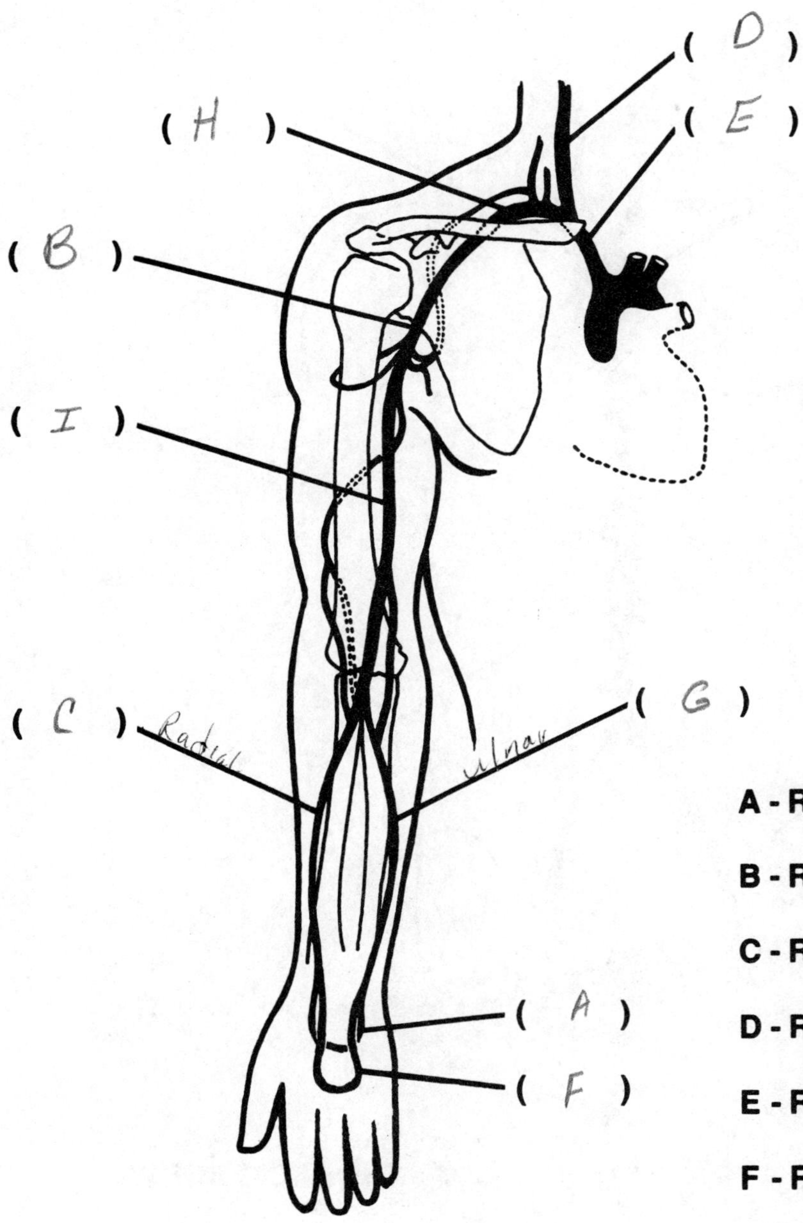

ANTERIOR VIEW

A - RIGHT DEEP PALMAR

B - RIGHT AXILLARY

C - RIGHT RADIAL

D - RIGHT COMMON CAROTID

E - RIGHT BRACHIOCEPHALIC

F - RIGHT SUPERFICIAL PALMAR

G - RIGHT ULNAR

H - RIGHT SUBCLAVIAN

I - RIGHT BRACHIAL

LESSON 11 — WORKSHEET
THE CARDIOVASCULAR SYSTEM
PRINCIPAL DIVISIONS OF AORTA

PRINT THE CORRECT LETTER WITHIN THE PARENTHESES

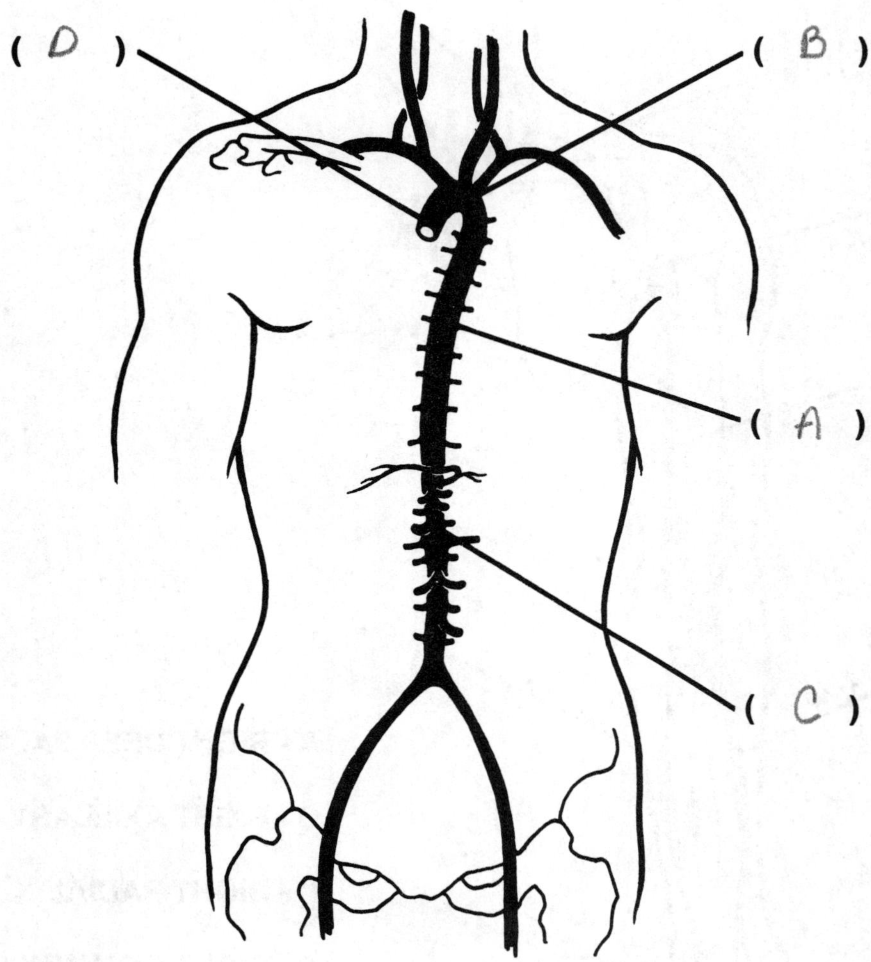

A - THORACIC AORTA

B - ARCH OF AORTA

C - ABDOMINAL AORTA

D - ASCENDING AORTA

LESSON 11 — WORKSHEET
THE CARDIOVASCULAR SYSTEM
PRINCIPAL ARTERIES OF PELVIS AND RIGHT LOWER EXTREMITY

PRINT THE CORRECT LETTER WITHIN THE PARENTHESES

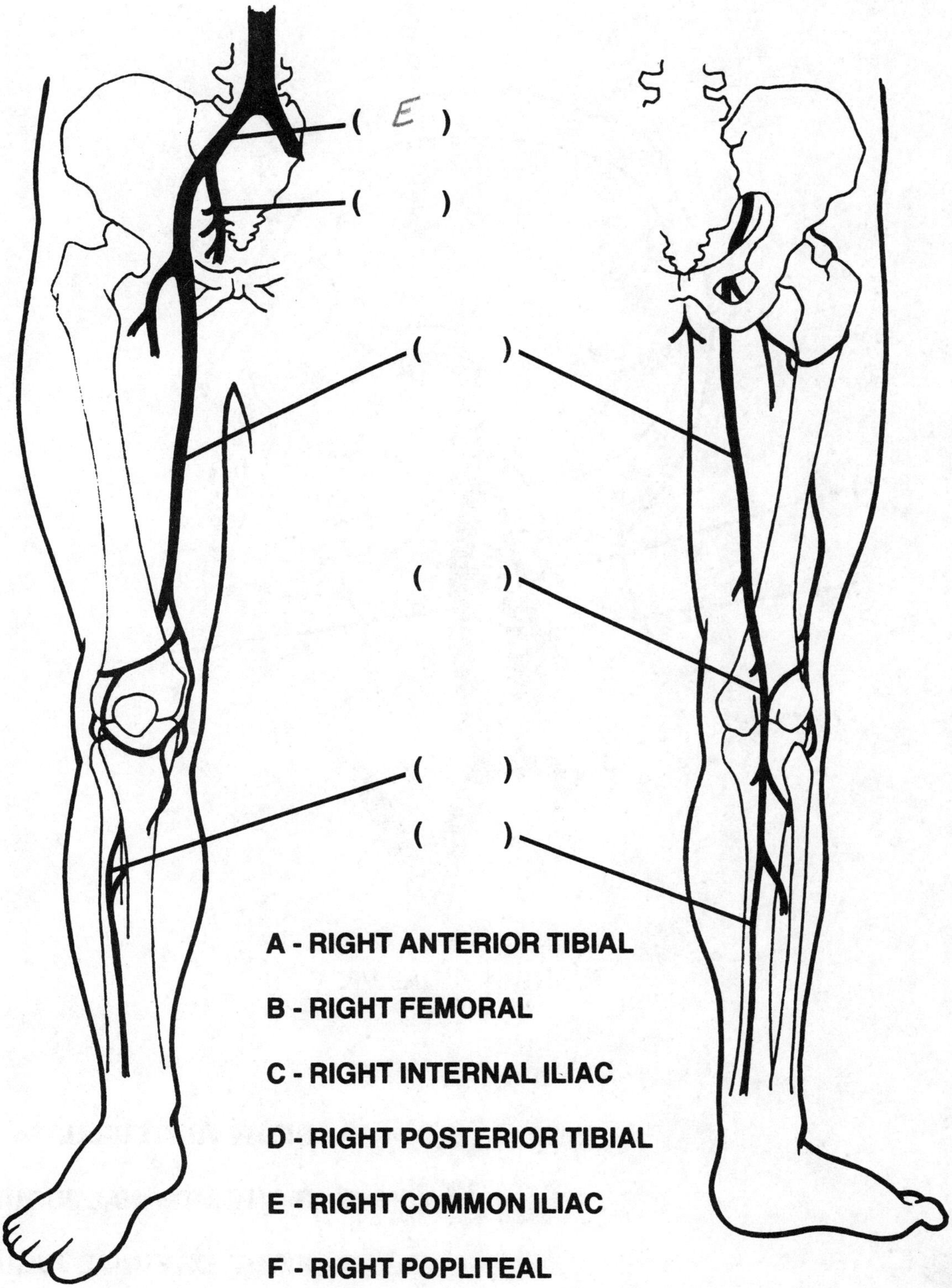

A - RIGHT ANTERIOR TIBIAL

B - RIGHT FEMORAL

C - RIGHT INTERNAL ILIAC

D - RIGHT POSTERIOR TIBIAL

E - RIGHT COMMON ILIAC

F - RIGHT POPLITEAL

ANTERIOR VIEW **POSTERIOR VIEW**

LESSON 11 — WORKSHEET
THE CARDIOVASCULAR SYSTEM
PRINCIPAL VEINS OF THE HEAD AND NECK

PRINT THE CORRECT LETTER WITHIN THE PARENTHESES

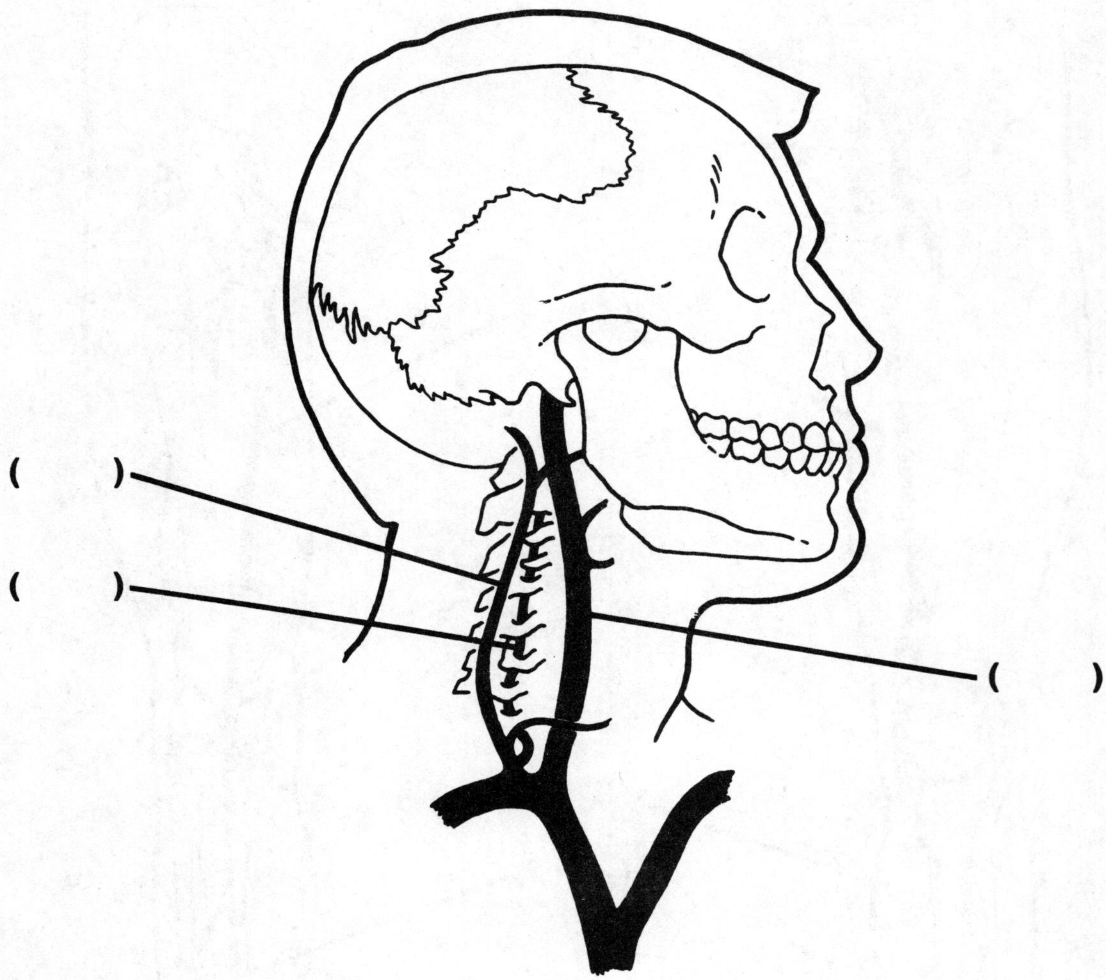

RIGHT LATERAL VIEW

A - RIGHT VERTEBRAL

B - RIGHT INTERNAL JUGULAR

C - RIGHT EXTERNAL JUGULAR

LESSON 11 — WORKSHEET
THE CARDIOVASCULAR SYSTEM
PRINCIPAL VEINS OF THE RIGHT UPPER EXTREMITY

PRINT THE CORRECT LETTER WITHIN THE PARENTHESES

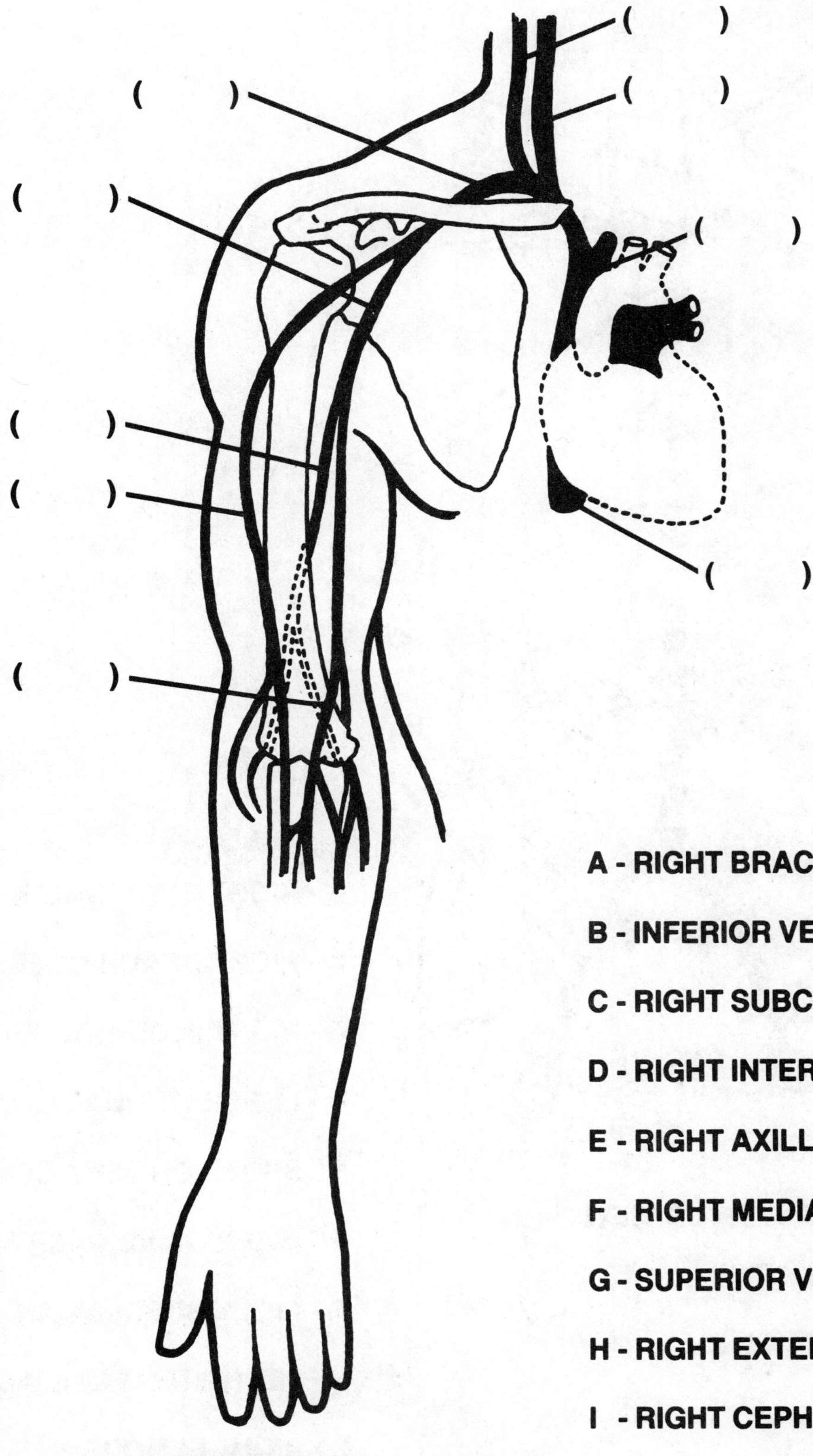

A - RIGHT BRACHIAL

B - INFERIOR VENA CAVA

C - RIGHT SUBCLAVIAN

D - RIGHT INTERNAL JUGULAR

E - RIGHT AXILLARY

F - RIGHT MEDIAN CUBITAL

G - SUPERIOR VENA CAVA

H - RIGHT EXTERNAL JUGULAR

I - RIGHT CEPHALIC

ANTERIOR VIEW

LESSON 11 — WORKSHEET
THE CARDIOVASCULAR SYSTEM
PRINCIPAL VEINS OF THE THORAX, ABDOMEN, AND PELVIS

PRINT THE CORRECT LETTER WITHIN THE PARENTHESES

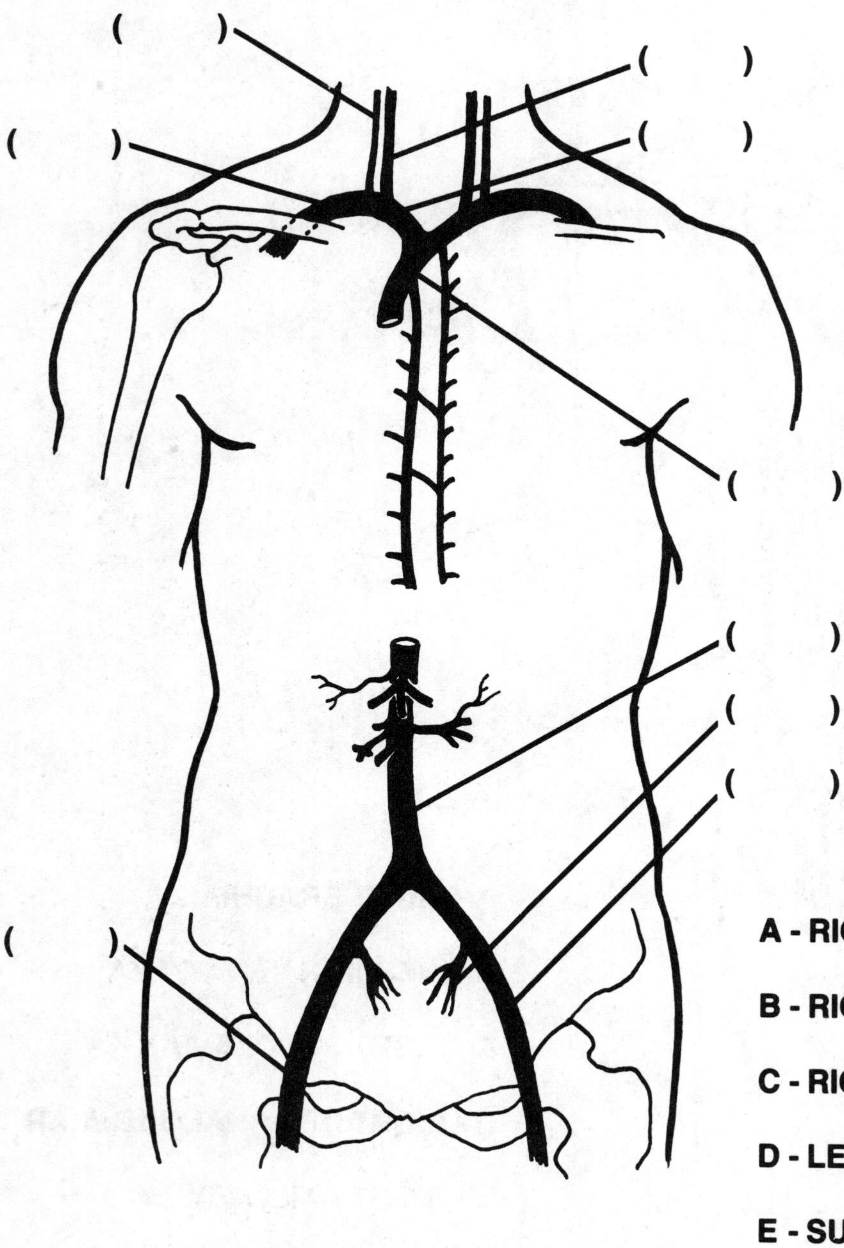

ANTERIOR VIEW

A - RIGHT EXTERNAL JUGULAR

B - RIGHT BRACHIOCEPHALIC

C - RIGHT INTERNAL JUGULAR

D - LEFT EXTERNAL ILIAC

E - SUPERIOR VENA CAVA

F - INFERIOR VENA CAVA

G - RIGHT SUBCLAVIAN

H - LEFT INTERNAL ILIAC

I - RIGHT FEMORAL

LESSON 11 — WORKSHEET
THE CARDIOVASCULAR SYSTEM
PRINCIPAL VEINS OF THE PELVIS AND RIGHT LOWER EXTREMITY

PRINT THE CORRECT LETTER WITHIN THE PARENTHESES

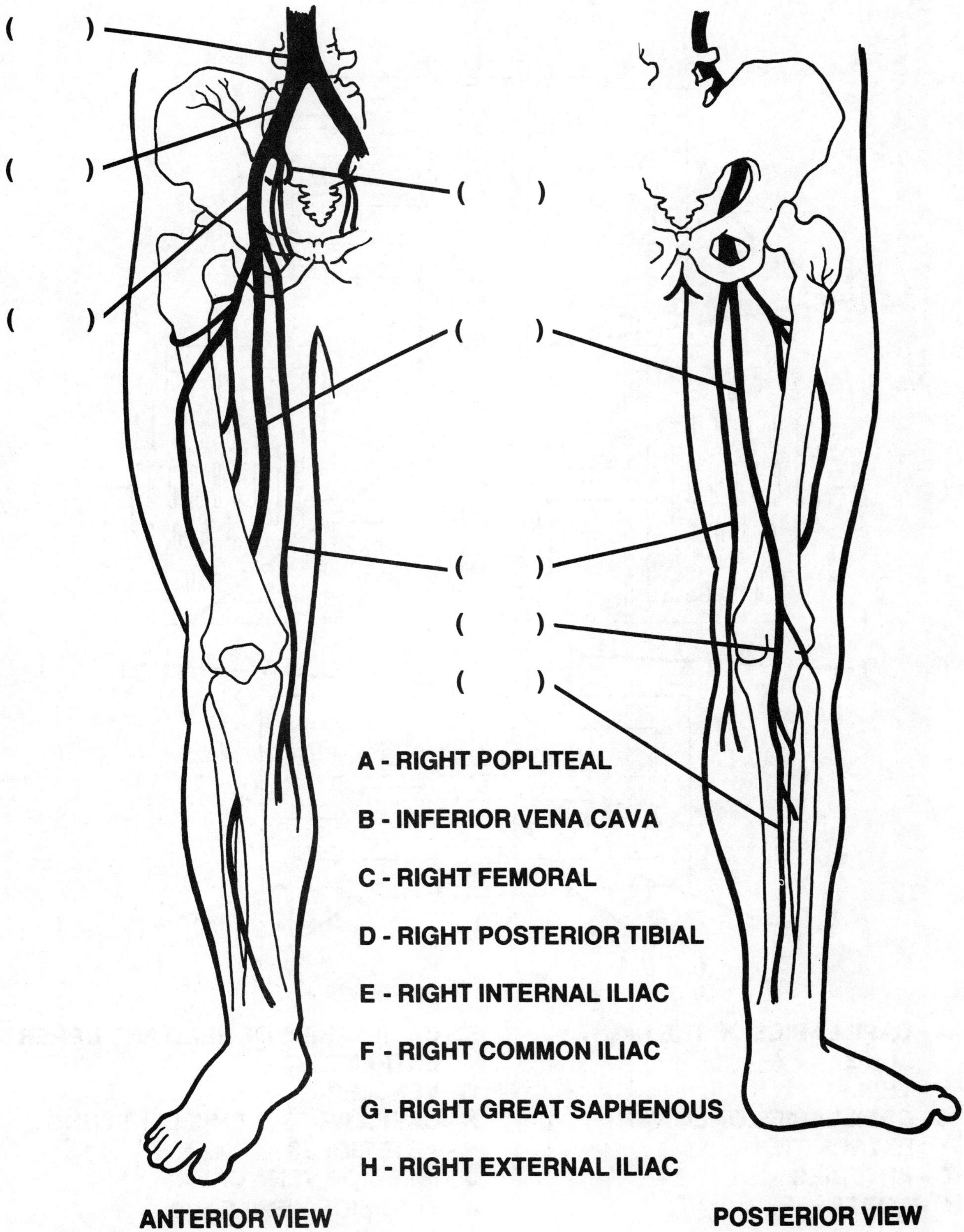

A - RIGHT POPLITEAL

B - INFERIOR VENA CAVA

C - RIGHT FEMORAL

D - RIGHT POSTERIOR TIBIAL

E - RIGHT INTERNAL ILIAC

F - RIGHT COMMON ILIAC

G - RIGHT GREAT SAPHENOUS

H - RIGHT EXTERNAL ILIAC

LESSON 11 — WORKSHEET
THE CARDIOVASCULAR SYSTEM
STRUCTURAL RELATIONSHIP OF VESSELS

PRINT THE CORRECT LETTER WITHIN THE PARENTHESES

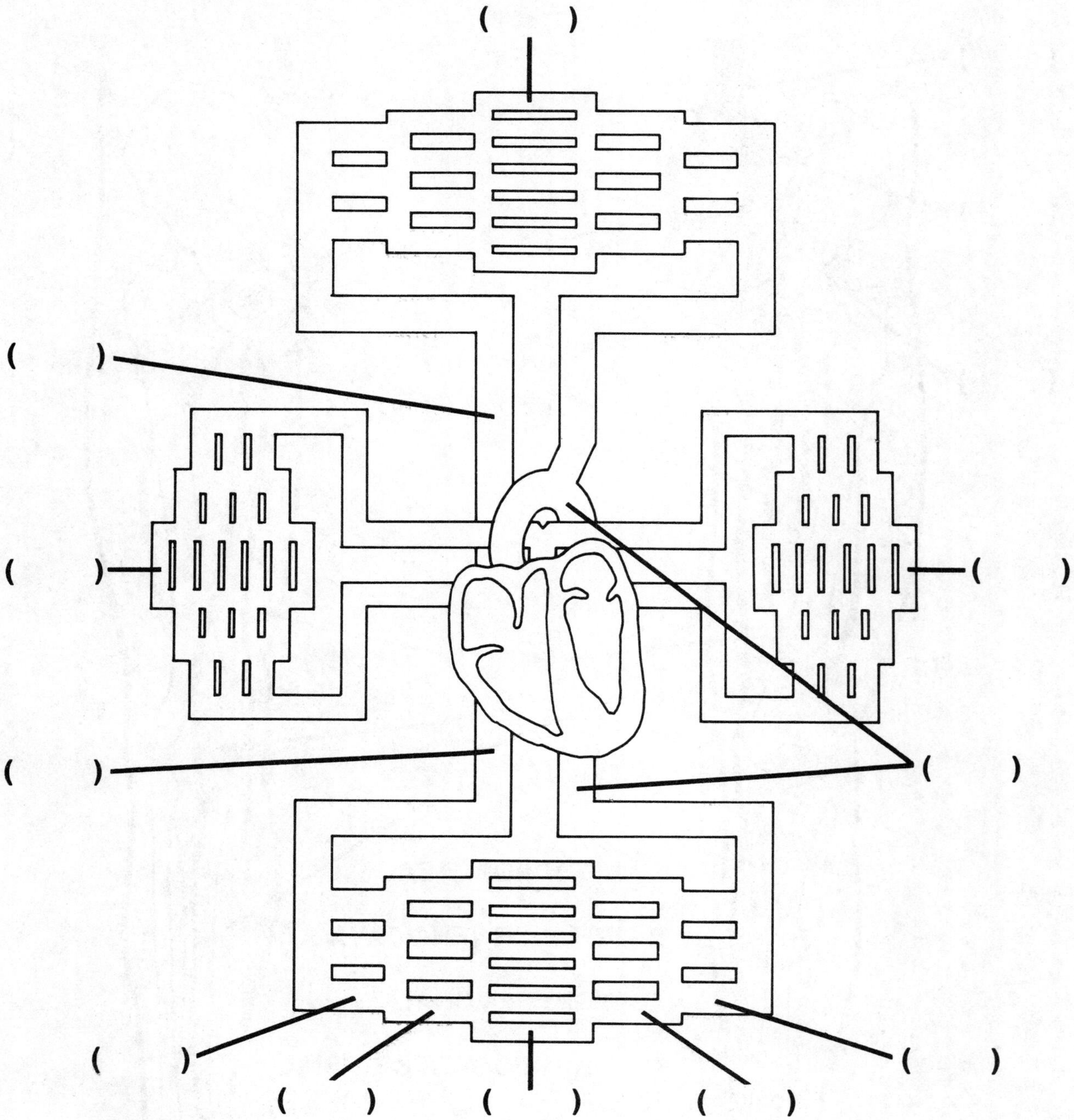

A - CAPILLARIES OF THE RIGHT LUNG
B - VEINS
C - CAPILLARIES OF LOWER EXTREMITIES
D - ARTERIES
E - AORTA
F - CAPILLARIES OF HEAD AND UPPER EXTREMITIES
G - VENULES
H - CAPILLARIES OF THE LEFT LUNG
I - ARTERIOLES
J - INFERIOR VENA CAVA
K - SUPERIOR VENA CAVA

LESSON 11 — WORKSHEET
THE CARDIOVASCULAR SYSTEM
THE HEART

PRINT THE CORRECT LETTER WITHIN THE PARENTHESES

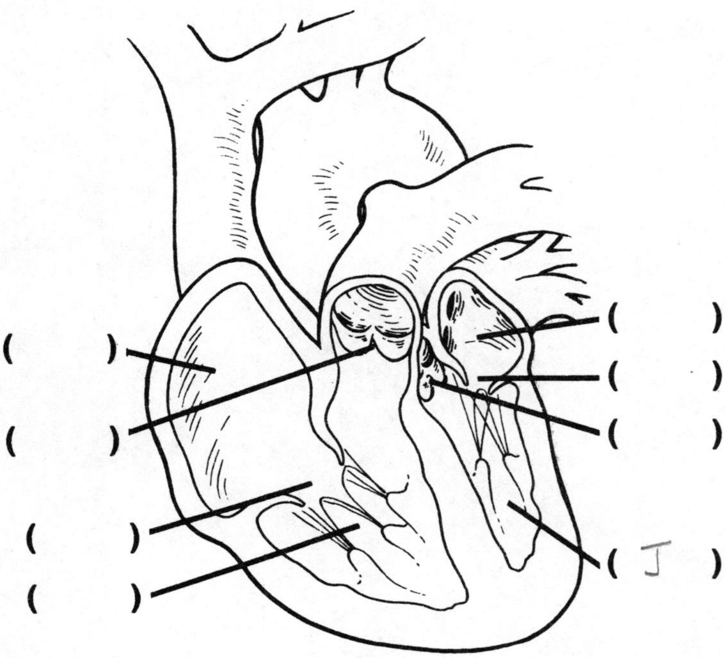

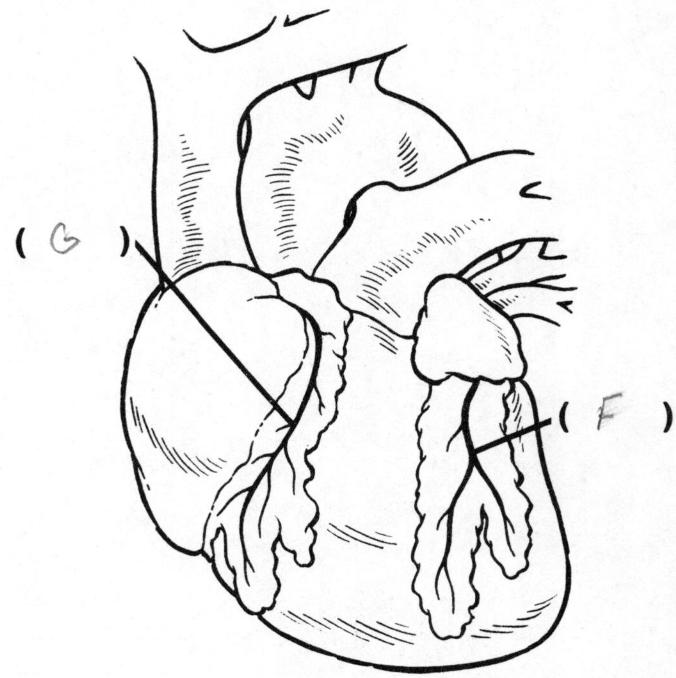

A - AORTIC SEMILUNAR VALVE	**F - LEFT CORONARY ARTERY**
B - RIGHT VENTRICLE	**G - RIGHT CORONARY ARTERY**
C - PULMONARY SEMILUNAR VALVE	**H - BICUSPID VALVE**
D - LEFT ATRIUM	**I - RIGHT ATRIUM**
E - TRICUSPID VALVE	**J - LEFT VENTRICLE**

PRINT THE CORRECT LETTER WITHIN THE PARENTHESES

( ) **MICROSCOPIC BLOOD VESSELS**

( ) **THE LARGEST ARTERY**

( ) **THE LARGEST VEIN ABOVE THE HEART**

( ) **SMALL ARTERIES**

( ) **LARGEST VEIN BELOW THE HEART**

( ) **SMALL VEINS**

A - INFERIOR VENA CAVA	**D - AORTA**
B - CAPILLARIES	**E - SUPERIOR VENA CAVA**
C - VENULES	**F - ARTERIOLES**

LESSON 12

THE LYMPHATIC SYSTEM

- ORGANS OF THE LYMPHATIC SYSTEM
- STRUCTURAL RELATIONSHIP OF VESSELS
- NAMES AND LOCATIONS OF PRINCIPAL LYMPH NODES

REMEMBER!

1st **Pronounce** *the name of the body part or term*
2nd **Recall** *and* **pronounce** *the audionym*
3rd **For body parts: visualize** *the audionym in place*
For terms: visualize *the association*
4th **Pronounce** *the name of the body part or term again.*

LESSON 12 — REVIEW
THE LYMPHATIC SYSTEM

AUDIONYMS

WORD	AUDIONYM
CAPILLARY	CAP
VESSEL	VASE
NODE	NOTE
TRUNK	TRUNK
DUCT	DUCK
THORACIC DUCT	DRAWER/AX/DUCK
RIGHT LYMPHATIC DUCT	RHINO/LIMB/DUCK
TONSILS	TINSEL
THYMUS	THUMBS
SPLEEN	SPOON

LESSON 12 — REVIEW
THE LYMPHATIC SYSTEM
ORGANS OF THE LYMPHATIC SYSTEM

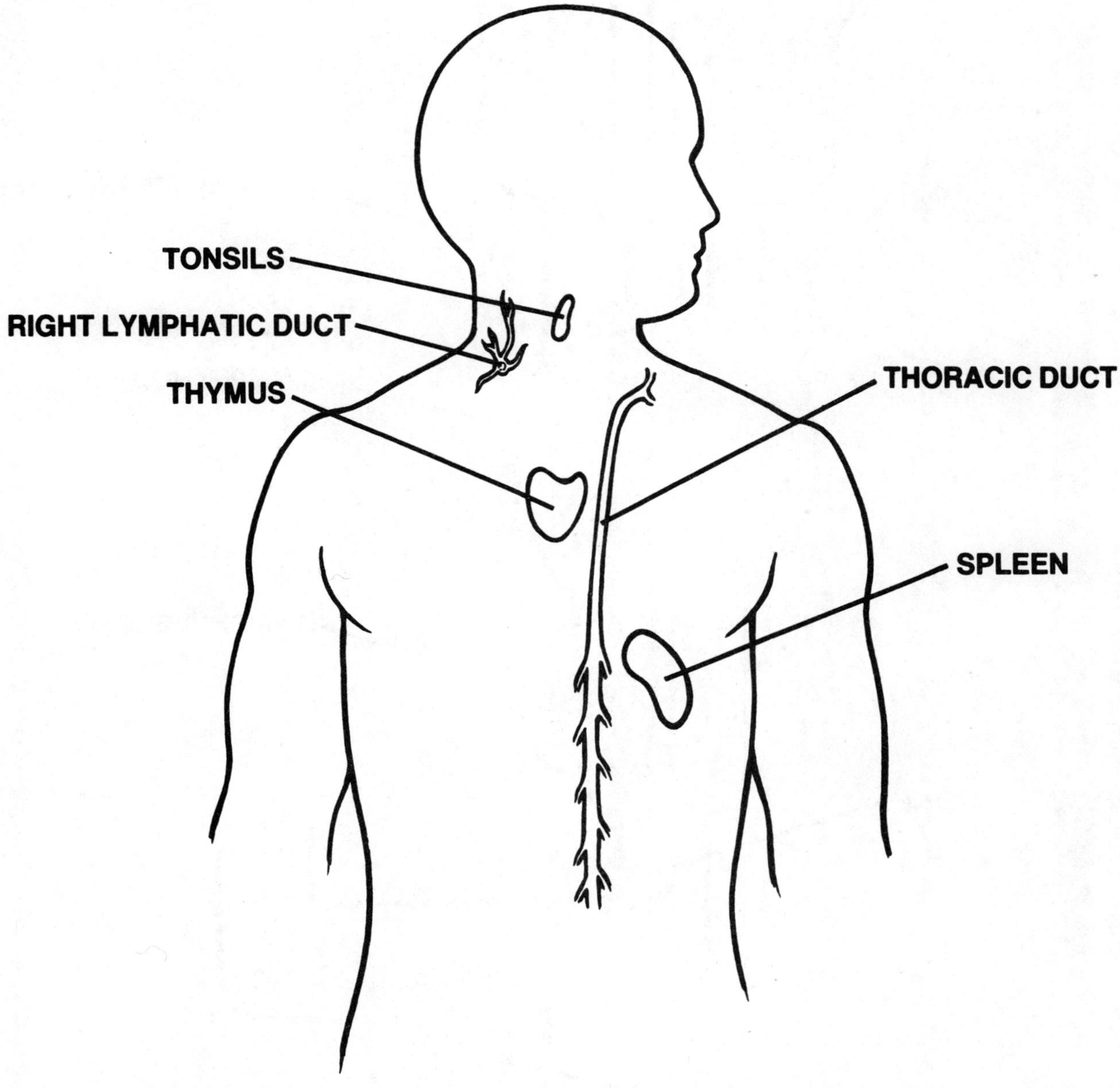

LESSON 12 — REVIEW
THE LYMPHATIC SYSTEM
STRUCTURAL RELATIONSHIP OF LYMPHATIC VESSELS

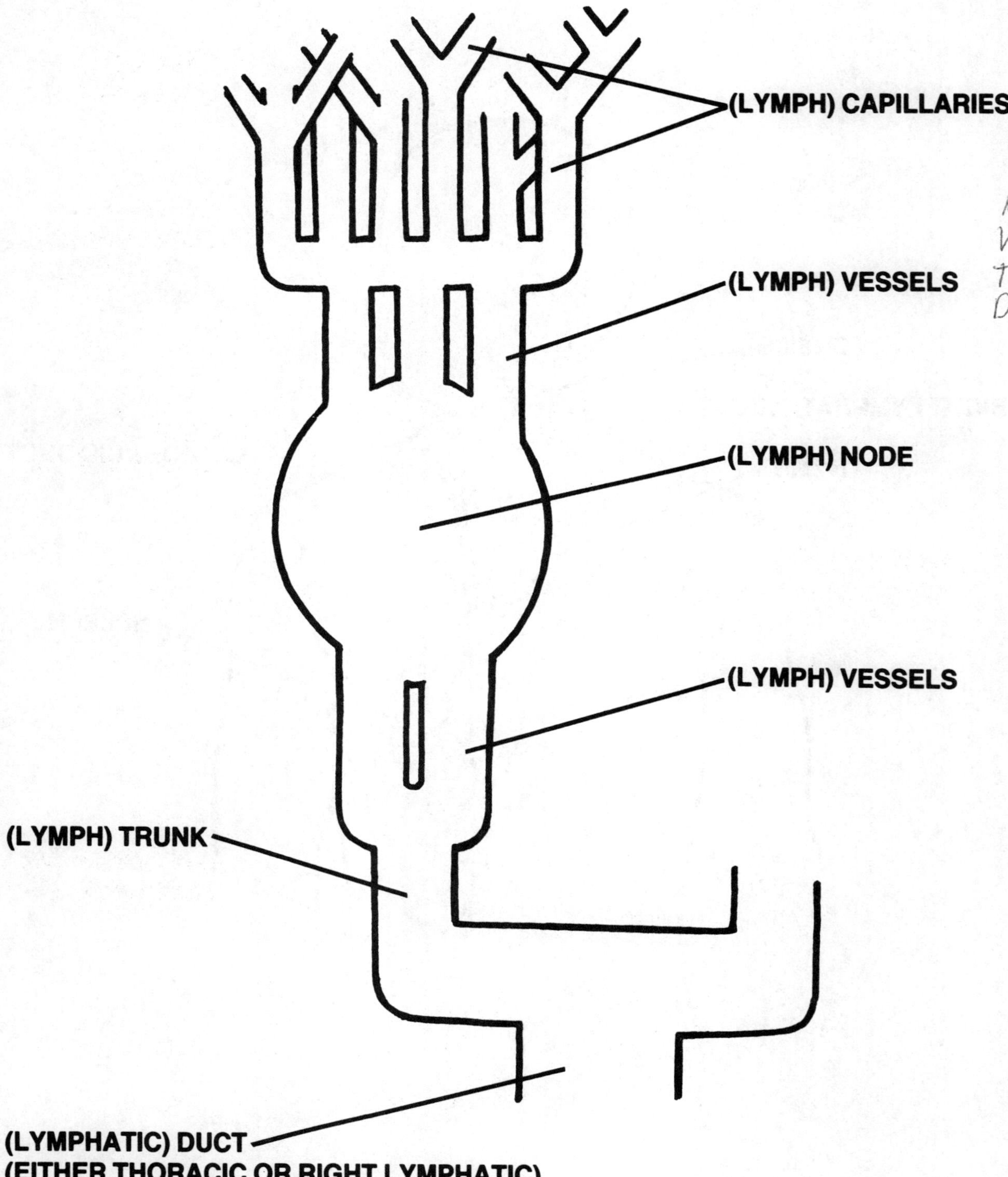

LESSON 12 — REVIEW
THE LYMPHATIC SYSTEM
LYMPH NODES

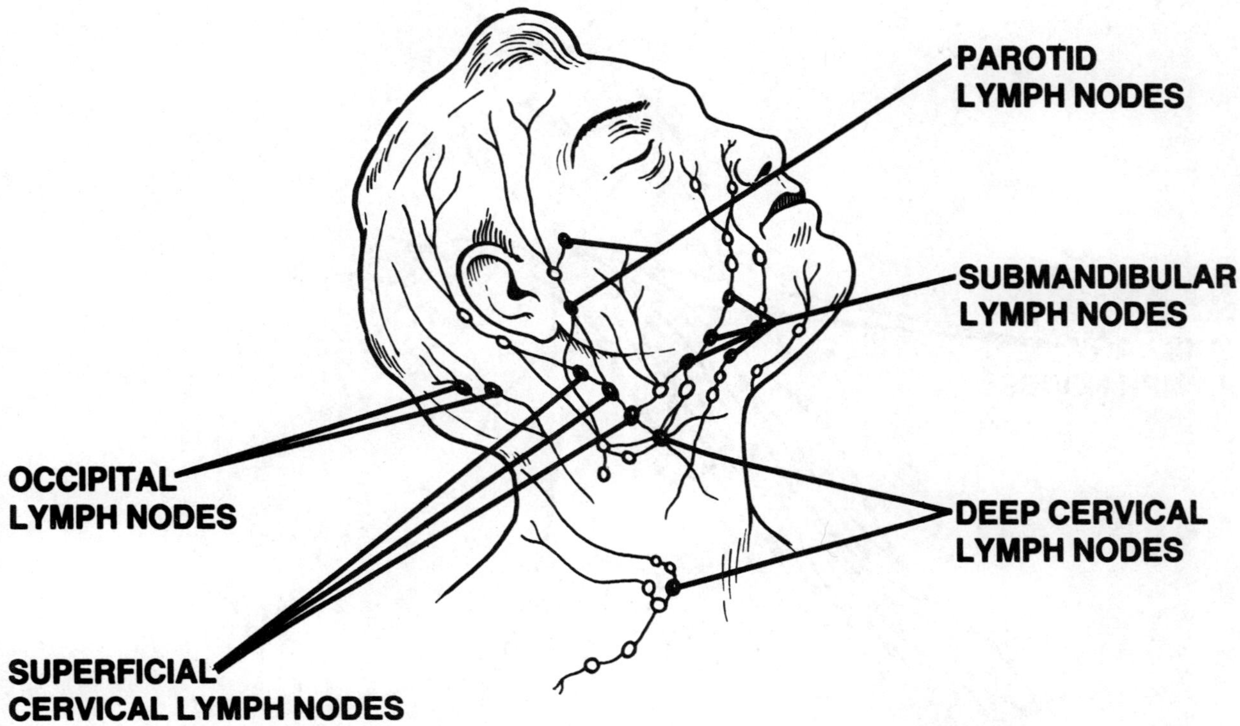

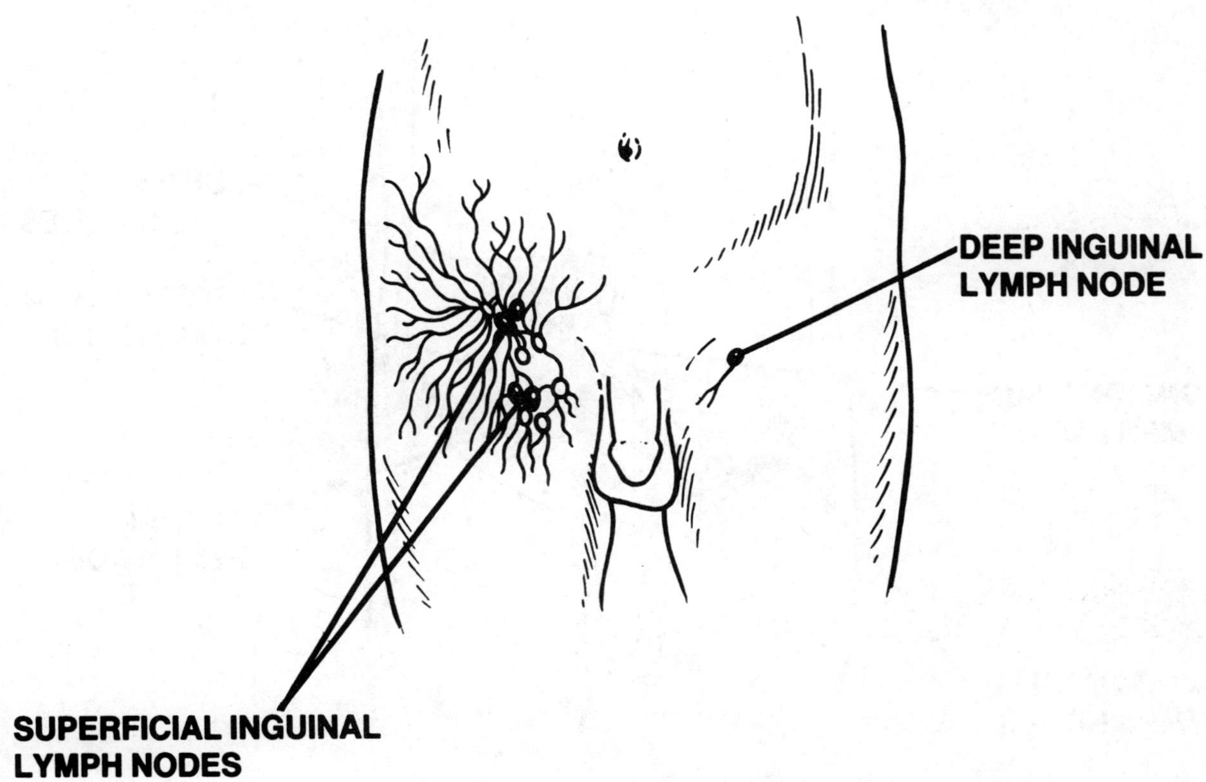

LESSON 12 — REVIEW
THE LYMPHATIC SYSTEM
LYMPH NODES

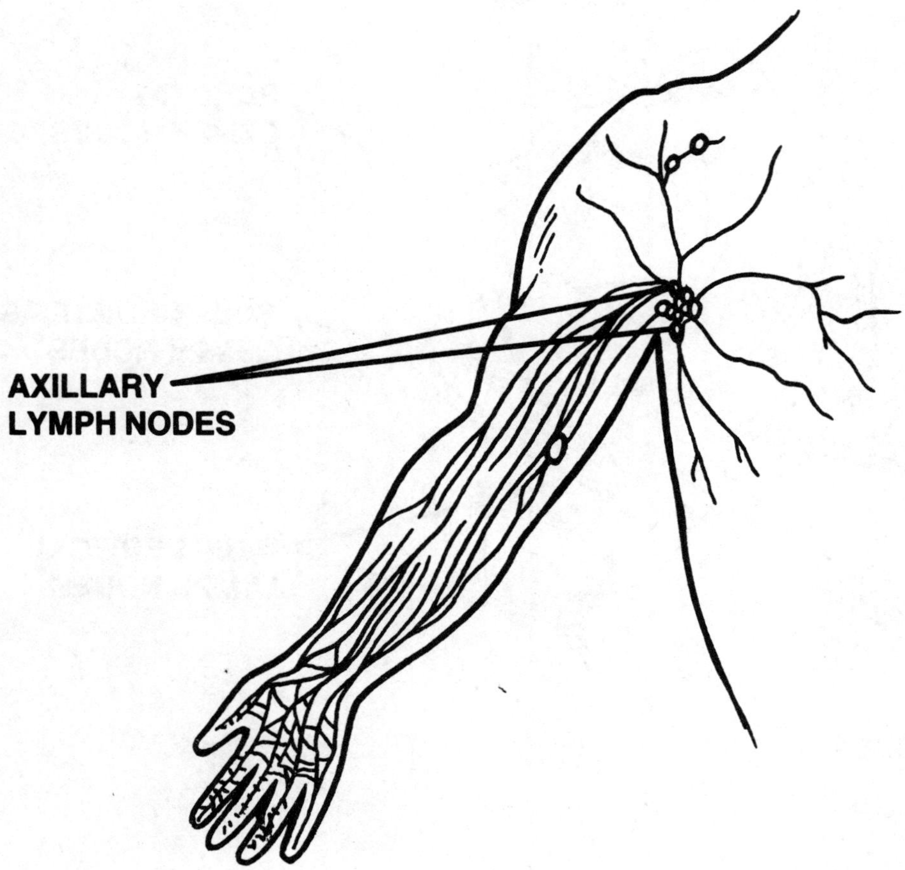

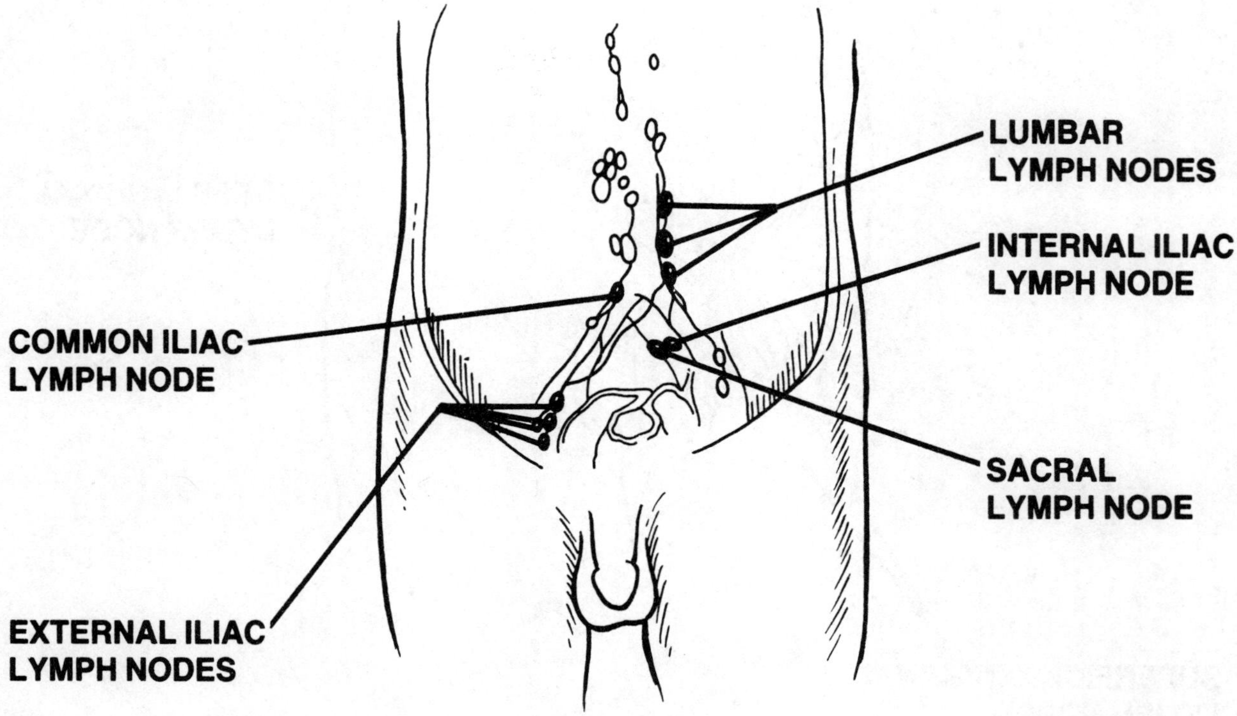

LESSON 12 — WORKSHEET
THE LYMPHATIC SYSTEM

COMPLETE THE BLANKS:

AUDIONYMS

WORD	AUDIONYM
CAPILLARY	Cap
VESSEL	Vase
NODE	Note
TRUNK	Trunk
DUCT	Duck
THORACIC DUCT	Drawer/Ax/duck
RIGHT LYMPHATIC DUCT	Rhino/Limb/Duck
TONSILS	Tinsel
THYMUS	Thumbs
SPLEEN	spoon

LESSON 12 — WORKSHEET
THE LYMPHATIC SYSTEM
ORGANS OF THE LYMPHATIC SYSTEM

PRINT THE CORRECT LETTER WITHIN THE PARENTHESES

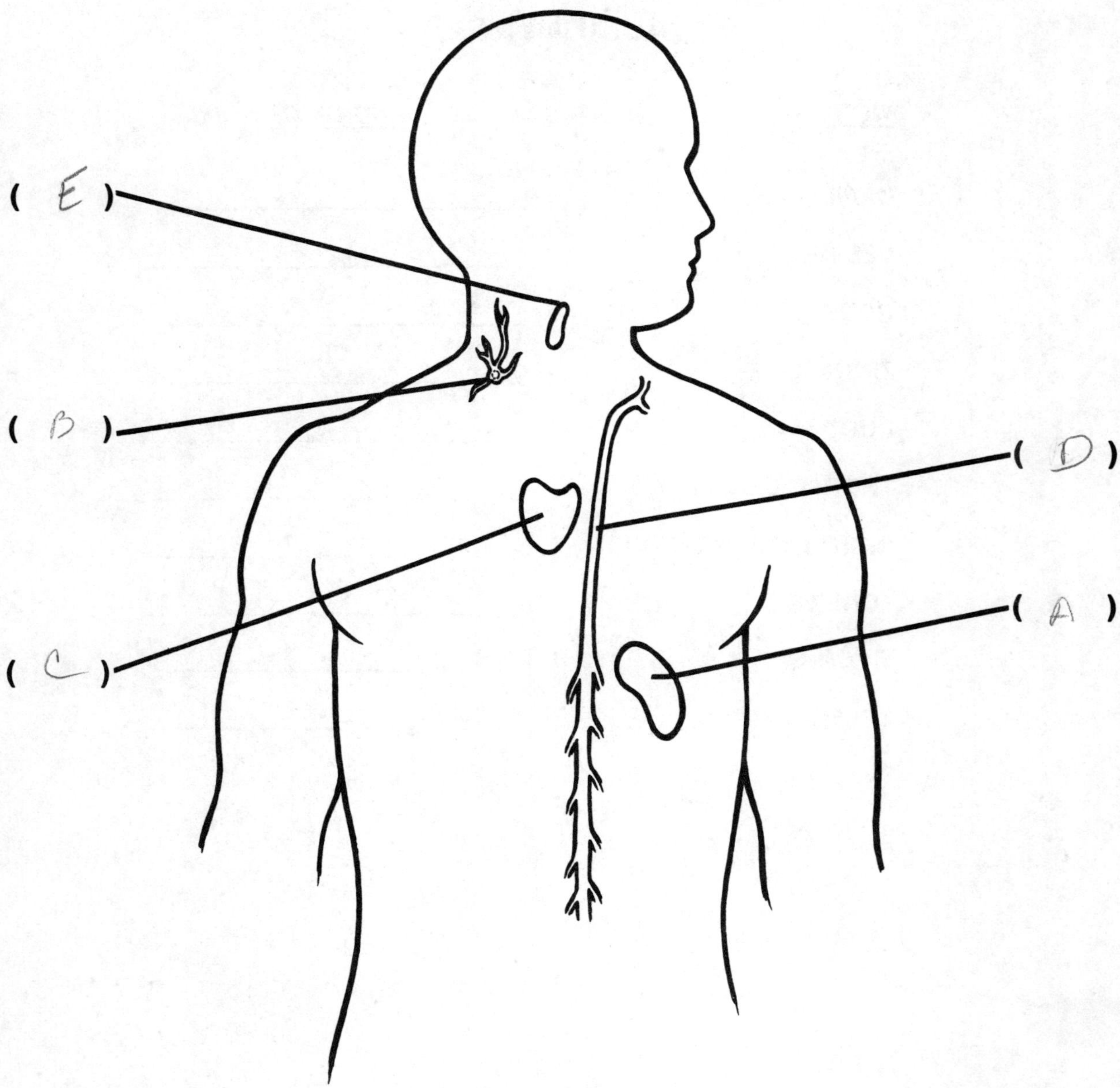

A - SPLEEN

B - RIGHT LYMPHATIC DUCT

C - THYMUS

D - THORACIC DUCT

E - TONSILS

LESSON 12 — WORKSHEET
THE LYMPHATIC SYSTEM
STRUCTURAL RELATIONSHIPS OF LYMPHATIC VESSELS

PRINT THE CORRECT LETTER WITHIN THE PARENTHESES

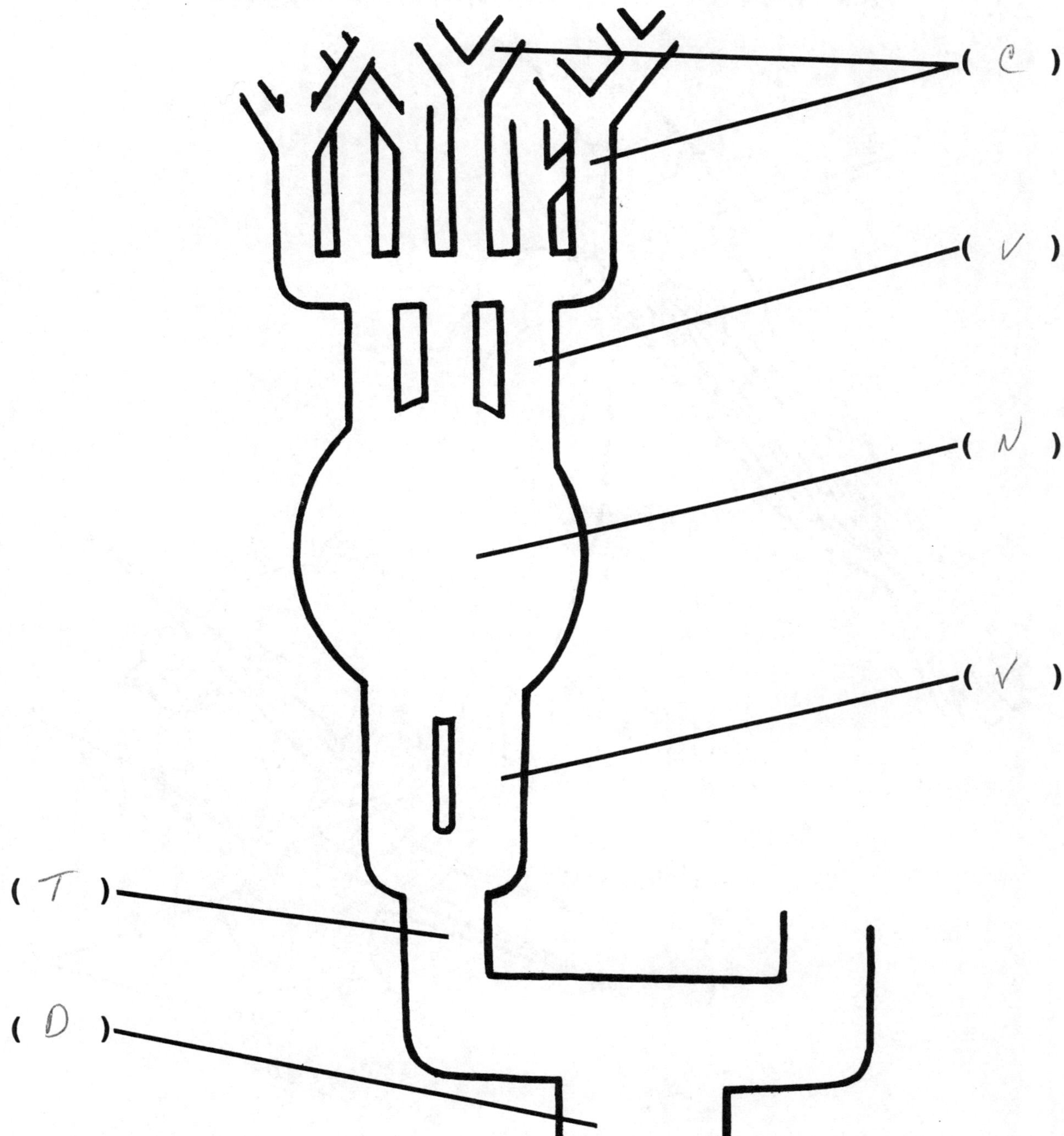

A - (LYMPH) TRUNK

B - (LYMPH) CAPILLARIES

C - (LYMPH) VESSELS

D - (LYMPHATIC) DUCT (EITHER THORACIC OR RIGHT LYMPHATIC)

E - (LYMPH) NODE

F - (LYMPH) VESSELS

LESSON 12 — WORKSHEET
THE LYMPHATIC SYSTEM
LYMPH NODES

PRINT THE CORRECT LETTER WITHIN THE PARENTHESES

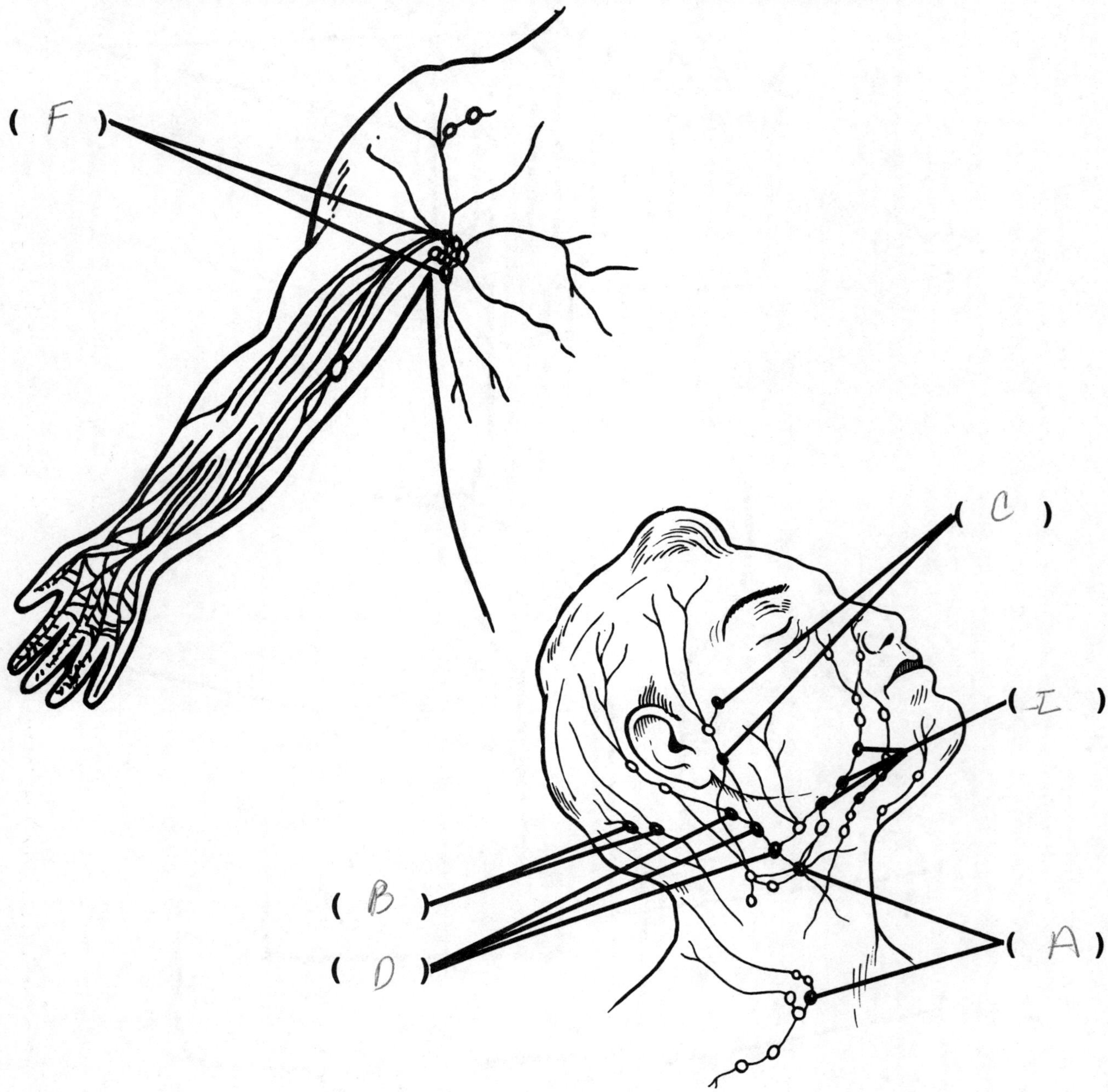

A - DEEP CERVICAL LYMPH NODES

B - OCCIPITAL LYMPH NODES

C - PAROTID LYMPH NODES

D - SUPERFICIAL CERVICAL LYMPH NODES

E - SUBMANDIBULAR CERVICAL LYMPH NODES

F - AXILLARY LYMPH NODES

LESSON 12 — WORKSHEET
THE LYMPHATIC SYSTEM
LYMPH NODES

PRINT THE CORRECT LETTER WITHIN THE PARENTHESES

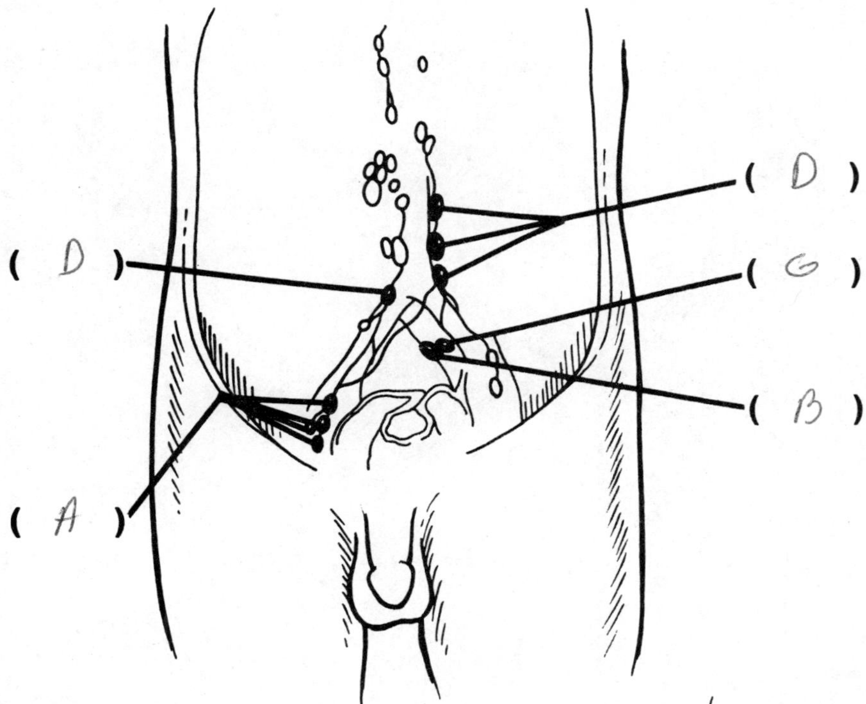

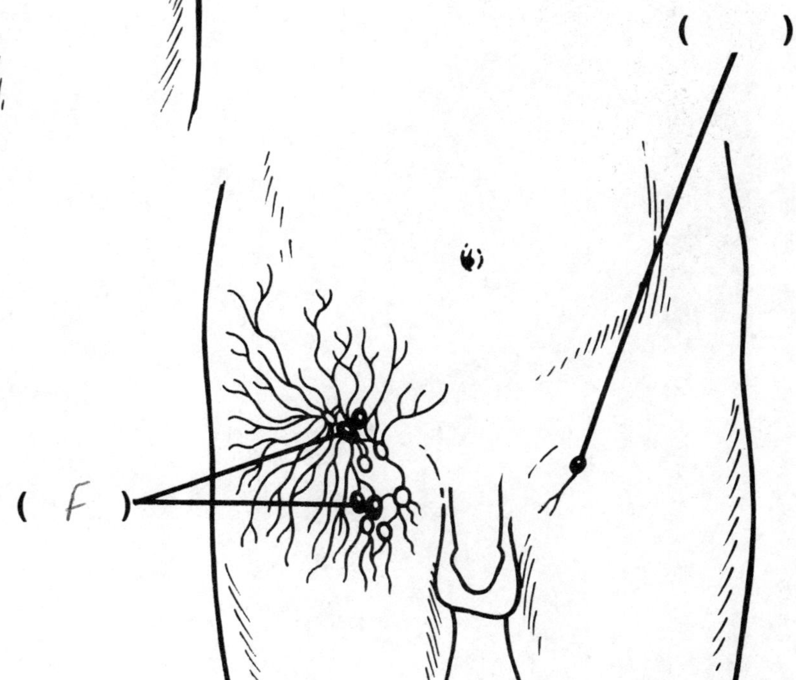

A - EXTERNAL ILIAC LYMPH NODES

B - SACRAL LYMPH NODE

C - DEEP INGUINAL LYMPH NODES

D - COMMON ILIAC LYMPH NODE

E - LUMBAR LYMPH NODES

F - SUPERFICIAL INGUINAL LYMPH NODES

G - INTERNAL ILIAC LYMPH NODE

LESSON 13

THE ENDOCRINE SYSTEM

GLANDS OF THE ENDOCRINE SYSTEM

	NUMBER
● PITUITARY	1
● THYROID	1
● PARATHYROID	4
● ADRENAL	2
● PANCREAS	1
● OVARIES	2
● TESTES	2
● PINEAL	1
● THYMUS	1

REMEMBER!

1st ***Pronounce*** *the name of the body part or term*
2nd ***Recall*** *and* ***pronounce*** *the audionym*
3rd ***For body parts: visualize*** *the audionym in place*
For terms: visualize *the association*
4th ***Pronounce*** *the name of the body part or term again.*

LESSON 13 — REVIEW
THE ENDOCRINE SYSTEM

AUDIONYMS

WORD	AUDIONYM
PITUITARY	PITCHER
THYROID	TIE/ROAD
PARATHYROID	PARROT/TIE/ROAD
ADRENAL	A DRAIN
PANCREAS	PAN
OVARY	OVAL TREE
TESTES	TESTS
PINEAL	PIN/EEL
THYMUS	THUMBS

LESSON 13 — REVIEW
THE ENDOCRINE SYSTEM
GLANDS OF THE ENDOCRINE SYSTEM

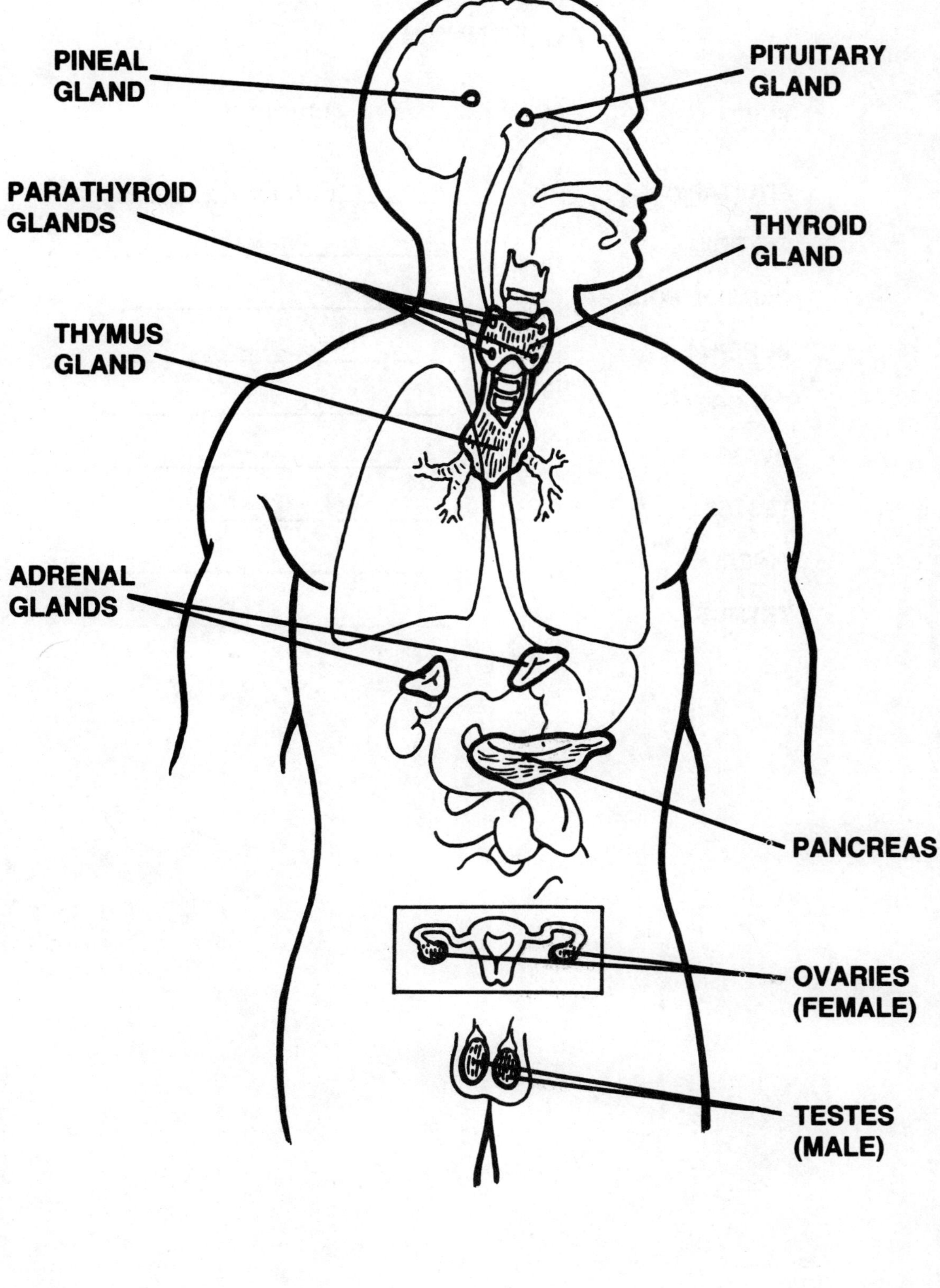

LESSON 13 — WORKSHEET
THE ENDOCRINE SYSTEM

COMPLETE THE BLANKS:

AUDIONYMS

WORD	AUDIONYM
PITUITARY	Pitcher
THYROID	Tie / road
PARATHYROID	Parrot / Tie / Road
ADRENAL	A drain
PANCREAS	Pan
OVARY	oval Tree
TESTES	Tests
PINEAL	pin / EEL
THYMUS	Thumbs

LESSON 13 — WORKSHEET
THE ENDOCRINE SYSTEM
GLANDS OF THE ENDOCRINE SYSTEM

PRINT THE CORRECT LETTER WITHIN THE PARENTHESES

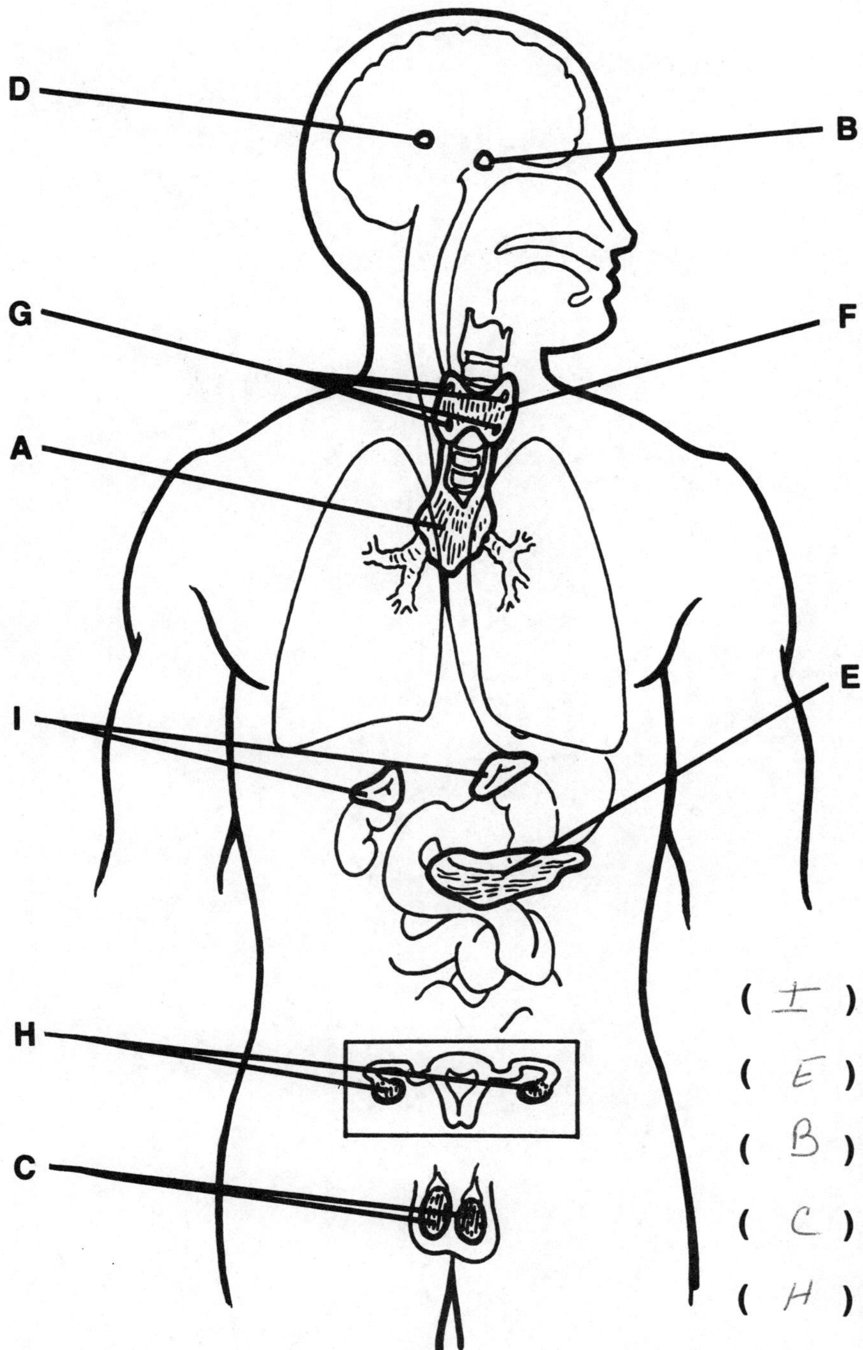

(I) **ADRENAL GLANDS**

(E) **PANCREAS**

(B) **PITUITARY GLAND**

(C) **TESTES**

(H) **OVARIES**

(A) **THYMUS GLAND**

(D) **PINEAL GLAND**

(G) **PARATHYROID GLANDS**

(F) **THYROID GLAND**

LESSON 14

THE URINARY SYSTEM

ORGANS OF THE URINARY SYSTEM

	NUMBER
● KIDNEY	2
● URETER	2
● URINARY BLADDER	1
● URETHRA	1

REMEMBER!

1st **Pronounce** *the name of the body part or term*
2nd **Recall** *and* **pronounce** *the audionym*
3rd **For body parts: visualize** *the audionym in place*
For terms: visualize *the association*
4th **Pronounce** *the name of the body part or term again.*

LESSON 14 — REVIEW
THE URINARY SYSTEM

AUDIONYMS

WORD	AUDIONYM
KIDNEY	KID/KNEE
URETER	"U" RUDDER
URINARY BLADDER	UKELELE PLATTER
URETHRA	"U" WREATH

LESSON 14 — REVIEW
THE URINARY SYSTEM
ORGANS OF THE URINARY SYSTEM

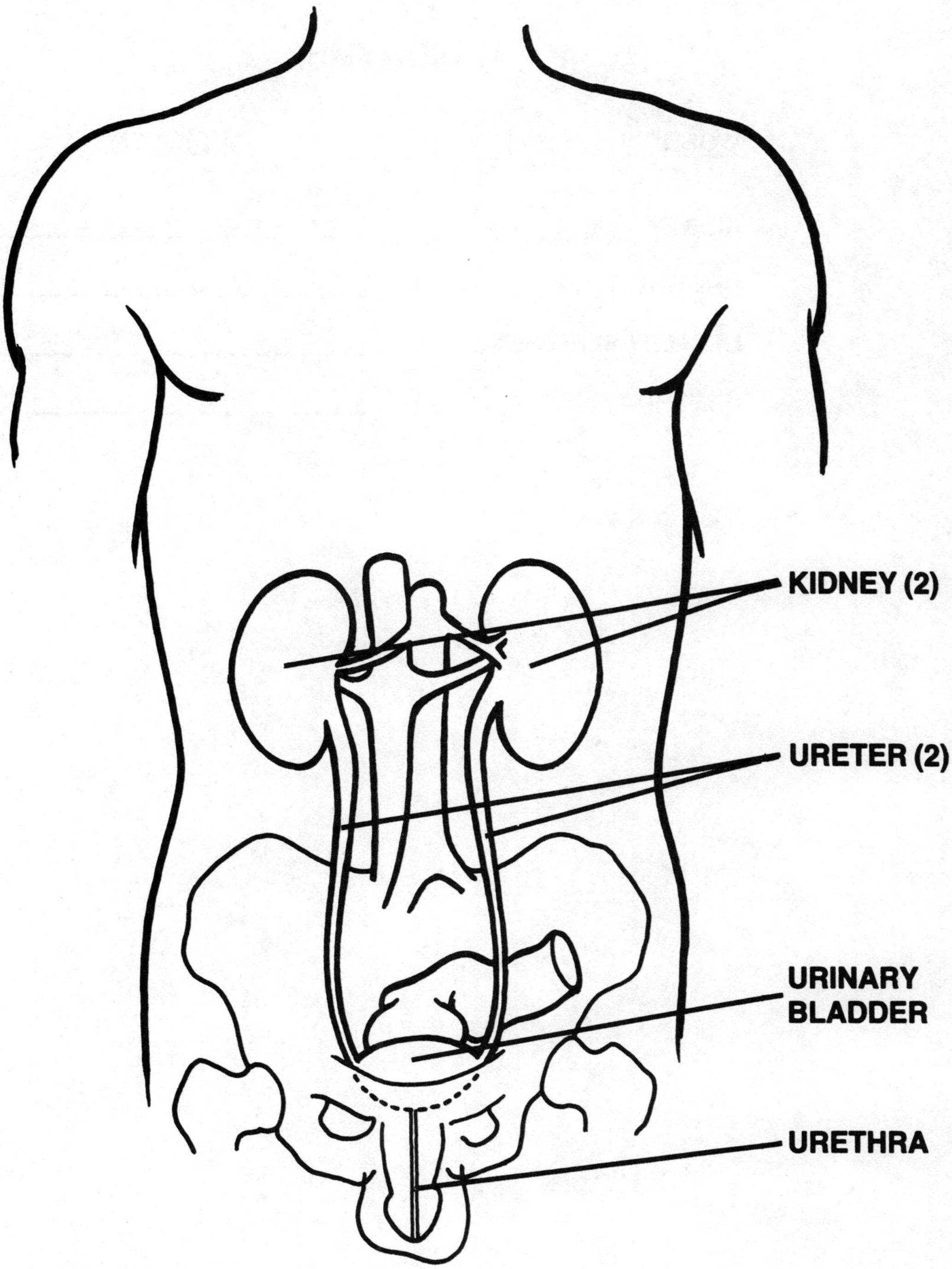

LESSON 14 — WORKSHEET
THE URINARY SYSTEM

COMPLETE THE BLANKS:

AUDIONYMS

WORD	AUDIONYM
KIDNEY	Kid Knee
URETER	"U" Rudder
URINARY BLADDER	Ukelele Platter
URETHRA	"U" wreath

LESSON 14 — WORKSHEET
THE URINARY SYSTEM
ORGANS OF THE URINARY SYSTEM

PRINT THE CORRECT LETTER WITHIN THE PARENTHESES

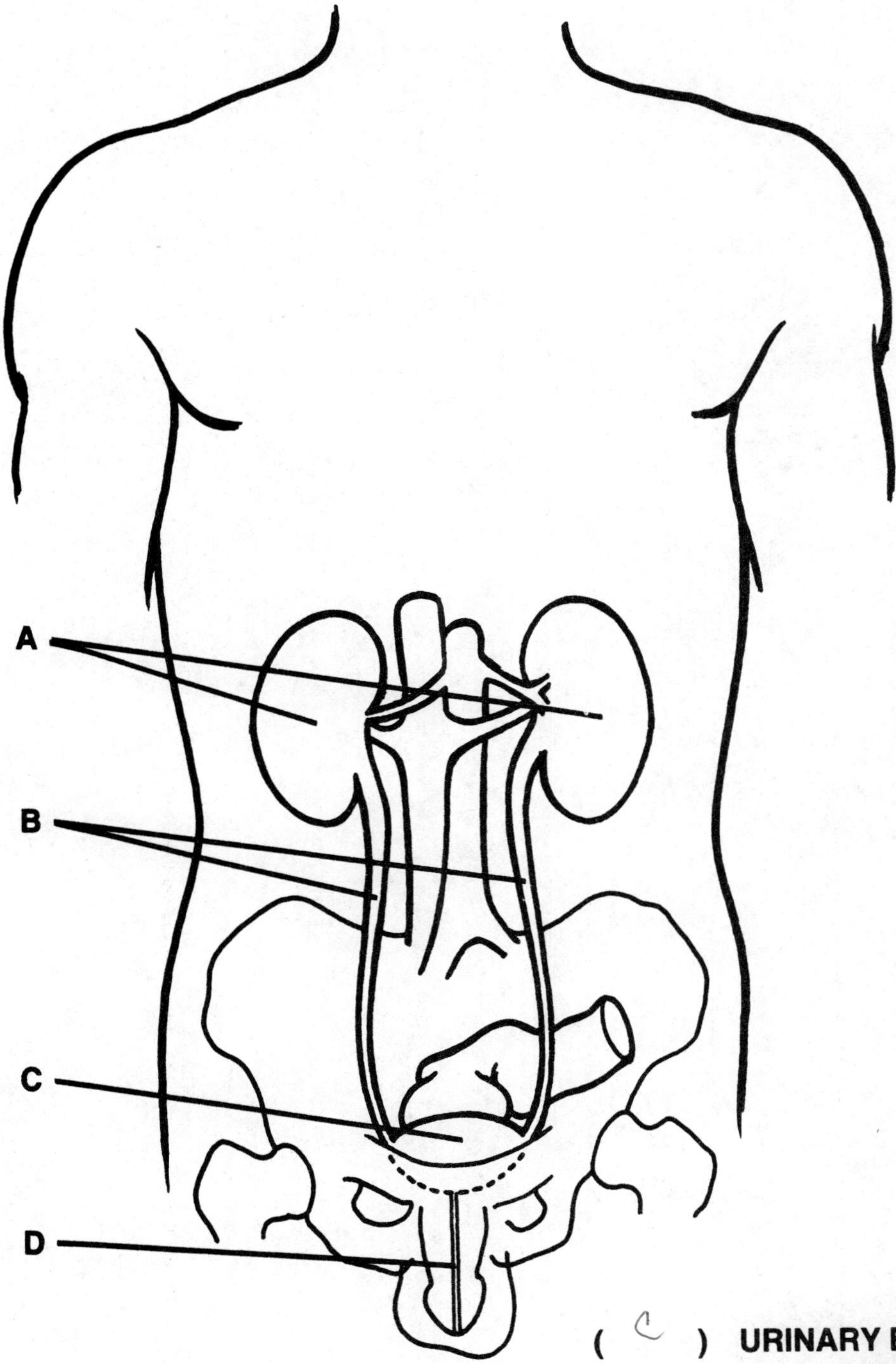

(C) **URINARY BLADDER**

(B) **URETER (2)**

(C) **URETHRA**

(A) **KIDNEY (2)**

LESSON 15

THE DIGESTIVE SYSTEM

- ORGANS OF THE ALIMENTARY CANAL
- MAJOR ACCESSORY ORGANS

REMEMBER!

1st **Pronounce** *the name of the body part or term*
2nd **Recall** *and* **pronounce** *the audionym*
3rd **For body parts: visualize** *the audionym in place*
For terms: visualize *the association*
4th **Pronounce** *the name of the body part or term again.*

LESSON 15 — REVIEW
THE DIGESTIVE SYSTEM

AUDIONYMS

WORD	AUDIONYM
ALIMENTARY CANAL	ELEMENTARY/CAN
ACCESSORY ORGANS	AX/ORGANS
MOUTH	MOUTH
PHARYNX	FIRE RINGS
ESOPHAGUS	A SOFT EGG
STOMACH	STOMACH
SMALL INTESTINE	SMALL TEST
LARGE INTESTINE	LARGE TEST
DUODENUM	DEW/DEN
JEJUNUM	JADE JUNEBUG
ILEUM	HELIUM
CECUM	SEA COMB
COLON	COLOGNE
RECTUM	WRECKER
ANUS	ANUS
SALIVARY (GLANDS)	SALAD
LIVER	LIVER
GALLBLADDER	GOLD PLATTER
PANCREAS	PAN
APPENDIX	A PEN

ASSOCIATIONS

WORD	AUDIONYM	VISUAL IMAGE / ASSOCIATION	MEANING
parotid	pirate	See the **pirate** who always wants to be **near the ear**!	near the ear
sub	sub	See the **sub under** the water!	under
lingu	language	See someone speaking many **languages** with many **tongues**!	tongue

LESSON 15 — REVIEW
THE DIGESTIVE SYSTEM
THE ALIMENTARY CANAL
ORGANS OF THE ALIMENTARY CANAL

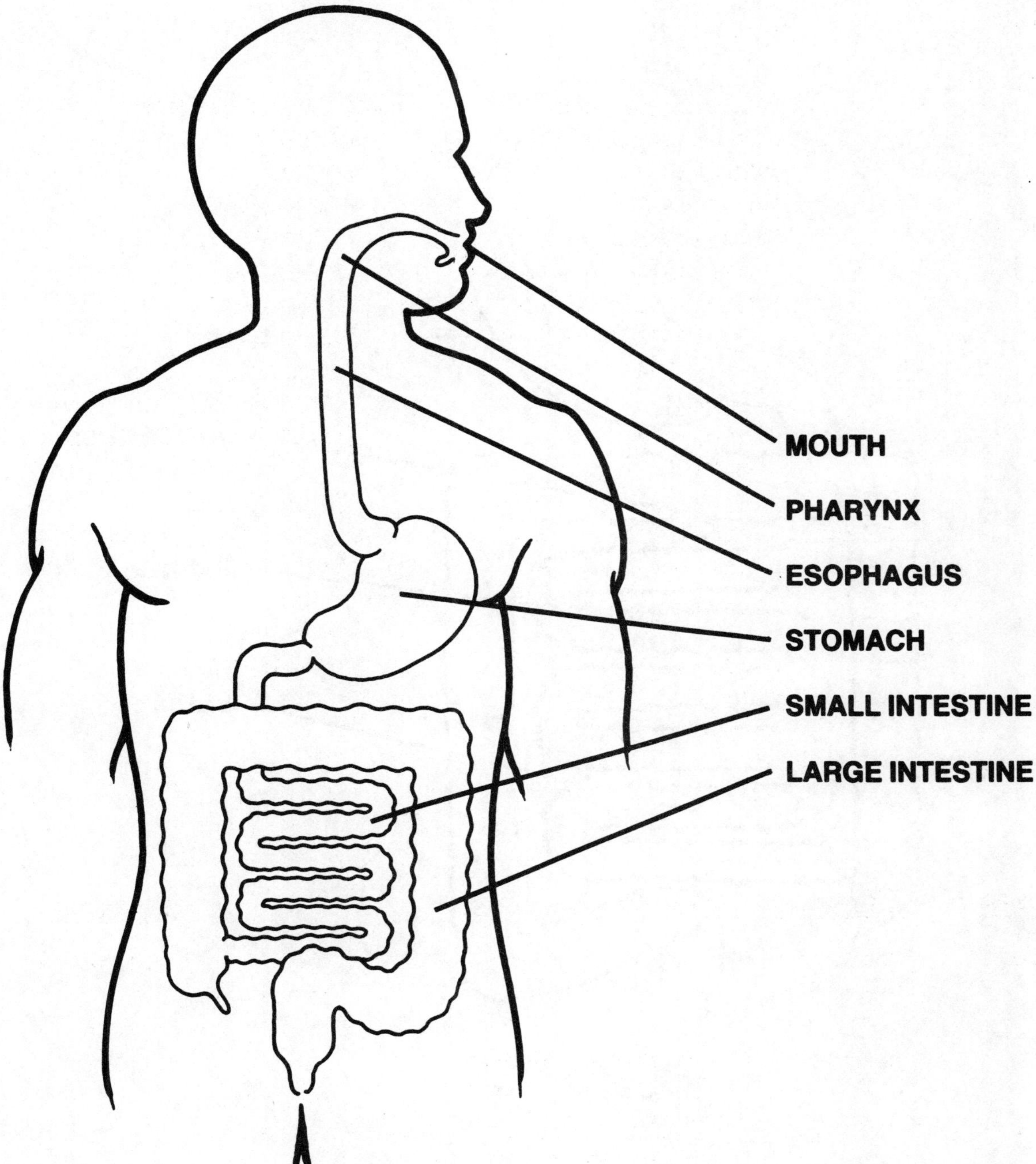

LESSON 15 — REVIEW
THE DIGESTIVE SYSTEM
THE ALIMENTARY CANAL
PARTS OF THE SMALL INTESTINE

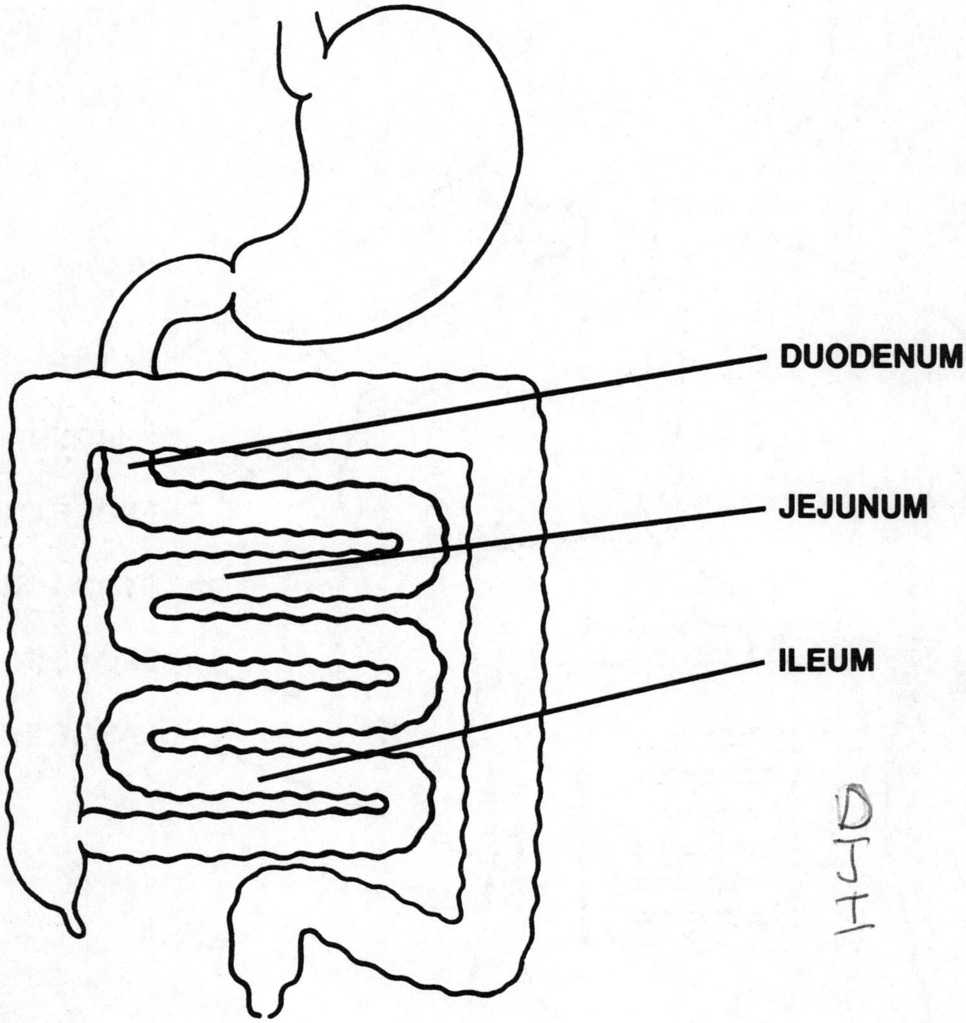

LESSON 15 — REVIEW
THE DIGESTIVE SYSTEM
ALIMENTARY CANAL
PARTS OF THE LARGE INTESTINE

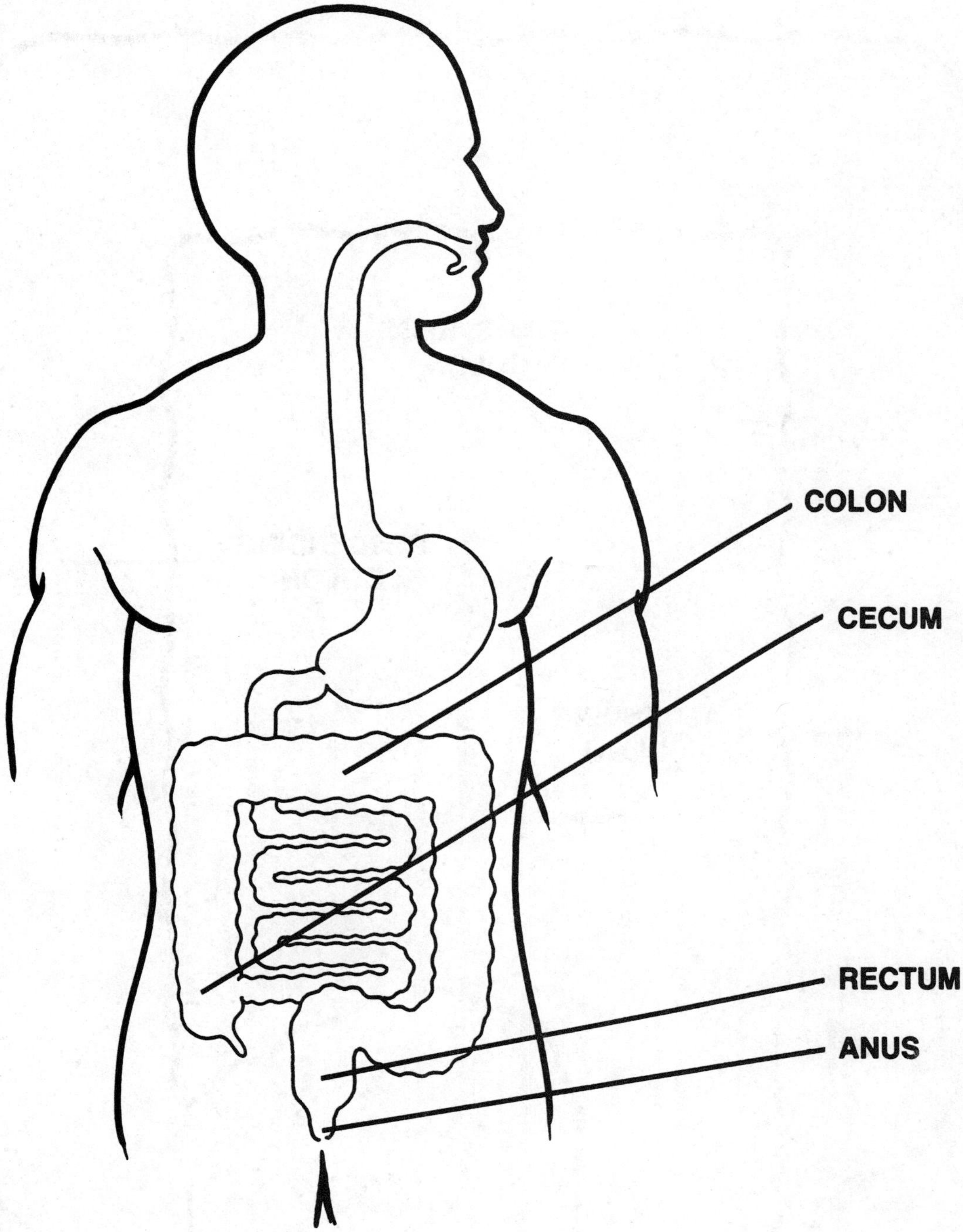

LESSON 15 — REVIEW
THE DIGESTIVE SYSTEM
SEGMENTS OF THE COLON

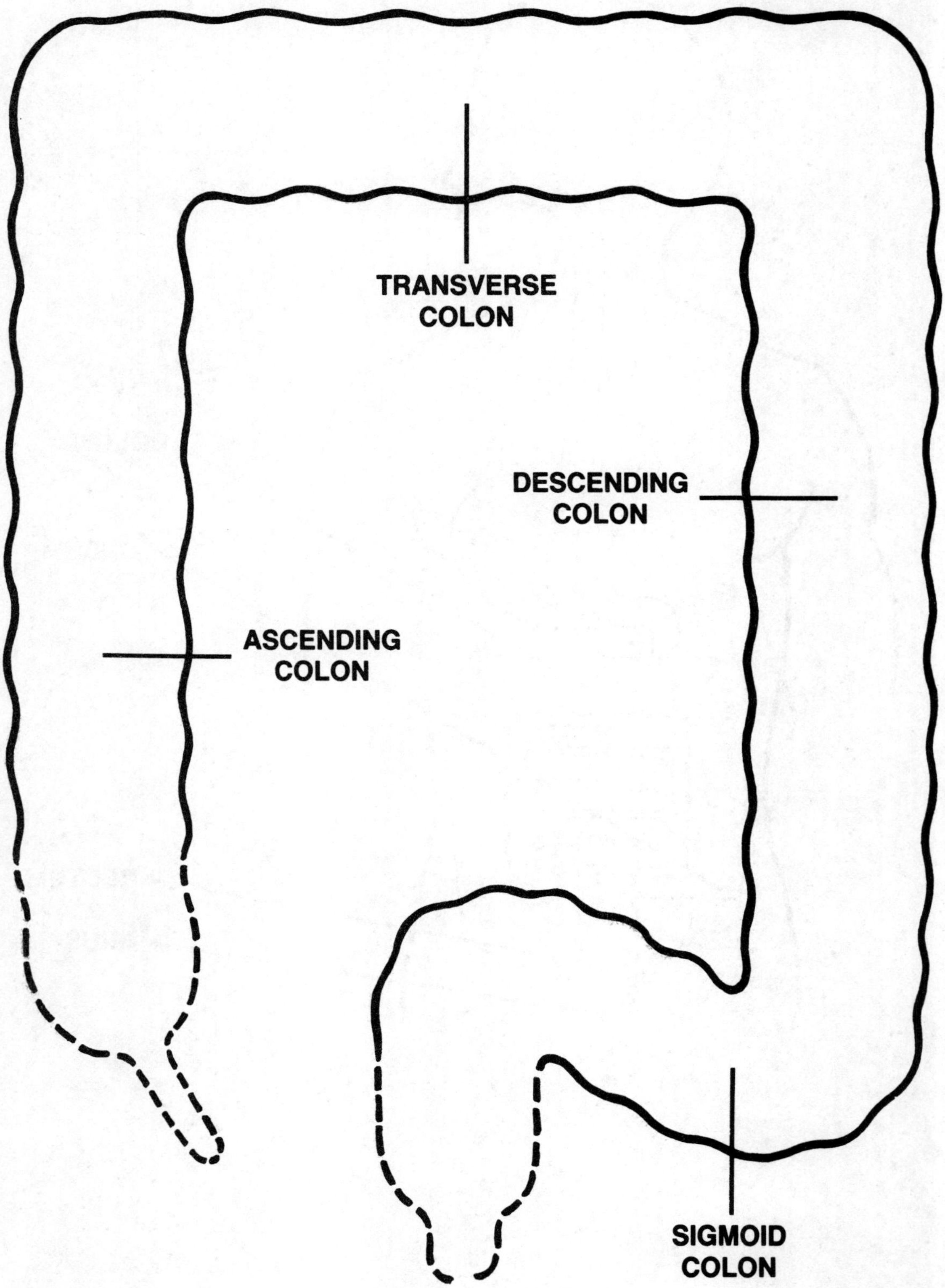

LESSON 15 — REVIEW
THE DIGESTIVE SYSTEM
MAJOR ACCESSORY ORGANS

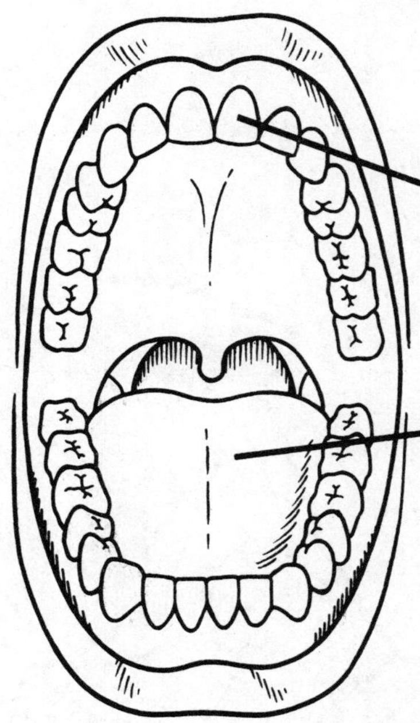

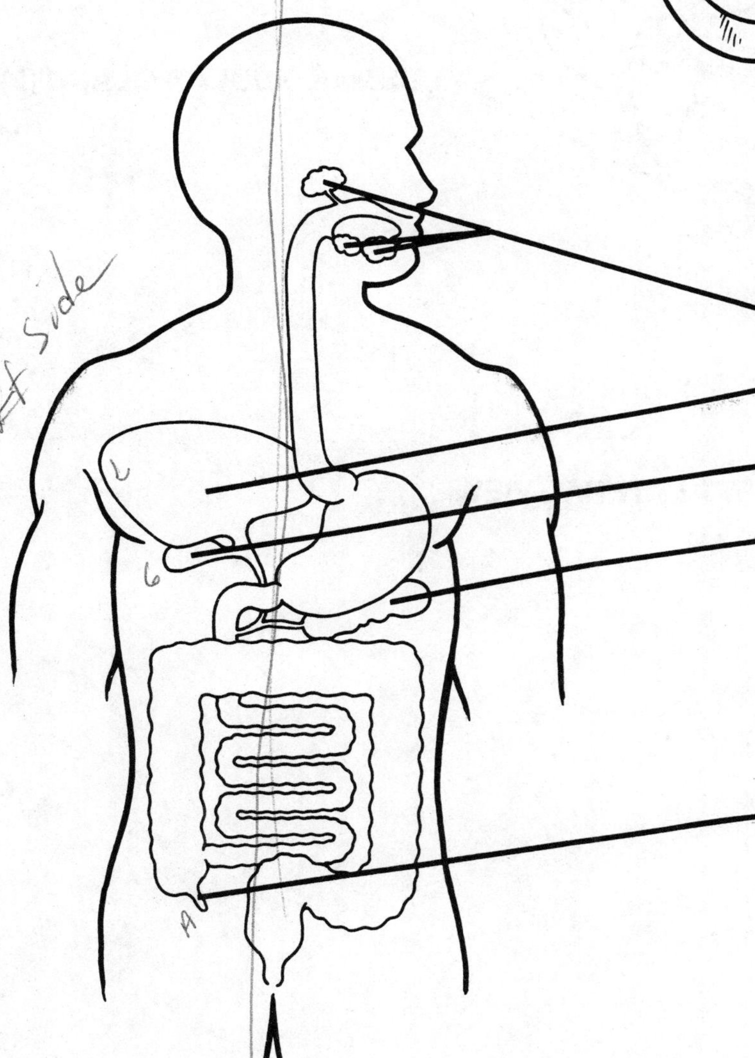

LESSON 15 — REVIEW
THE DIGESTIVE SYSTEM
THE ACCESSORY ORGANS
THE SALIVARY GLANDS

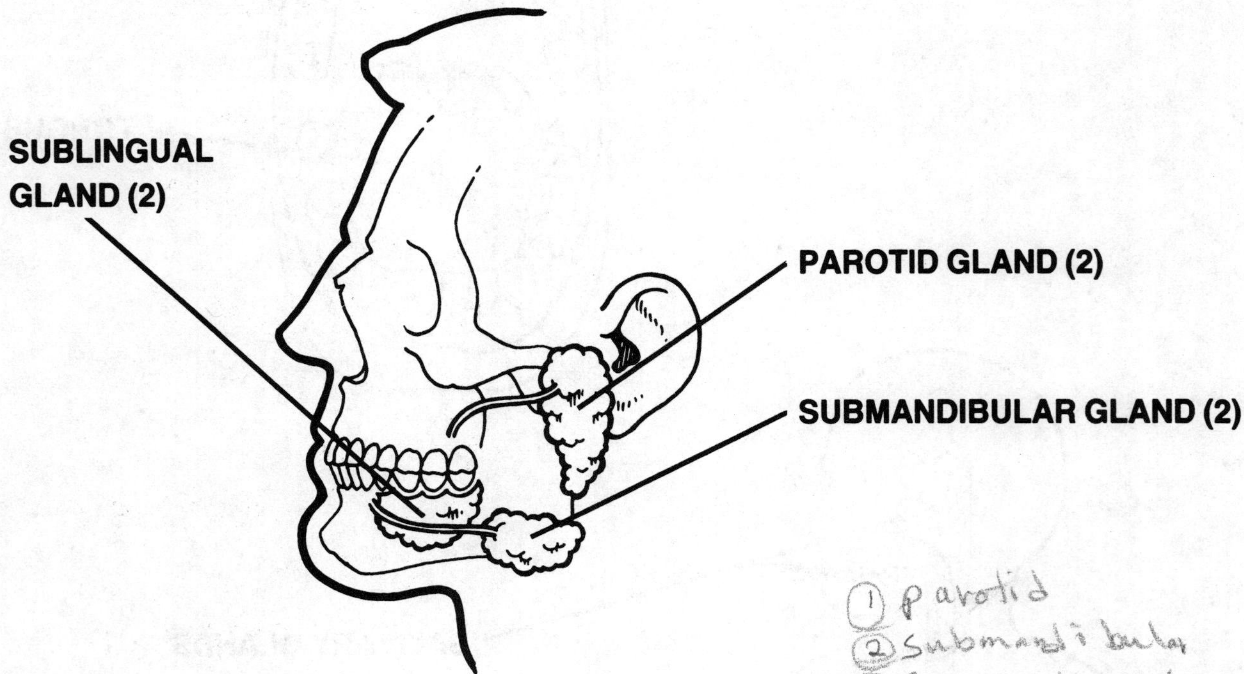

1 parotid
2 submandibular
3 sublingual

LEFT LATERAL VIEW

LESSON 15 — WORKSHEET
THE DIGESTIVE SYSTEM
COMPLETE THE BLANKS:

40

AUDIONYMS

WORD	AUDIONYM
ALIMENTARY CANAL	Elementary / can
ACCESSORY ORGANS	Ax / organs
MOUTH	mouth
PHARYNX	Five rings
ESOPHAGUS	A soft Egg
STOMACH	Stomach
SMALL INTESTINE	Small Test
LARGE INTESTINE	Large Test
DUODENUM	Dew Den
JEJUNUM	Jade Junebug
ILEUM	Helium
CECUM	Sea comb
COLON	Cologne
RECTUM	wrecker
ANUS	anus
SALIVARY (GLANDS)	salad
LIVER	Liver
GALLBLADDER	Gold platter
PANCREAS	pan
APPENDIX	a Pen

	MEANING
PAROTID	Near The ear
SUB-	under
LINGU-	Tongue

LESSON 15 — WORKSHEET
THE DIGESTIVE SYSTEM
THE ALIMENTARY CANAL
ORGANS OF THE ALIMENTARY CANAL

PRINT THE CORRECT LETTER WITHIN THE PARENTHESES

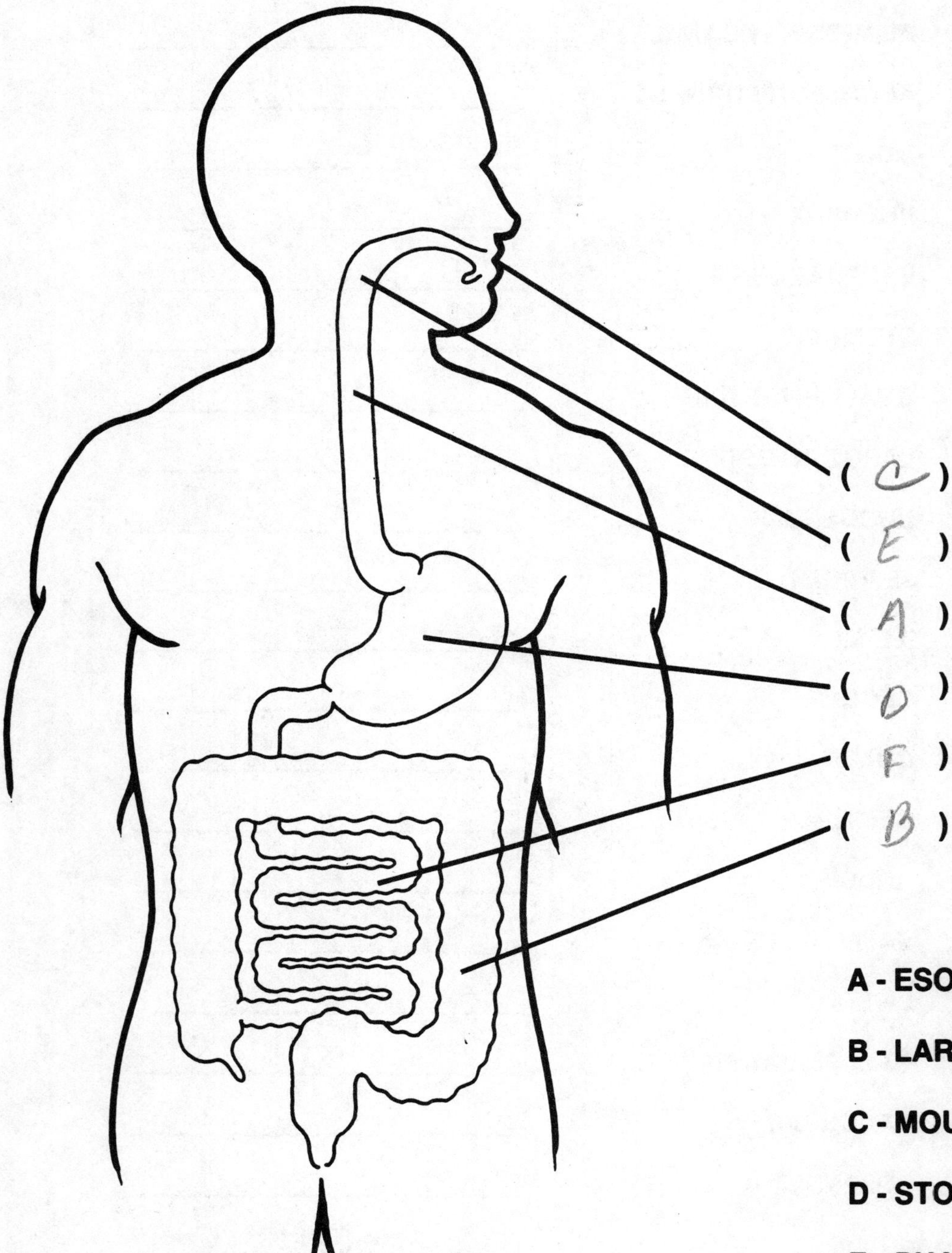

A - ESOPHAGUS

B - LARGE INTESTINE

C - MOUTH

D - STOMACH

E - PHARYNX

F - SMALL INTESTINE

LESSON 15 — WORKSHEET
THE DIGESTIVE SYSTEM
THE ALIMENTARY CANAL
PARTS OF THE SMALL INTESTINE

PRINT THE CORRECT LETTER WITHIN THE PARENTHESES

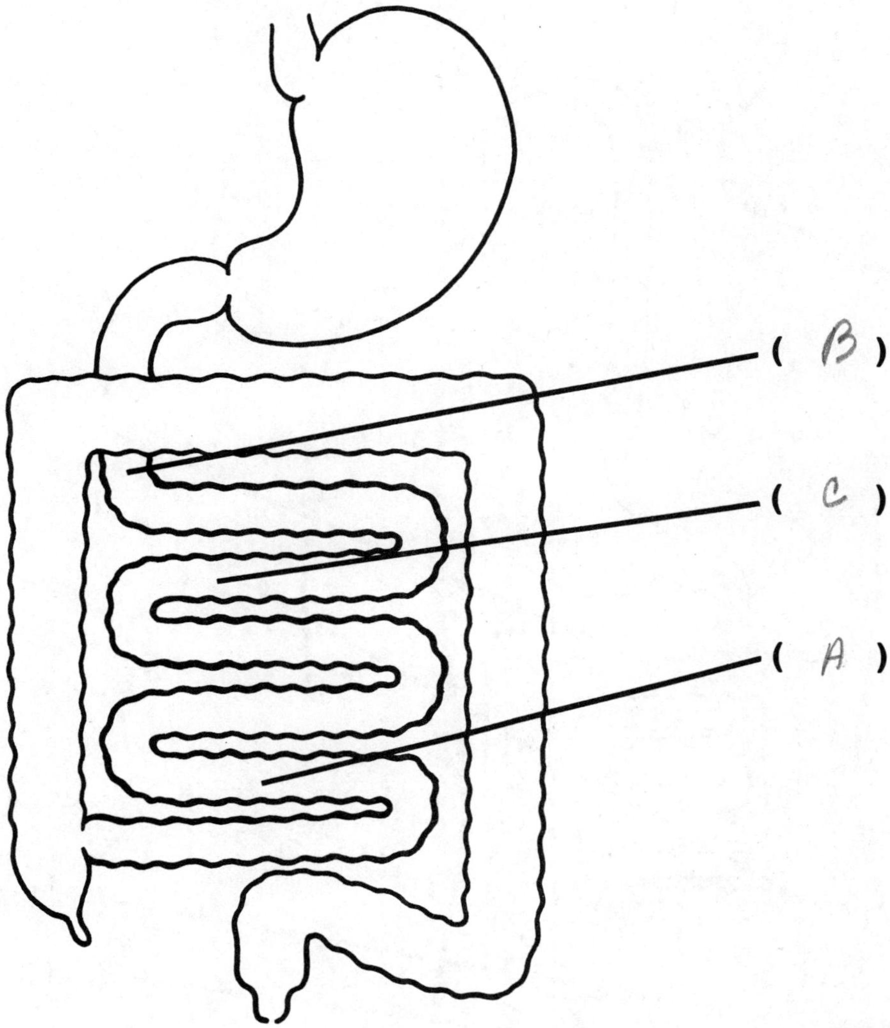

A - ILEUM

B - DUODENUM

C - JEJUNUM

LESSON 15 — WORKSHEET
THE DIGESTIVE SYSTEM
THE ALIMENTARY CANAL
PARTS OF THE LARGE INTESTINE

PRINT THE CORRECT LETTER WITHIN THE PARENTHESES

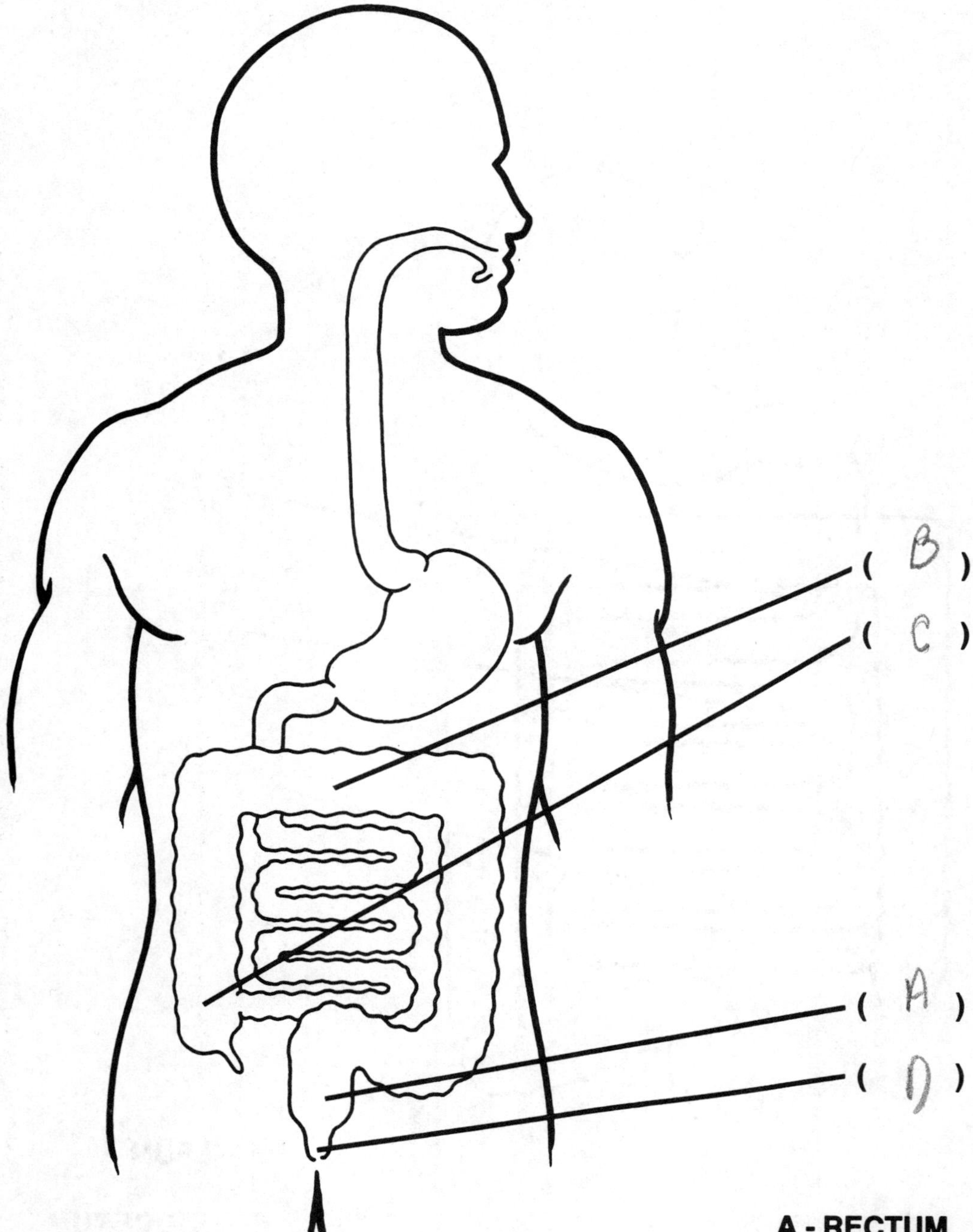

A - RECTUM

B - COLON

C - CECUM

D - ANUS

LESSON 15 — WORKSHEET
THE DIGESTIVE SYSTEM
THE ALIMENTARY CANAL
SEGMENTS OF THE COLON

PRINT THE CORRECT LETTER WITHIN THE PARENTHESES

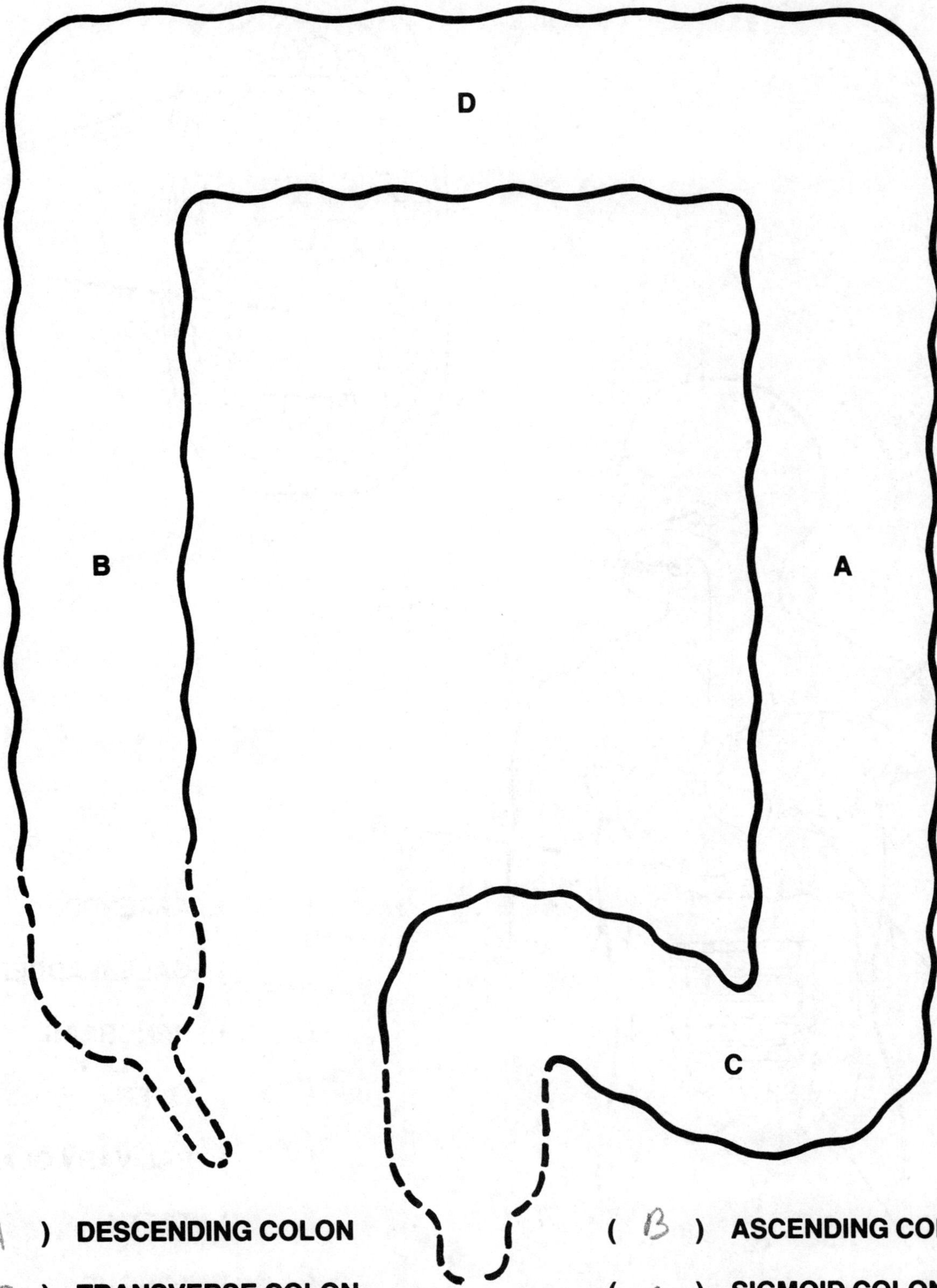

(A) **DESCENDING COLON**

(B) **ASCENDING COLON**

(D) **TRANSVERSE COLON**

(C) **SIGMOID COLON**

LESSON 15 — WORKSHEET
THE DIGESTIVE SYSTEM
MAJOR ACCESSORY ORGANS

PRINT THE CORRECT LETTER WITHIN THE PARENTHESES

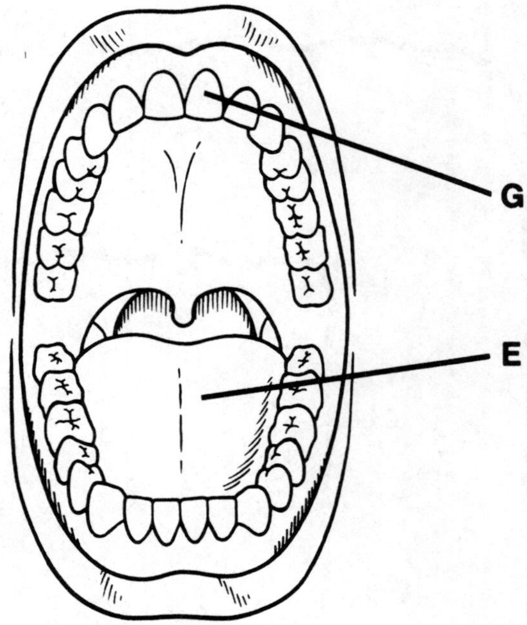

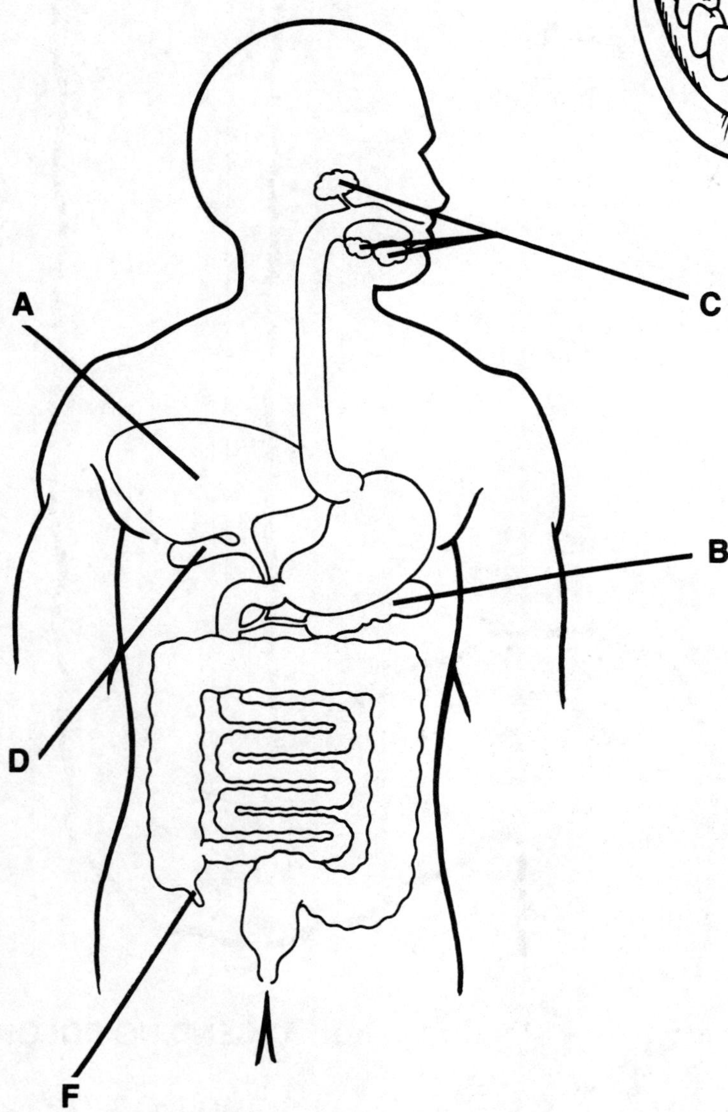

(F) **APPENDIX**

(D) **GALLBLADDER**

(B) **PANCREAS**

(A) **LIVER**

(C) **SALIVARY GLANDS**

(G) **TEETH**

(E) **TONGUE**

LESSON 15 — WORKSHEET
THE DIGESTIVE SYSTEM
THE SALIVARY GLANDS

PRINT THE CORRECT LETTER WITHIN THE PARENTHESES

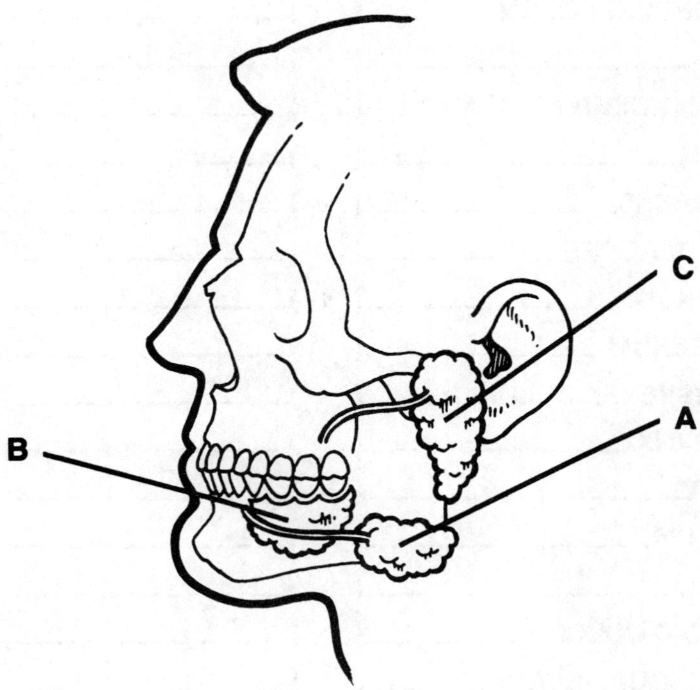

(A) **SUBMANDIBULAR GLAND**

(C) **PAROTID GLAND**

(B) **SUBLINGUAL GLAND**

LESSON 15 — WORKSHEET
THE DIGESTIVE SYSTEM

Mark an "X" under the appropriate heading to indicate whether the body part is a part of the alimentary canal or is an accessory organ.

ALIMENTARY CANAL		ACCESSORY ORGAN	LOCATION
(X)	DESCENDING COLON	( )	(D)
(X)	CECUM	( )	( )
(X)	ASCENDING COLON	( )	(K)
(X)	ANUS	( )	(O)
( )	SUBMANDIBULAR GLAND	(X)	(N)
( )	TEETH	(X)	( )
( )	PANCREAS	(X)	( )
( )	GALLBLADDER	(X)	( )
( )	APPENDIX	(X)	( )
(X)	DUODENUM	( )	(G)
(X)	TRANSVERSE COLON	( )	(H)
(X)	PHARYNX	( )	(C)
( )	LIVER	(X)	( )
(X)	RECTUM	( )	(I)
(X)	ILEUM	( )	(E)
(X)	SIGMOID COLON	( )	(F)
( )	SUBLINGUAL GLAND	(X)	(M)
( )	TONGUE	(X)	( )
( )	PAROTID GLAND	(X)	(L)
(X)	JEJUNUM	( )	(B)
(X)	STOMACH	( )	(J)
(X)	MOUTH	( )	(P)
(X)	ESOPHAGUS	( )	(A)

PRINT THE CORRECT LETTER WITHIN THE PARENTHESES UNDER THE HEADING - LOCATION

A- LOCATED BETWEEN THE PHARYNX AND STOMACH
B- LOCATED BETWEEN THE DUODENUM AND ILEUM
C- LOCATED BETWEEN THE MOUTH AND ESOPHAGUS
D- LOCATED BETWEEN THE TRANSVERSE AND SIGMOID COLON
E- LOCATED BETWEEN THE JEJUNUM AND ASCENDING COLON
F- LOCATED BETWEEN THE DESCENDING COLON AND RECTUM
G- LOCATED BETWEEN THE STOMACH AND JEJUNUM
H- LOCATED BETWEEN THE ASCENDING AND DESENDING COLON
I- LOCATED BETWEEN THE SIGMOID COLON AND ANUS
J- LOCATED BETWEEN THE ESOPHAGUS AND DUODENUM
K- LOCATED BETWEEN THE ILEUM AND TRANSVERSE COLON
L- A SALIVARY GLAND LOCATED NEAR THE EAR
M- A SALIVARY GLAND LOCATED UNDER THE TONGUE
N- A SALIVARY GLAND LOCATED UNDER THE MANDIBLE
O- THE TERMINAL OPENING OF THE ALIMENTARY CANAL
P- THE BEGINNING OF THE ALIMENTARY CANAL

LESSON 16

THE REPRODUCTIVE SYSTEM

PART A

- ORGANS OF THE MALE REPRODUCTIVE SYSTEM

REMEMBER!

1st **Pronounce** *the name of the body part or term*
2nd **Recall** *and* **pronounce** *the audionym*
3rd **For body parts: visualize** *the audionym in place*
For terms: visualize *the association*
4th **Pronounce** *the name of the body part or term again.*

LESSON 16 — REVIEW
REPRODUCTIVE SYSTEM
PART A
ORGANS OF MALE REPRODUCTIVE SYSTEM

AUDIONYMS

WORD	AUDIONYM
TESTES	TESTS
SCROTUM	SCROLL
PENIS	PEANUTS
GLANS PENIS	GLANDS/PEANUTS
SEMINAL VESICLE	SEAMAN/VEST
BULBOURETHRAL GLAND	BULB/"U" WREATH/GLAND
PROSTATE GLAND	PRETZEL/GLAND
EPIDIDYMIS	A PEA/DYNAMITE
DUCTUS DEFERENS	DUCK/DEAF EARS
EJACULATORY DUCT	EJECTION SEAT/DUCK
MEMBRANOUS URETHRA	MAN'S BRAINS/"U" WREATH
SPONGY URETHRA	SPONGE/"U" WREATH
URETHRAL ORIFICE	"U" WREATH/OFFICE
PROSTATIC URETHRA	SEE NOTE

NOTE: The prostatic urethra is located within the prostate gland, from which it takes its name. It is the beginning of the urethra which continues as the membranous urethra, the spongy urethra, and terminates at the urethral orifice.

LESSON 16 — REVIEW
THE REPRODUCTIVE SYSTEM
PART A
ORGANS AND STRUCTURES OF THE MALE REPRODUCTIVE SYSTEM

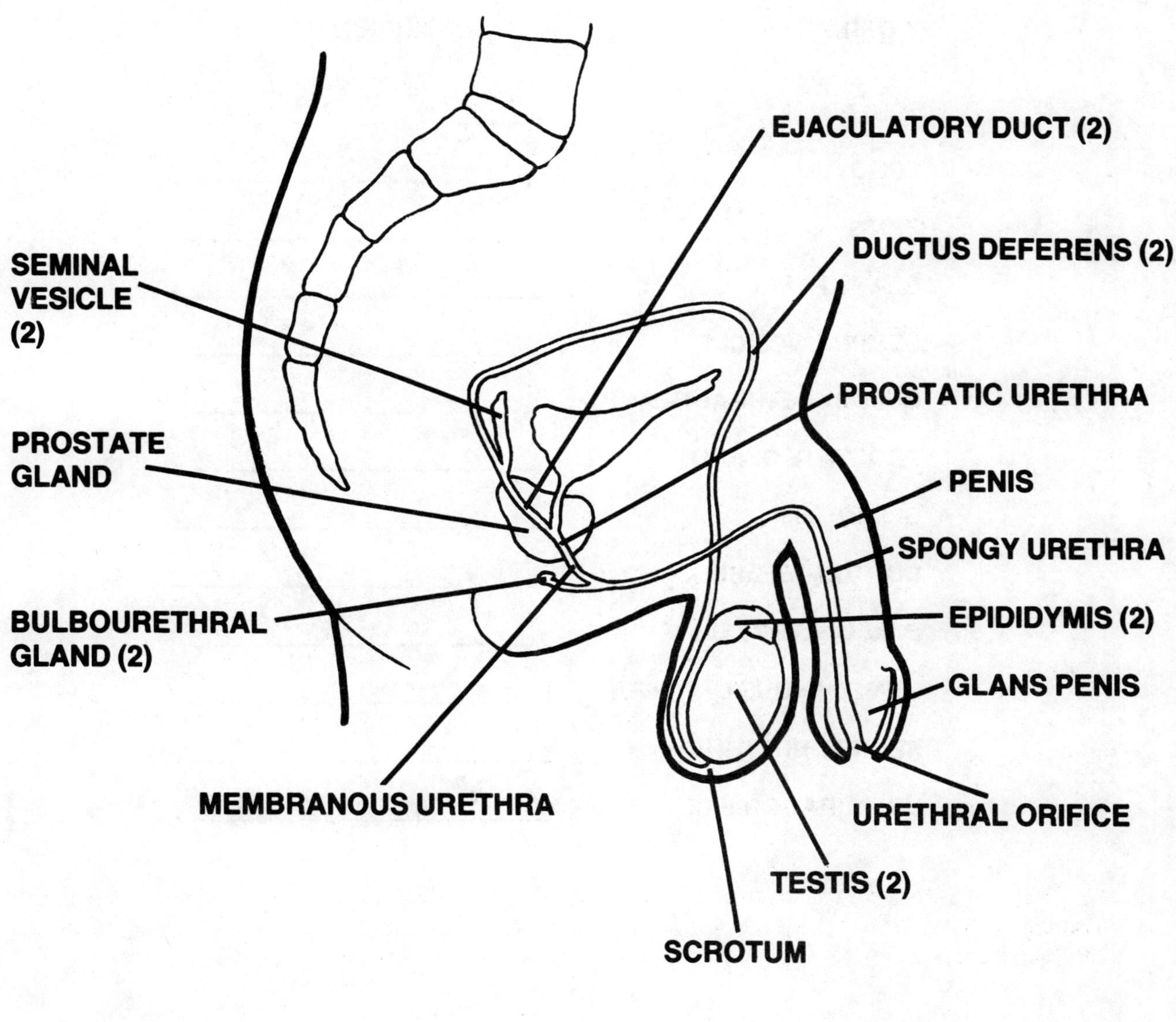

LESSON 16 — WORKSHEET
THE REPRODUCTIVE SYSTEM
PART A
ORGANS AND STRUCTURES OF THE MALE REPRODUCTIVE SYSTEM

COMPLETE THE BLANKS:

AUDIONYMS

WORD	AUDIONYM
TESTES	Tests
SCROTUM	SCroll
PENIS	Peanuts
GLANS PENIS	Glands / Peanuts
SEMINAL VESICLE	Seman / Vest
BULBOURETHRAL GLAND	Bulb / u / wreath / Gland
PROSTATE GLAND	Pretzel Gland
EPIDIDYMIS	a pea / dynamite
DUCTUS DEFERENS	Duck deaf ears
EJACULATORY DUCT	Ejection seat Duck
MEMBRANOUS URETHRA	mans brain u wreath
SPONGY URETHRA	Sponge u wreath
URETHRAL ORIFICE	u wreath office

LESSON 16 — WORKSHEET
THE REPRODUCTIVE SYSTEM
PART A
ORGANS AND STRUCTURES OF THE MALE REPRODUCTIVE SYSTEM

PRINT THE CORRECT LETTER WITHIN THE PARENTHESES

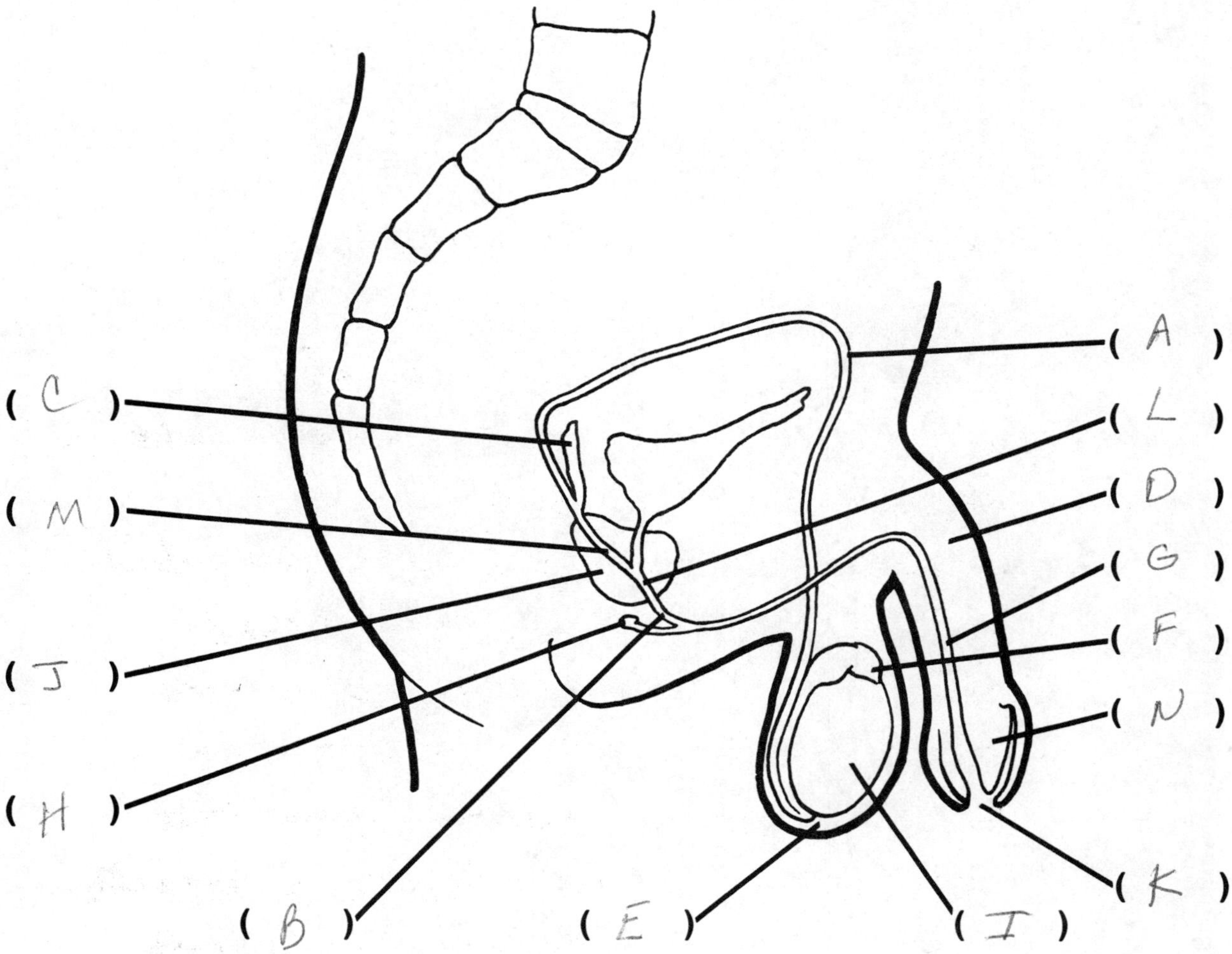

A - DUCTUS DEFERENS

B - MEMBRANOUS URETHRA

C - SEMINAL VESICLE

D - PENIS

E - SCROTUM

F - EPIDIDYMIS

G - SPONGY URETHRA

H - BULBOURETHRAL GLAND

I - TESTIS

J - PROSTATE GLAND

K - URETHRAL ORIFICE

L - PROSTATIC URETHRA

M - EJACULATORY DUCT

N - GLANS PENIS

LESSON 16

THE REPRODUCTIVE SYSTEM

PART B

- ORGANS OF THE FEMALE REPRODUCTIVE SYSTEM

REMEMBER!

1st ***Pronounce*** *the name of the body part or term*
2nd ***Recall*** *and* ***pronounce*** *the audionym*
3rd ***For body parts: visualize*** *the audionym in place*
For terms: visualize *the association*
4th ***Pronounce*** *the name of the body part or term again.*

LESSON 16 — REVIEW
THE REPRODUCTIVE SYSTEM
PART B
ORGANS OF THE FEMALE REPRODUCTIVE SYSTEM

AUDIONYMS

WORD	AUDIONYM
OVARY	OVAL TREE
UTERINE TUBE	UDDERS IN TUBE
UTERUS	UDDERS
CERVIX (NECK OF UTERUS)	SERVE HIC'S/NECK TIE
VAGINA	"V" CHINA
CLITORIS	CLIPPERS
LABIUM MINOR	LAB (MINOR)
LABIUM MAJOR	LAB (MAJOR)
VULVA*	VELVET

ASSOCIATIONS

WORD	AUDIONYM	VISUAL IMAGE / ASSOCIATION	MEANING
mammary	mummy	See the **mummy** with **breasts**	breast

*NOTE: **Vulva** is a term used to designate the external genitalia of the female.

LESSON 16 — REVIEW
THE REPRODUCTIVE SYSTEM
ORGANS OF THE FEMALE REPRODUCTIVE SYSTEM

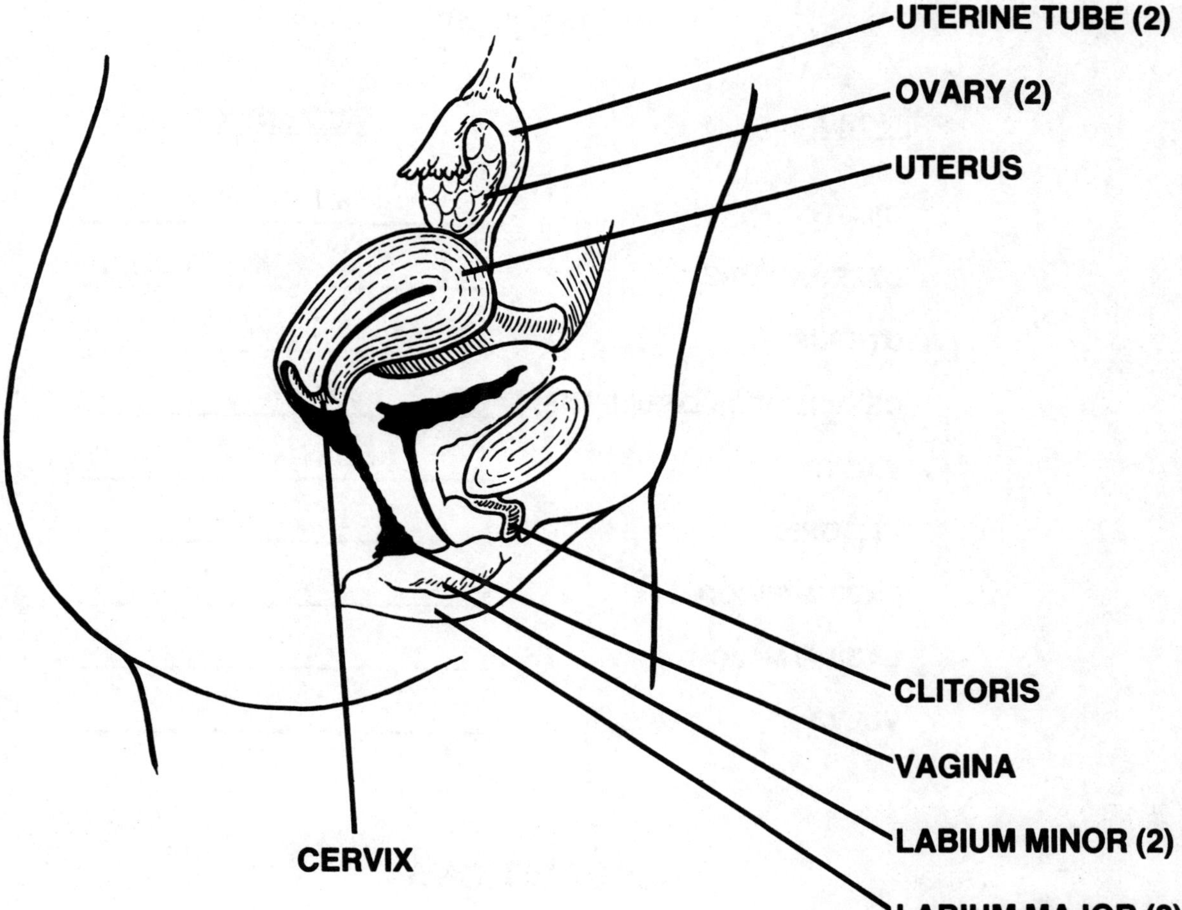

LESSON 16 — WORKSHEET
THE REPRODUCTIVE SYSTEM
PART B
ORGANS OF THE FEMALE REPRODUCTIVE SYSTEM

COMPLETE THE BLANKS:

AUDIONYMS

WORD	AUDIONYM
OVARY	oval Tree
UTERINE TUBE	udders in Tube
UTERUS	udders
CERVIX (NECK OF UTERUS)	Serve His neck Tie
VAGINA	V china
CLITORIS	Clippers
LABIUM MINOR	Lab minor
LABIUM MAJOR	Lab Major
VULVA	velvet

ASSOCIATIONS

WORD	AUDIONYM	MEANING
MAMMARY	mummy	breast

LESSON 16 — WORKSHEET
THE REPRODUCTIVE SYSTEM — FEMALE
PART B
ORGANS OF THE FEMALE REPRODUCTIVE SYSTEM

PRINT THE CORRECT LETTER WITHIN THE PARENTHESES

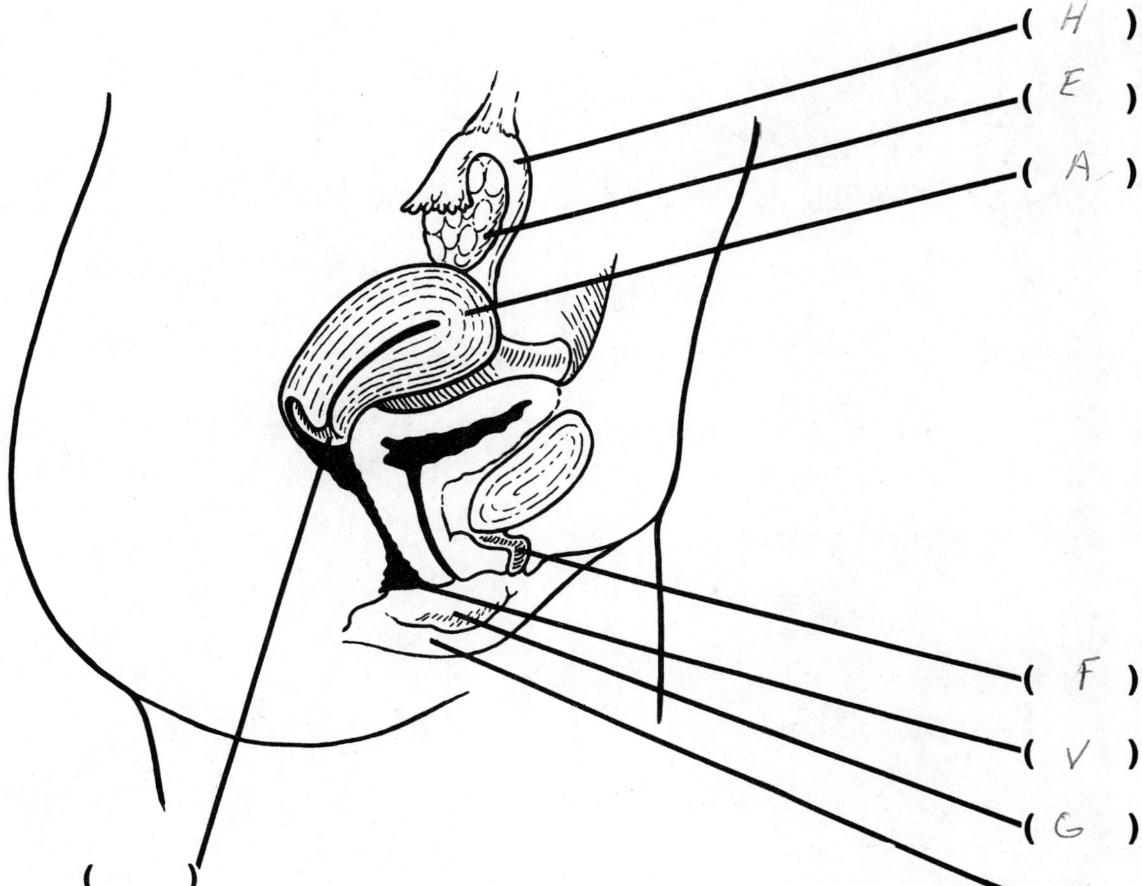

EXTERNAL GENITALIA OF THE FEMALE ( )

BREASTS ( )

A - UTERUS

B - CERVIX

C - VAGINA

D - VULVA

E - OVARY

F - CLITORIS

G - LABIUM MINOR

H - UTERINE TUBE

I - LABIUM MAJOR

J - MAMMARY GLANDS

SKELETAL SYSTEM SUPPLEMENT

INDIVIDUAL INSTRUCTION

(OPTIONAL)

THE INDIVIDUAL CARPAL AND TARSAL BONES

This section is included at the request of many organizations whose students/employees need to know the names and locations of the individual carpal and tarsal bones. It is designed as an optional section for individual learning. It includes a step-by-step learning process (not included in the audio-visual program) which will enable you to remember the names and locations of each of the bones.

Your instructor will advise you regarding the requirements of this optional section.

INDIVIDUAL INSTRUCTION

CARPALS
(Wrist Bones)

BONE NAME	NUMBER (left)	NUMBER (right)
SCAPHOID*	1	1
LUNATE	1	1
TRIANGULAR	1	1
PISIFORM	1	1
HAMATE	1	1
CAPITATE	1	1
TRAPEZOID	1	1
TRAPEZIUM	1	1

*alternate name: navicular

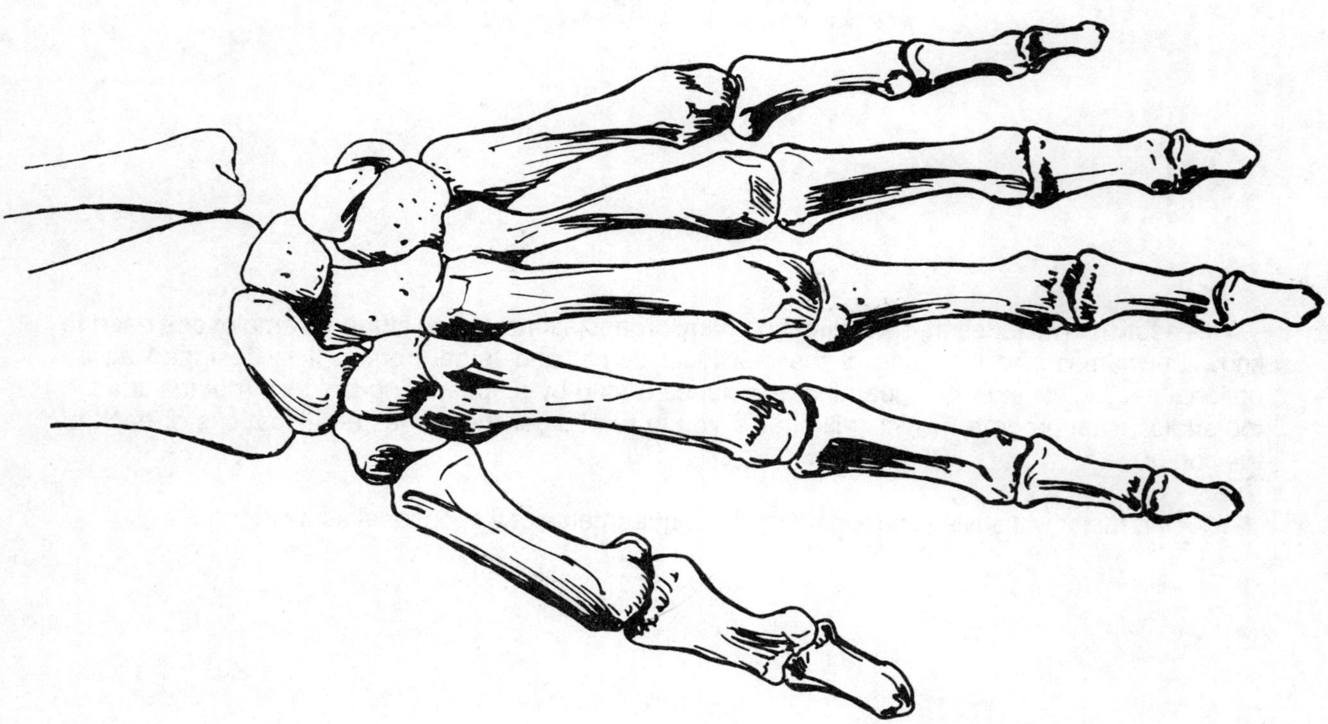

To learn the names and locations of the individual carpal bones, use the same learning system that was used for all the other bones:

1. Pronounce the name of the bone.
2. Create an audionym (sound-alike) for the bone name.
3. Picture the audionym (sound-alike object).
4. See the audionym instead of the bone on the skeleton.
5. Remember the location of the object on the skeleton and you will remember the name and location of the bone on the real skeleton.

The individual carpal bones will be learned by studying the back of the left hand in the following sequence starting on the thumb side:

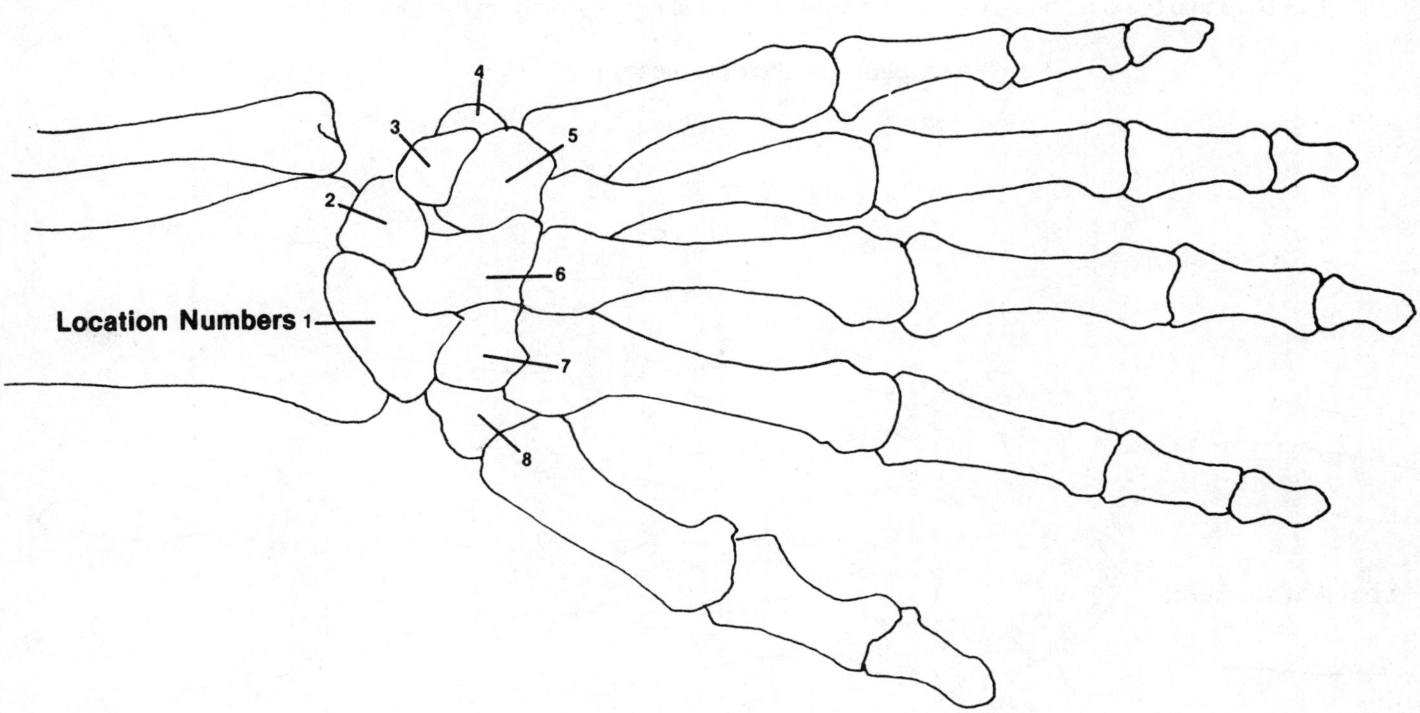

SCAPHOID

Pronunciation: scaff oid

Scaphoid sounds like: scaffold

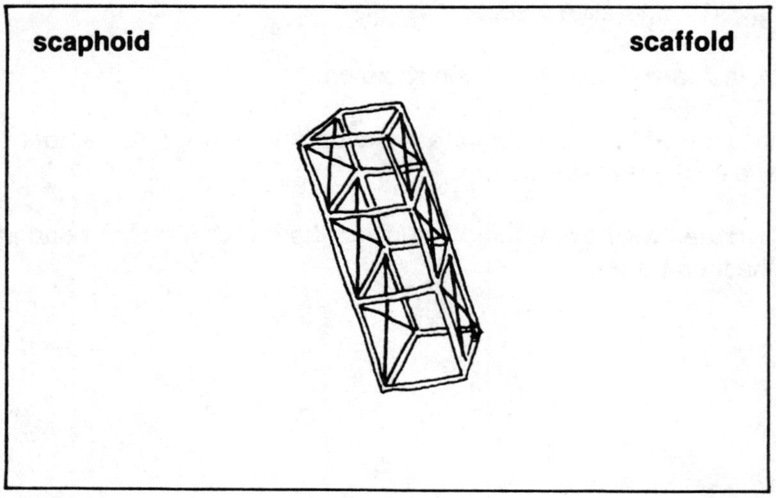

Pronounce it twice: scaphoid — scaffold
scaphoid — scaffold

The scaphoid bone (scaffold) is the first bone in the first row, starting on the thumb side.

See the scaphoid (scaffold) in place.

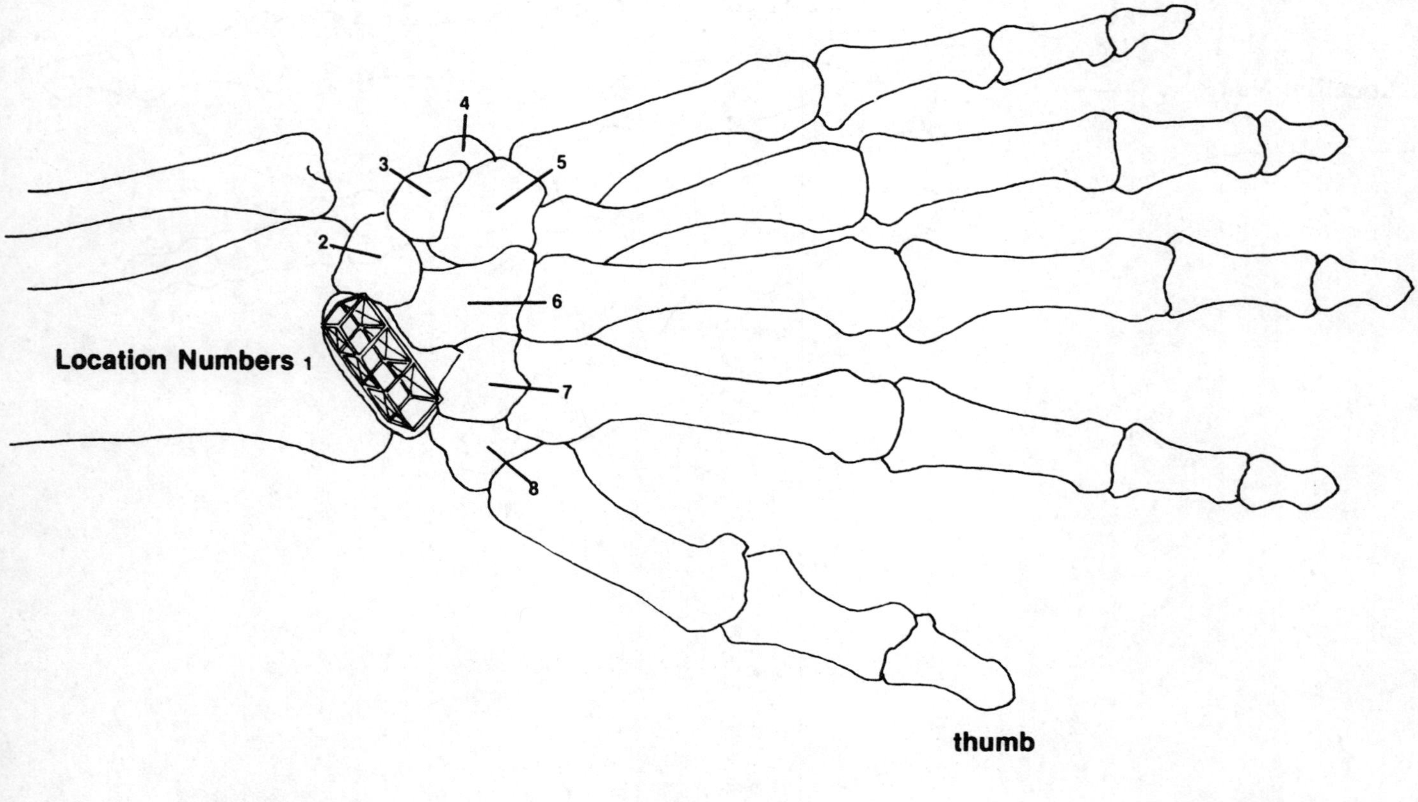

LUNATE

Pronunciation: loon ate

Lunate sounds like: lunatic

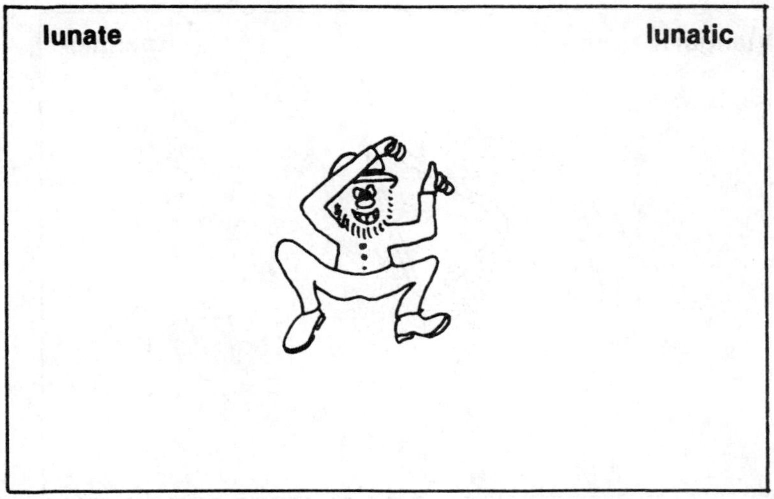

Pronounce it twice: lunate — lunatic
lunate — lunatic

The lunate bone (lunatic) is the second bone in the first row starting on the thumb side. Notice how the radius (radio) articulates only with the scaphoid (scaffold) and the lunate (lunatic).

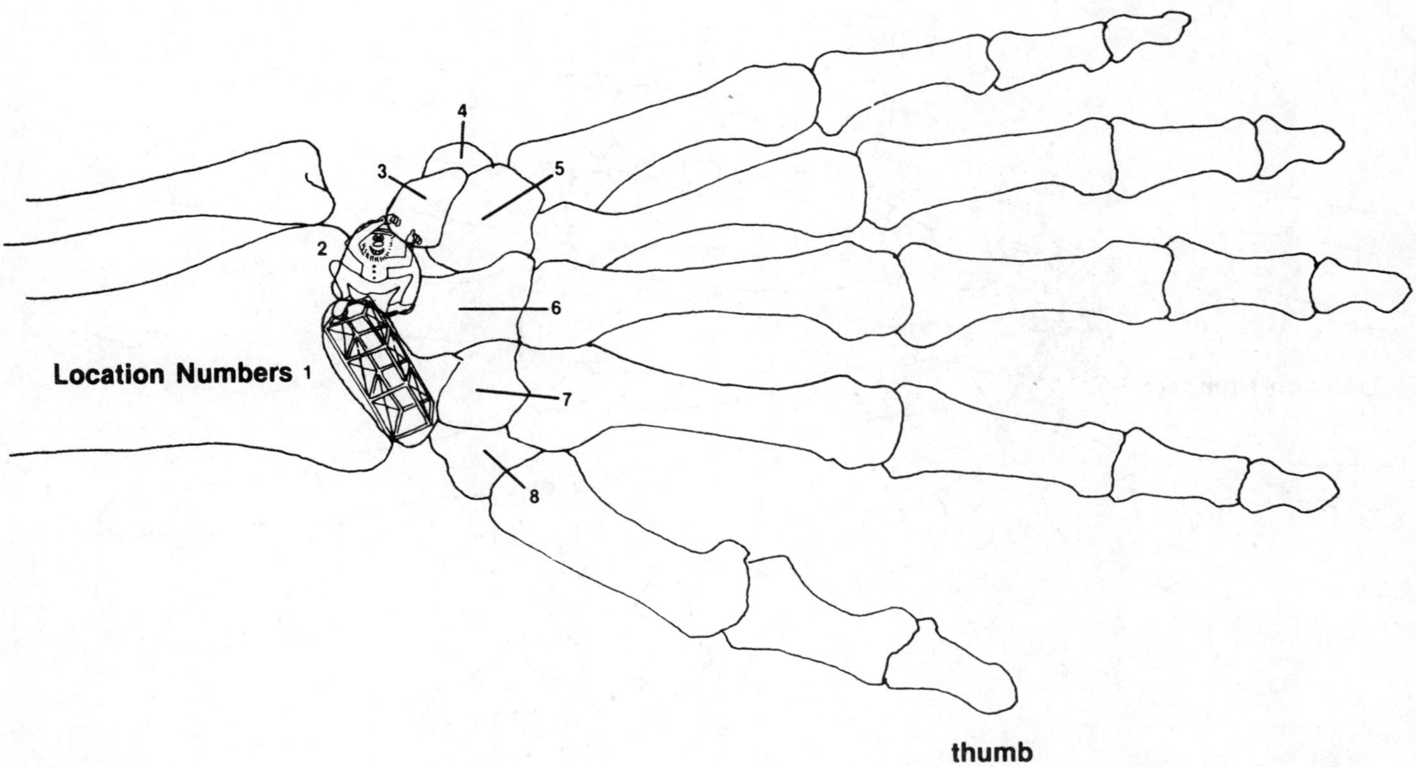

Begin to develop the sequence of the carpal bones:

1. See the scaffold (scaphoid).
2. On top of the scaffold is a lunatic (lunate).

TRIANGULAR

Pronunciation: try ang gue lar

Triangular sounds like: triangle

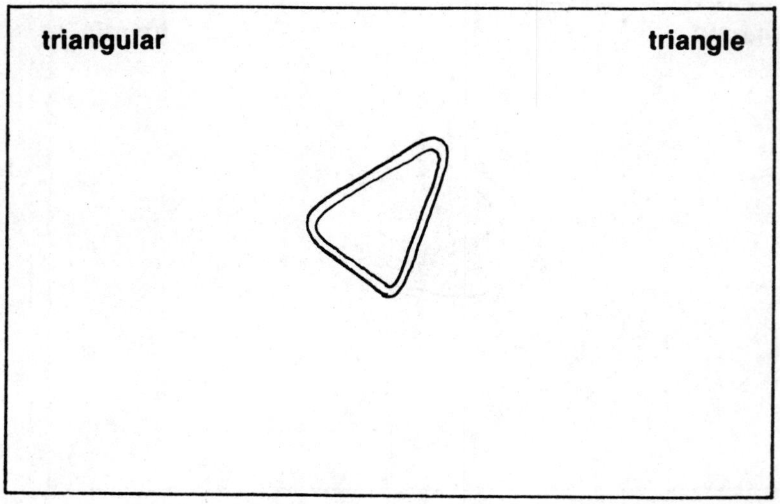

Pronounce it twice: triangular — triangle
triangular — triangle

The triangular bone (triangle) is the third bone in the first row starting on the thumb side.

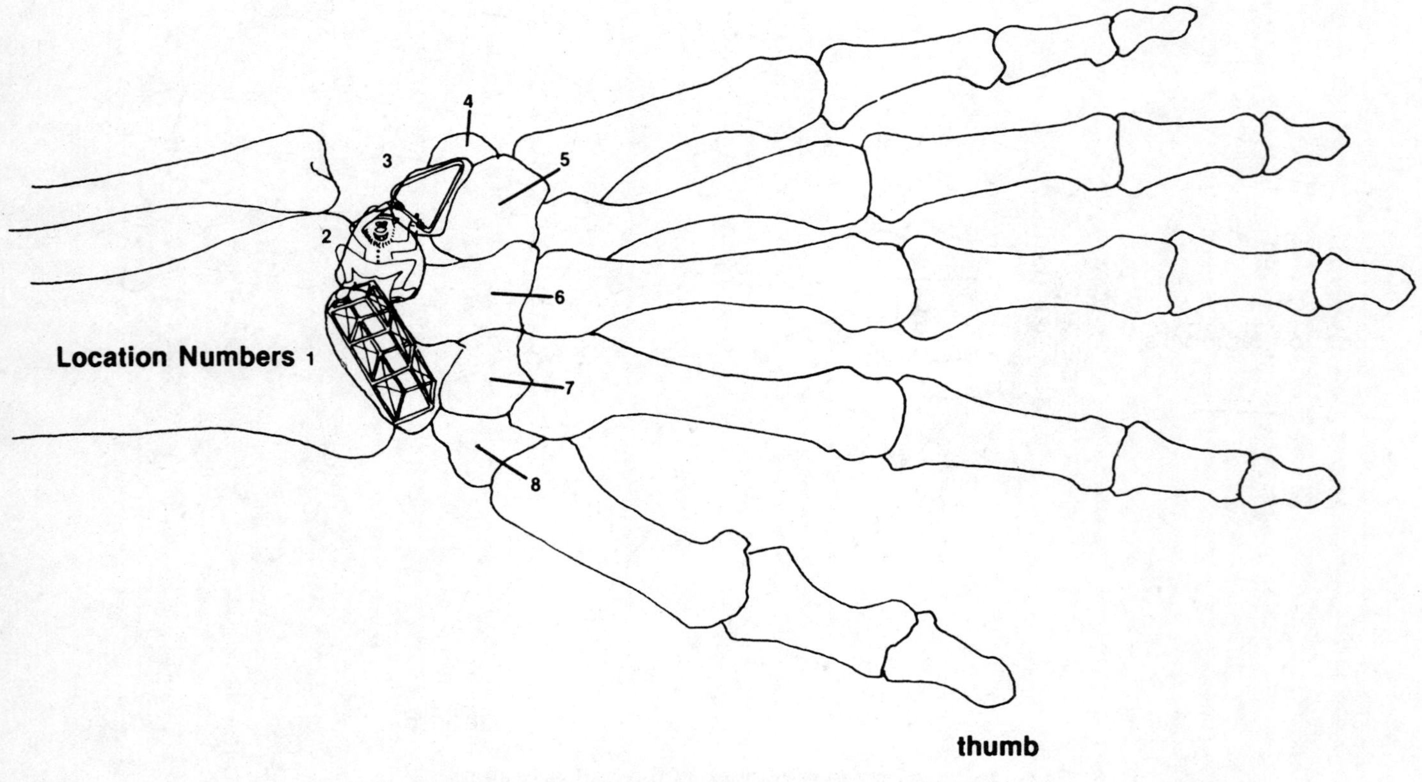

1. See the scaffold (scaphoid).
2. On top of the scaffold is a lunatic (lunate).
3. The lunatic is holding a triangle (triangular).

PISIFORM

Pronunciation: peace if orm

Pisiform sounds like: pizza farm

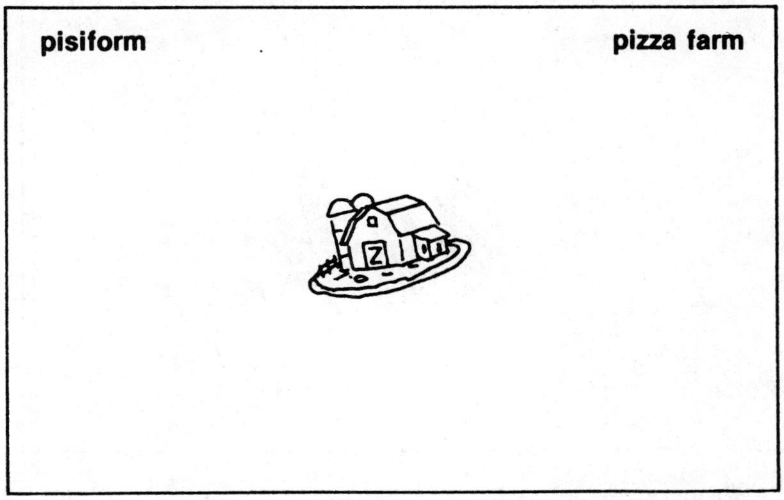

Here is a pizza with a farm on it.

Pronounce it twice: pisiform — pizza farm
pisiform — pizza farm

The pisiform bone (pizza farm) is the fourth bone in the first row starting on the thumb side.

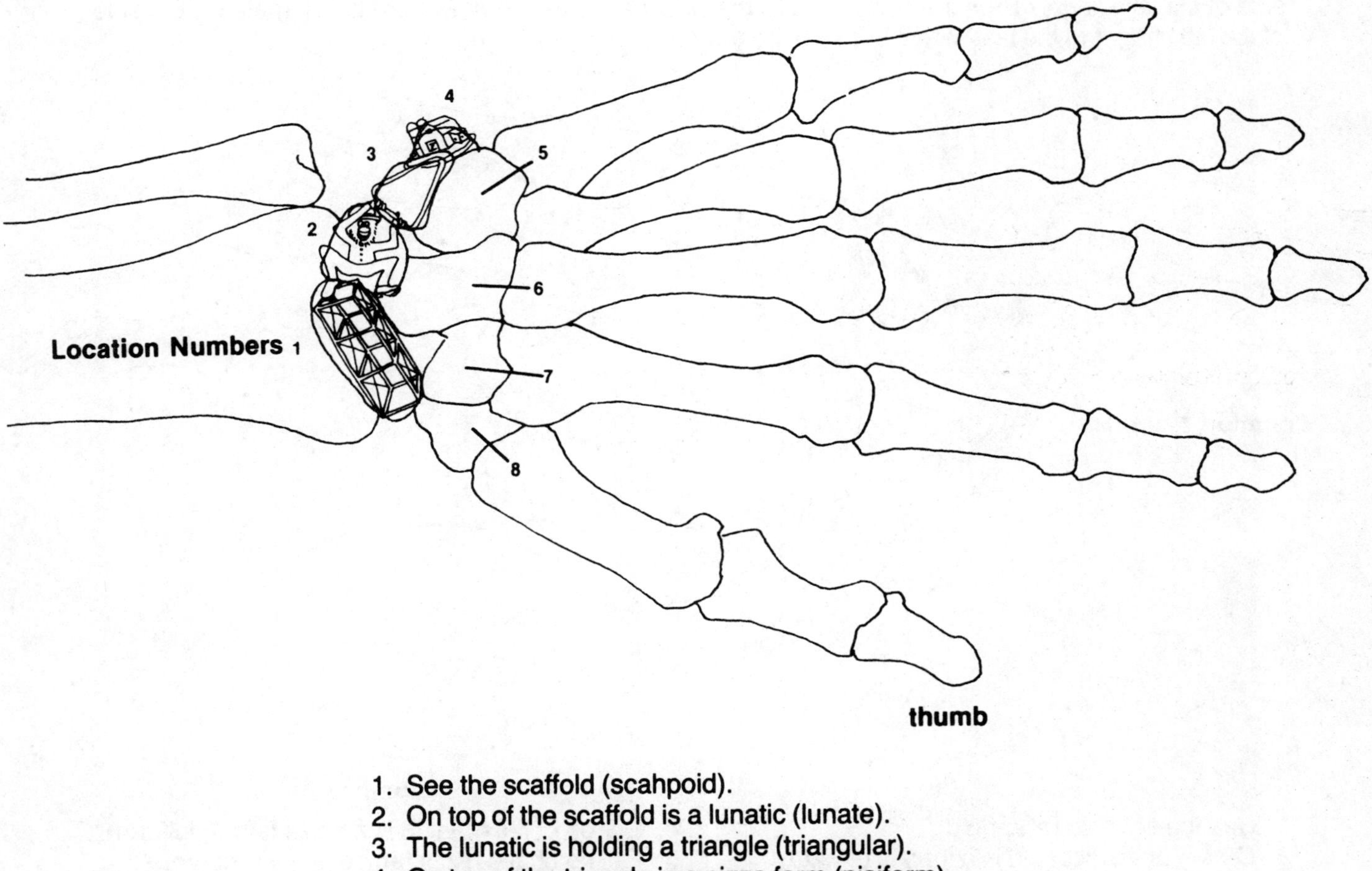

1. See the scaffold (scahpoid).
2. On top of the scaffold is a lunatic (lunate).
3. The lunatic is holding a triangle (triangular).
4. On top of the triangle is a pizza farm (pisiform).

HAMATE

Pronunciation: <u>ham</u> ate

Hamate sounds like: ham

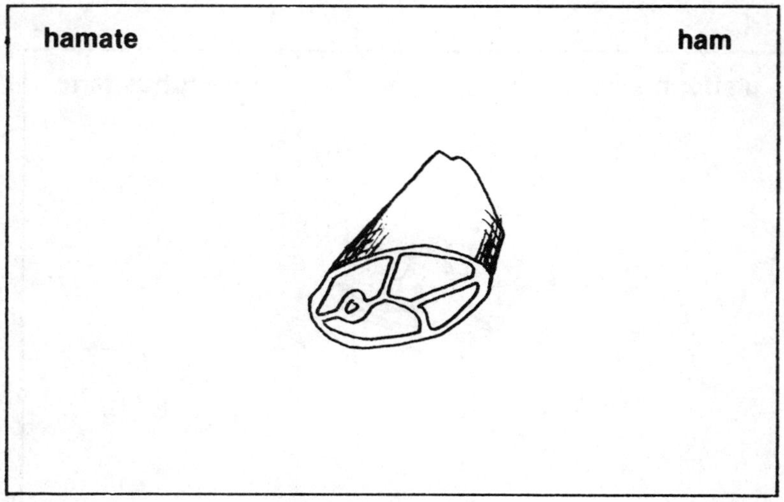

Pronounce it twice: hamate — ham
hamate — ham

The hamate bone (ham) is the fourth bone in the second row starting on the thumb side.

NOTE: To learn and remember the sequence of the carpal bones, continue to link the audionyms together. Start with the scaphoid in the first row on the thumb side and continue to the pisiform on the side of the little finger. Then start back across the wrist on the second row from the hamate on the side of the little finger to the last carpal bone on the thumb side.

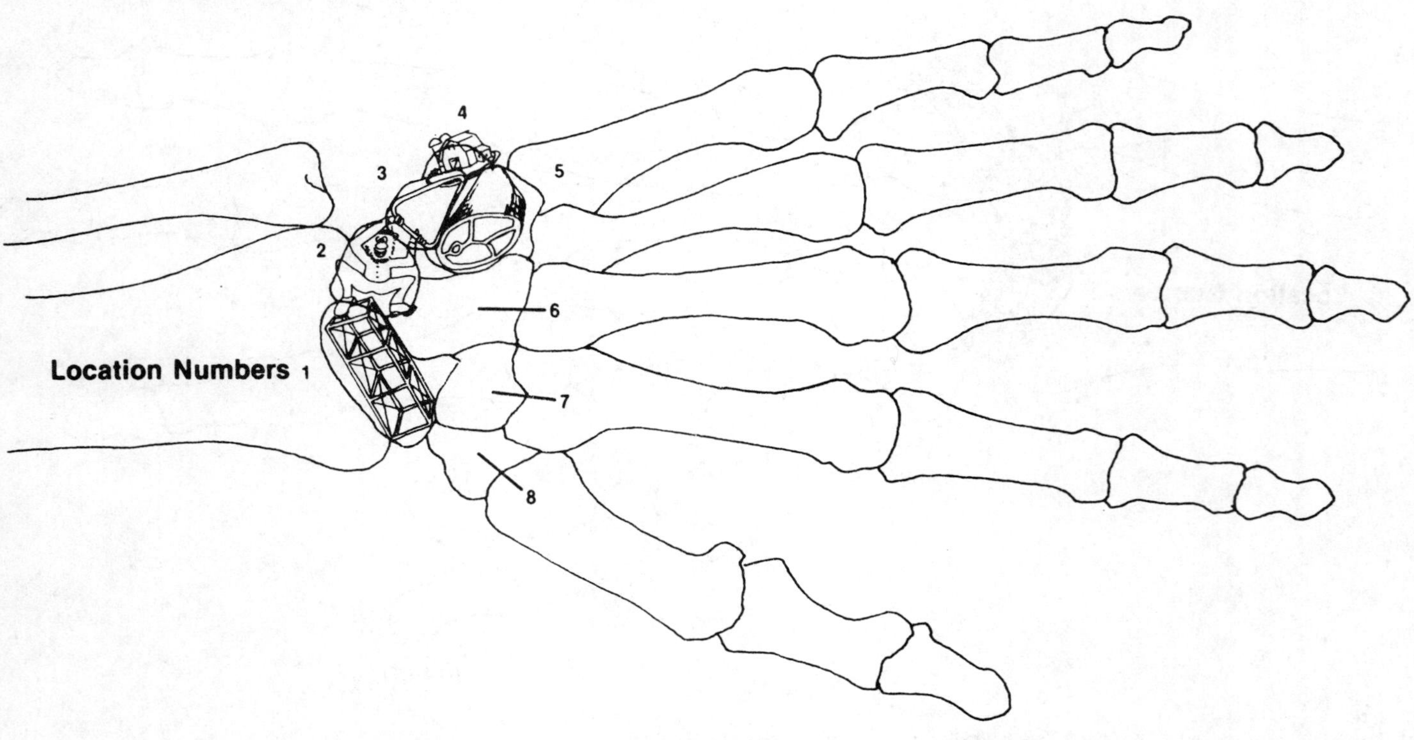

1. See the scaffold (scaphoid).
2. On top of the scaffold is a lunatic (lunate).
3. The lunatic is holding a triangle (triangular).
4. On top of the triangle is a pizza farm (pisiform).
5. Falling off the pizza farm is a ham (hamate).

CAPITATE

Pronunciation: <u>cap</u> it ate

Capitate sounds like: cap

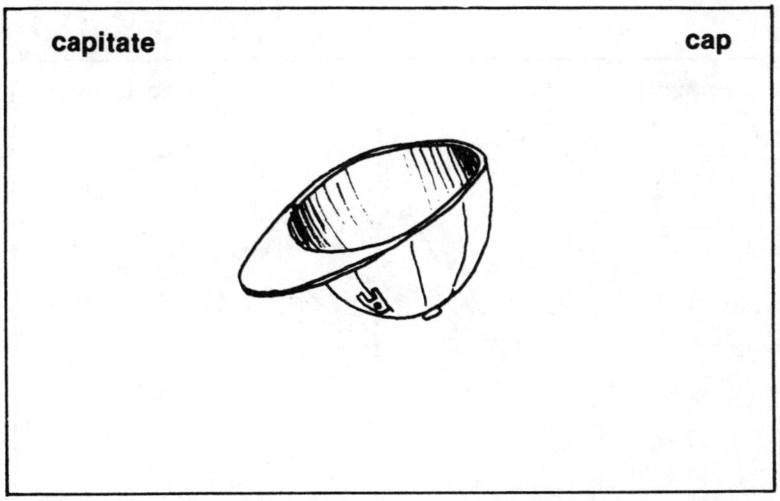

Pronounce it twice: capitate — cap
capitate — cap

The capitate bone (cap) is the third bone in the second row starting on the thumb side.

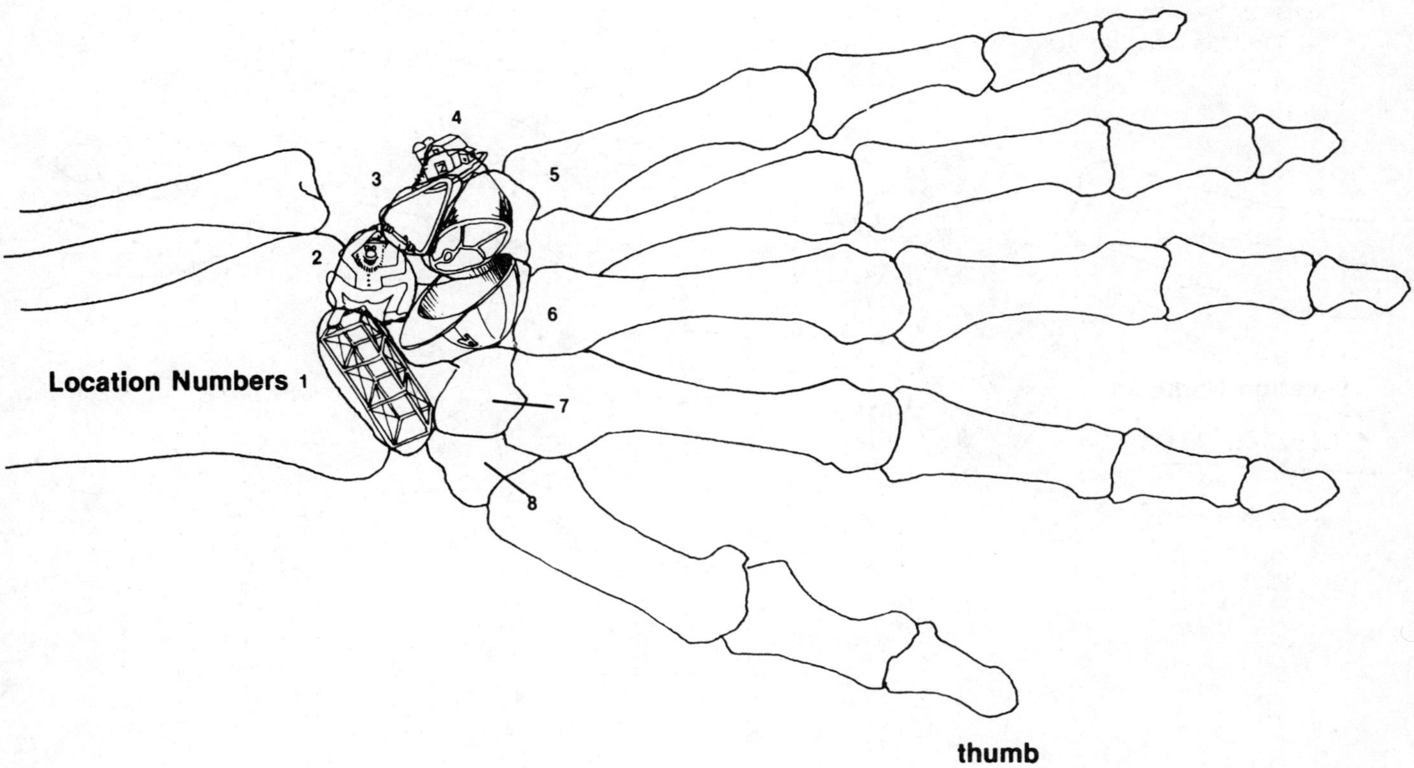

1. See the scaffold (scaphoid).
2. On top of the scaffold is a lunatic (lunate).
3. The lunatic is holding a triangle (triangular).
4. On top of the triangle is a pizza farm (pisiform).
5. Falling off the pizza farm is a ham (hamate).
6. The ham has a cap on the bottom of it (capitate).

TRAPEZOID

Pronunciation: trap is oid

Trapezoid sounds like: trap is oiled

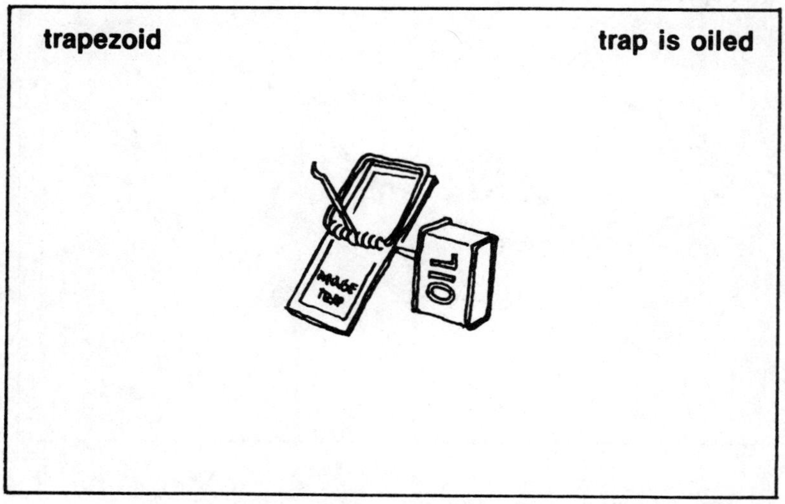

Pronounce it twice: trapezoid — trap is oiled
trapezoid — trap is oiled

The trapezoid bone (trap is oiled) is the second bone in the second row starting on the thumb side.

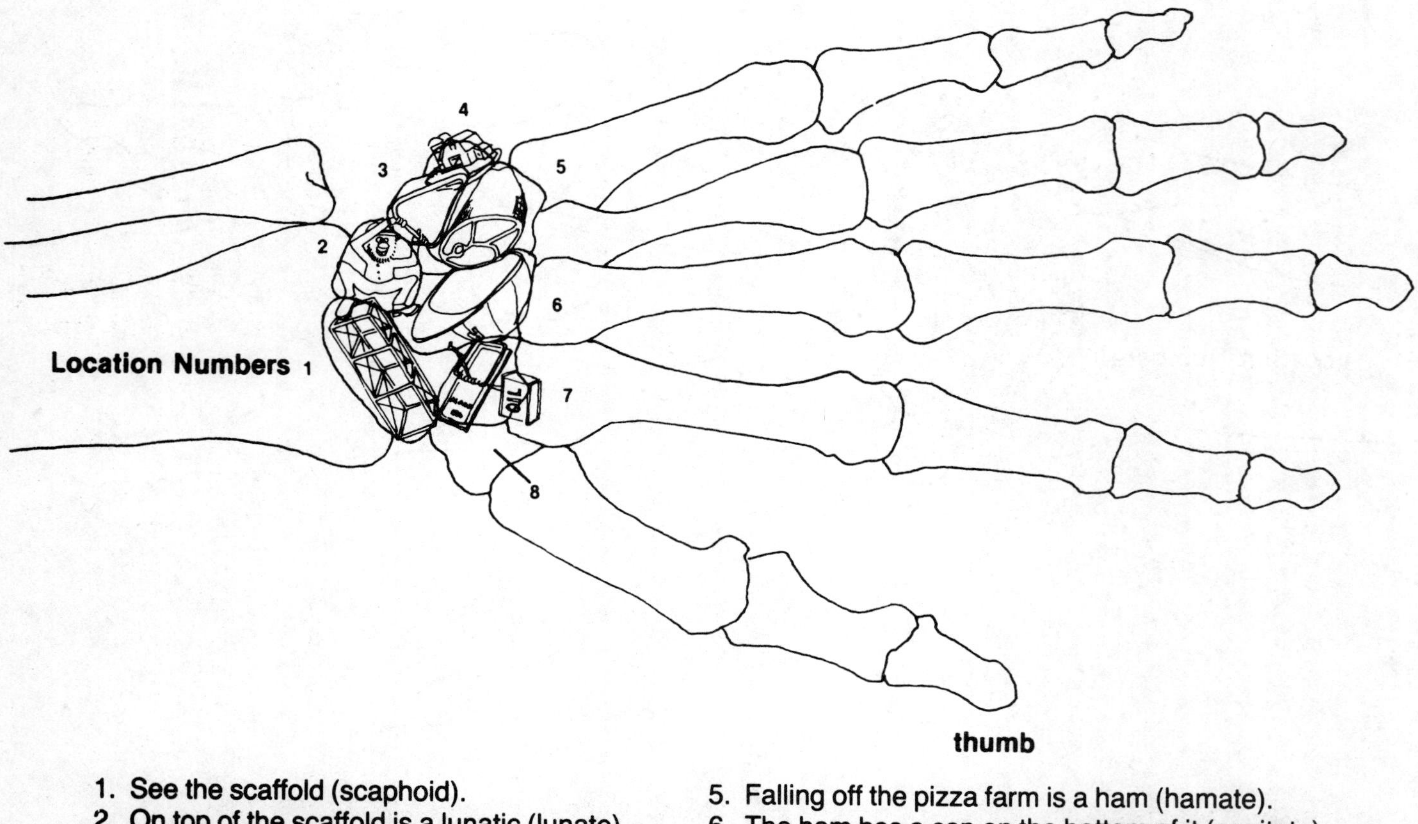

1. See the scaffold (scaphoid).
2. On top of the scaffold is a lunatic (lunate).
3. The lunatic is holding a triangle (triangular).
4. On top of the triangle is a pizza farm (pisiform).
5. Falling off the pizza farm is a ham (hamate).
6. The ham has a cap on the bottom of it (capitate).
7. The cap has a trap is oiled hanging on it (trapezoid).

TRAPEZIUM

Pronunciation: trap eez ee um

Trapezium sounds like: trapeze

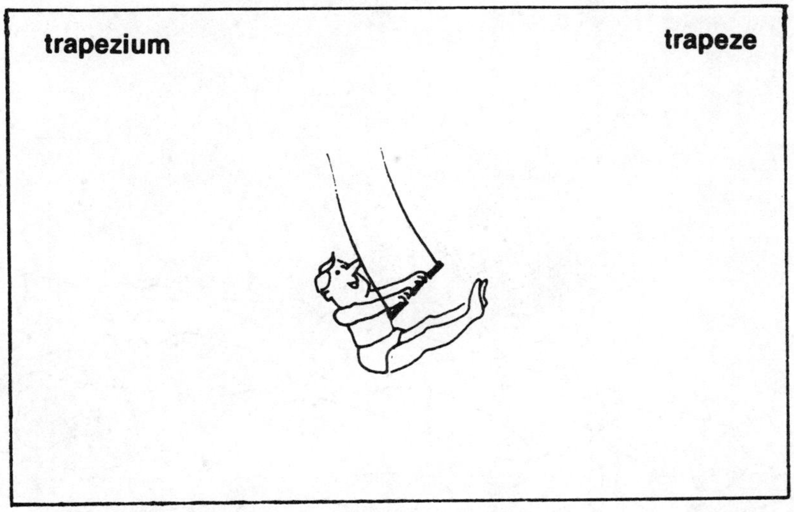

Pronounce it twice: trapezium — trapeze
trapezium — trapeze

The trapezium bone (trapeze) is the first bone in the second row starting on the thumb side.

Location Numbers

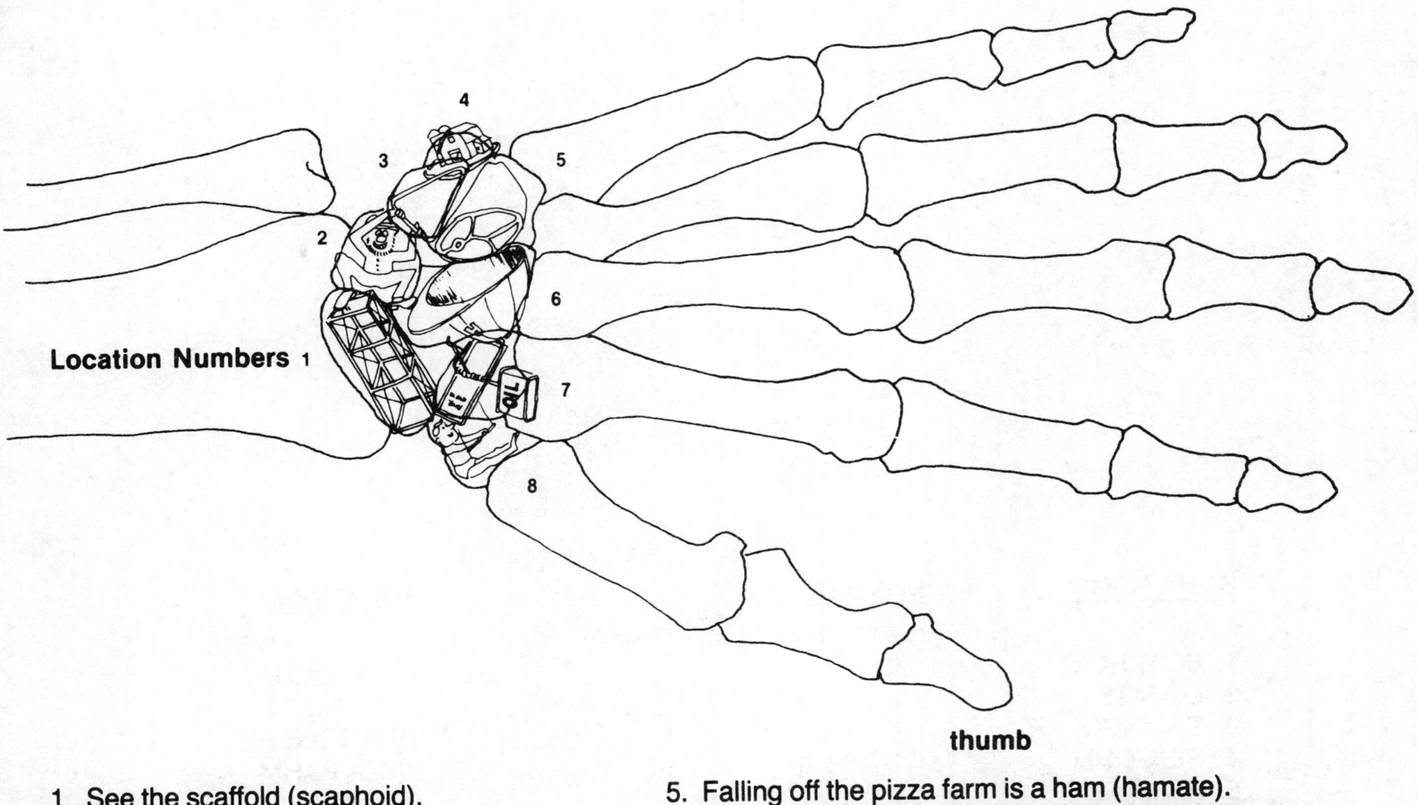

1. See the scaffold (scaphoid).
2. On top of the scaffold is a lunatic (lunate).
3. The lunatic is holding a triangle (triangular).
4. On top of the triangle is a pizza farm (pisiform).
5. Falling off the pizza farm is a ham (hamate).
6. The ham has a cap on the bottom of it (capitate).
7. The cap has a trap is oiled hanging on it (trapezoid).
8. The trap is oiled has a trapeze hanging on it (trapezium).

INDIVIDUAL INSTRUCTION
REVIEW
CARPALS

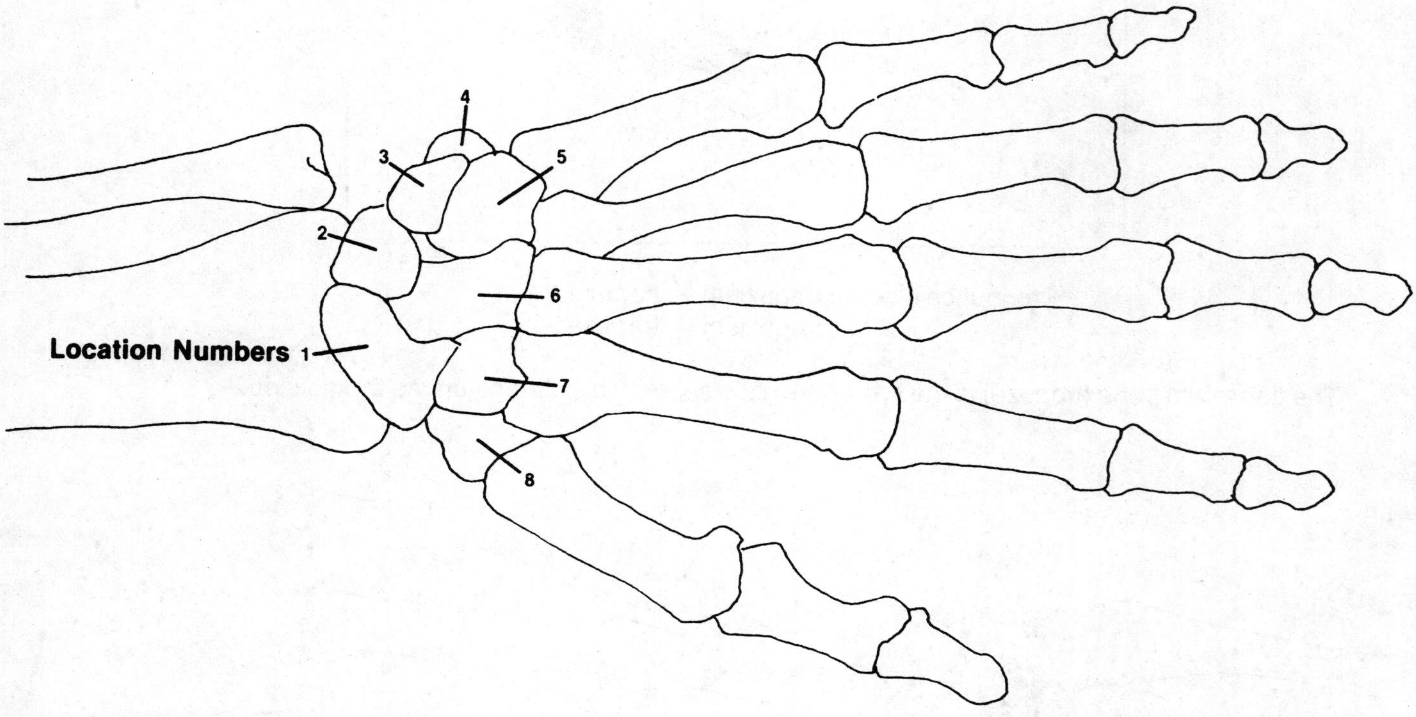

BONE NAME	NUMBER (left)	NUMBER (right)	AUDIONYM
1. SCAPHOID	1	1	SCAFFOLD
2. LUNATE	1	1	LUNATIC
3. TRIANGULAR	1	1	TRIANGLE
4. PISIFORM	1	1	PIZZA FARM
5. HAMATE	1	1	HAM
6. CAPITATE	1	1	CAP
7. TRAPEZOID	1	1	TRAP IS OILED
8. TRAPEZIUM	1	1	TRAPEZE

INDIVIDUAL INSTRUCTION
REVIEW
CARPALS

Important to Remember

1. There are sixteen carpal bones (wrist bones) — eight on each hand.

   a. Four in the first row (row toward the head)
   b. Four in the second row (row toward the fingers)

2. The radius articulates with only two of the carpal bones (the scaphoid and the lunate).

3. To remember the names and locations of all eight carpal bones, picture the four audionyms in the first row starting on the thumb side to the side of the little finger:

   a. See the scaffold (scaphoid).
   b. On top of the scaffold is a lunatic (lunate).
   c. The lunatic is holding a triangle (triangular).
   d. On top of the triangle is a pizza farm (pisiform).

   Then picture the four audionyms in the second row starting on the side of the little finger back to the thumb side:

   e. See the pizza farm with a ham falling off of it (hamate).
   f. The ham has a cap on the bottom of it (capitate).
   g. The cap has a trap is oiled hanging on it (trapezoid).
   h. The trap is oiled has a trapeze hanging on it (trapezium).

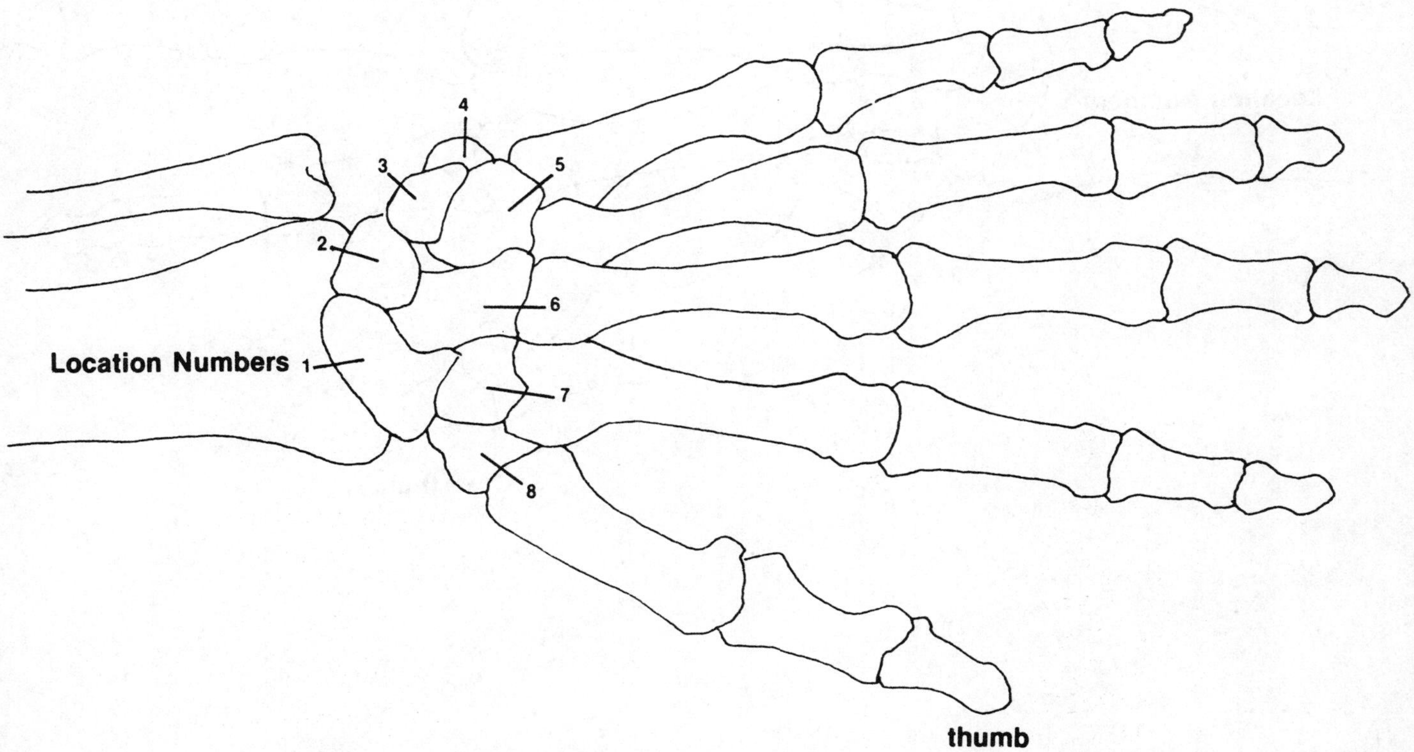

INDIVIDUAL INSTRUCTION
WORKSHEET
CARPALS

In the space provided, fill in the appropriate location number to correspond to the correct audionym.

_______ LUNATIC

_______ TRAP IS OILED

_______ CAP

_______ SCAFFOLD

_______ TRAPEZE

_______ PIZZA FARM

_______ HAM

_______ TRIANGLE

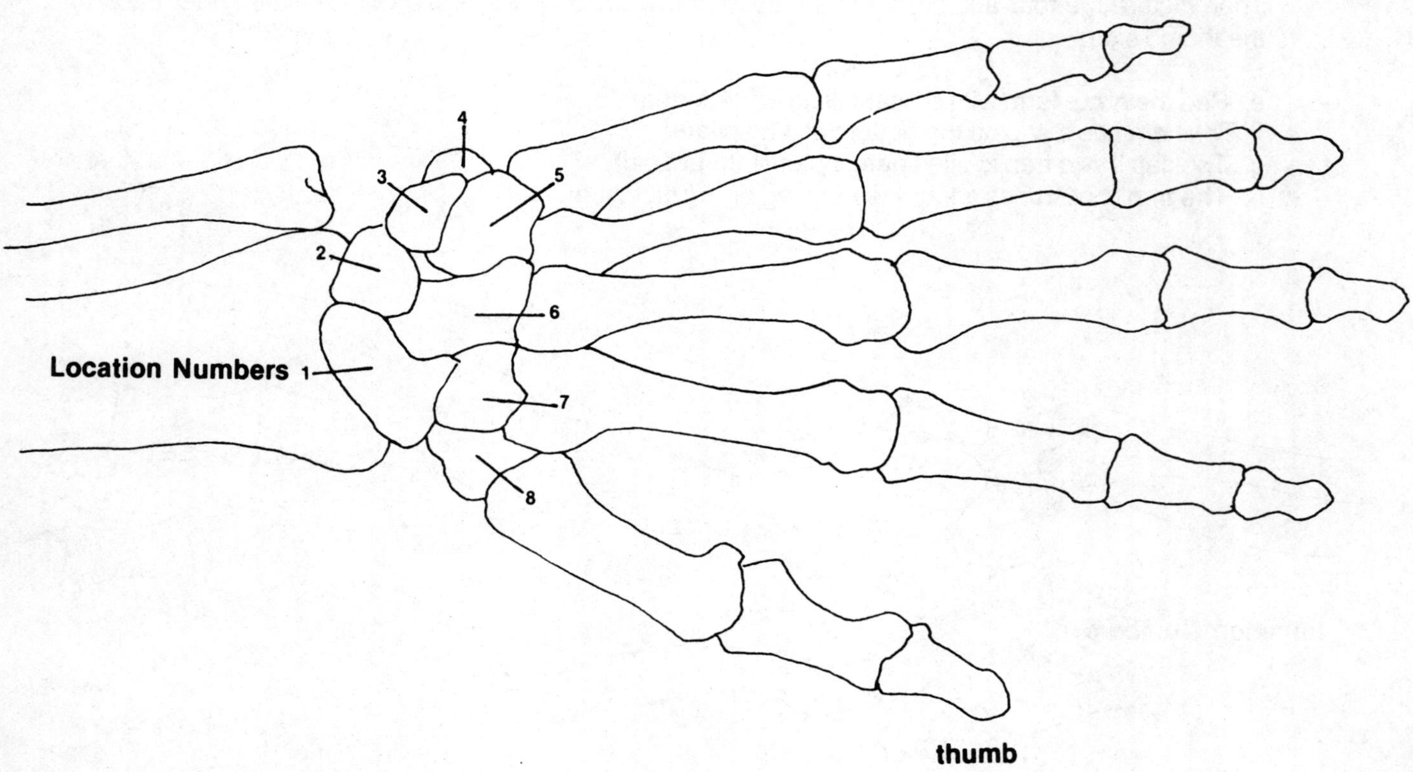

INDIVIDUAL INSTRUCTION
WORKSHEET
CARPALS

In the space provided, fill in the appropriate location number to correspond to the correct audionym.

_______ HAMATE

_______ LUNATE

_______ TRAPEZIUM

_______ PISIFORM

_______ TRIANGULAR

_______ TRAPEZOID

_______ SCAPHOID

_______ CAPITATE

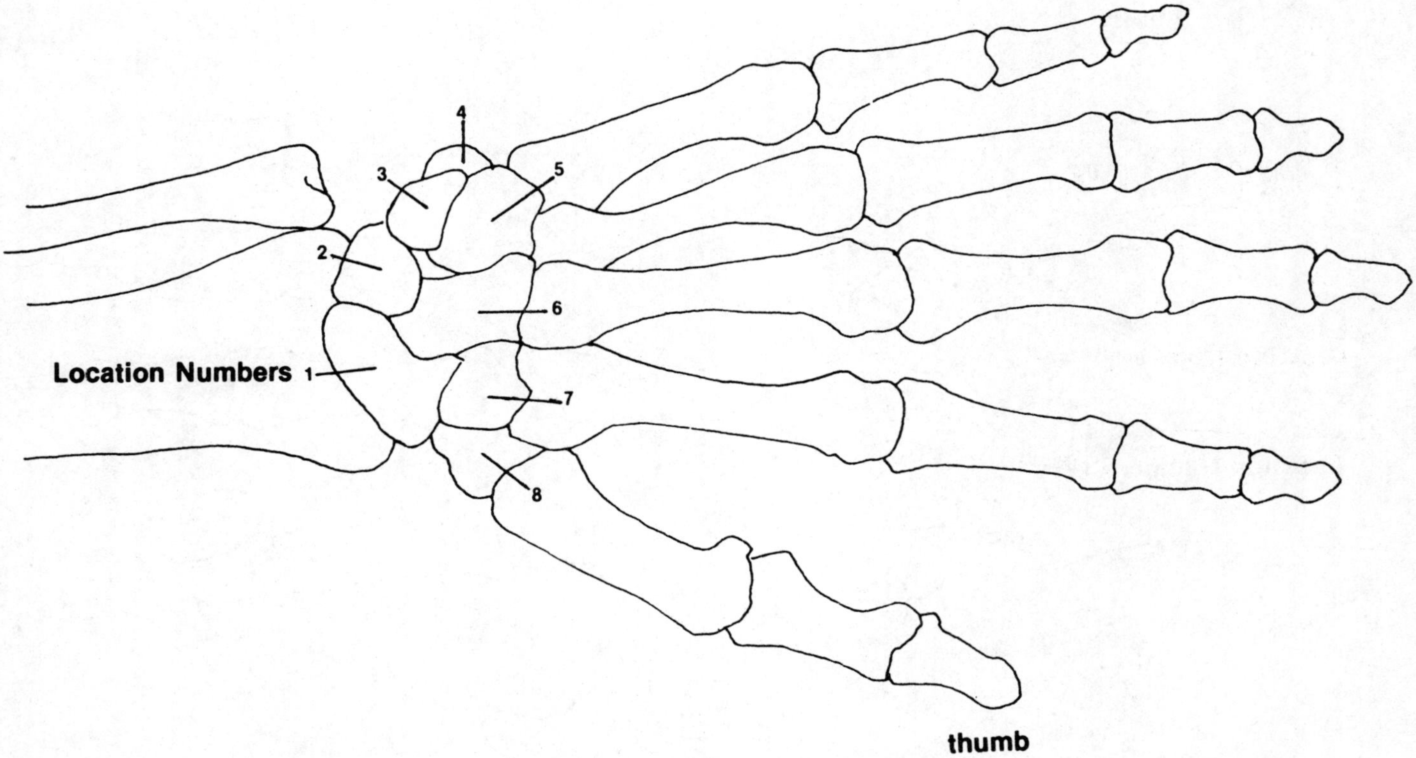

INDIVIDUAL INSTRUCTION
WORKSHEET
CARPALS

Fill in the appropriate audionym on the numbered line below which corresponds to the location number on the drawing.

1. ______________________________
2. ______________________________
3. ______________________________
4. ______________________________
5. ______________________________
6. ______________________________
7. ______________________________
8. ______________________________

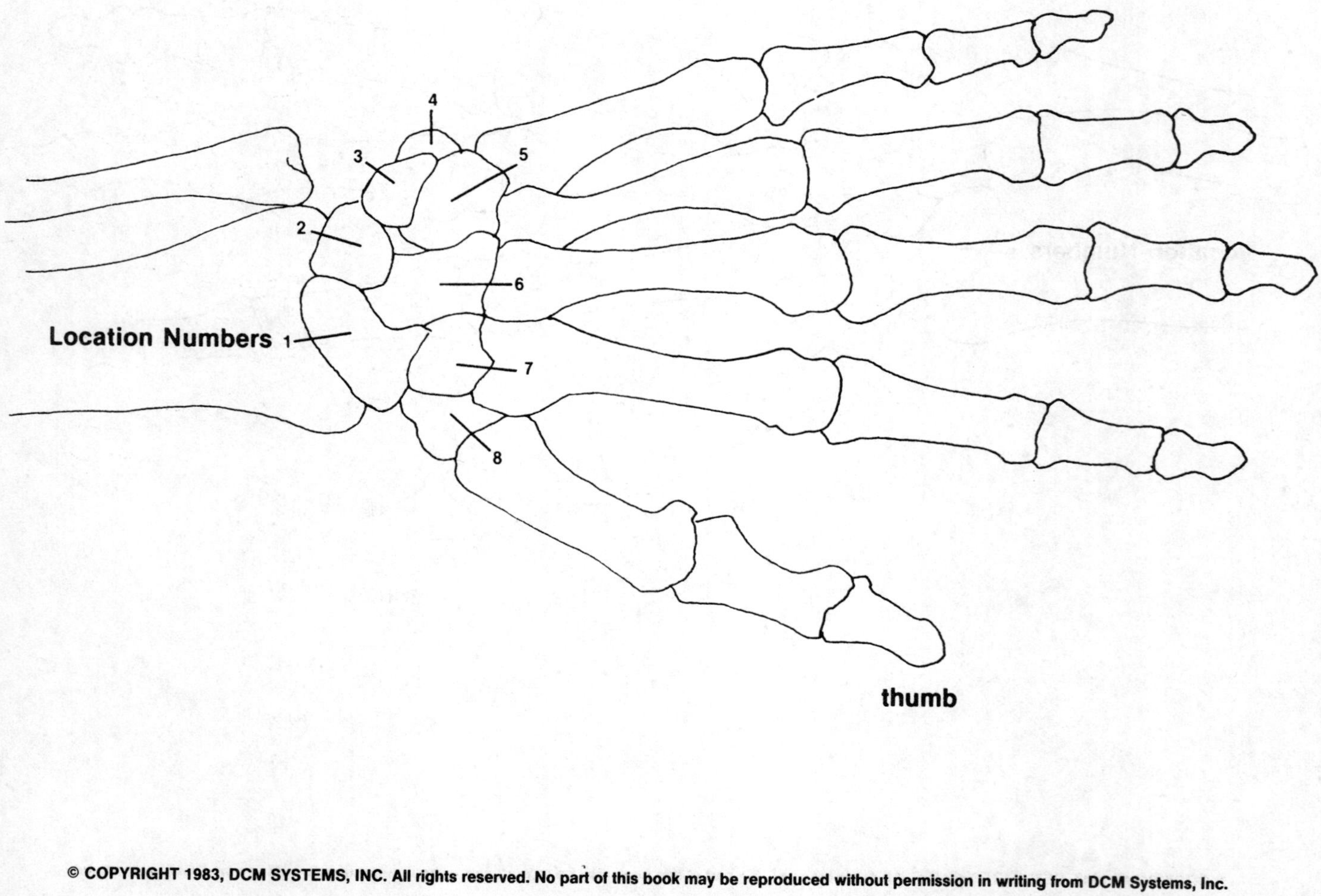

INDIVIDUAL INSTRUCTION
WORKSHEET
CARPALS

Fill in the appropriate bone name on the numbered line below which corresponds to the location number on the drawing.

1. ______________________________
2. ______________________________
3. ______________________________
4. ______________________________
5. ______________________________
6. ______________________________
7. ______________________________
8. ______________________________

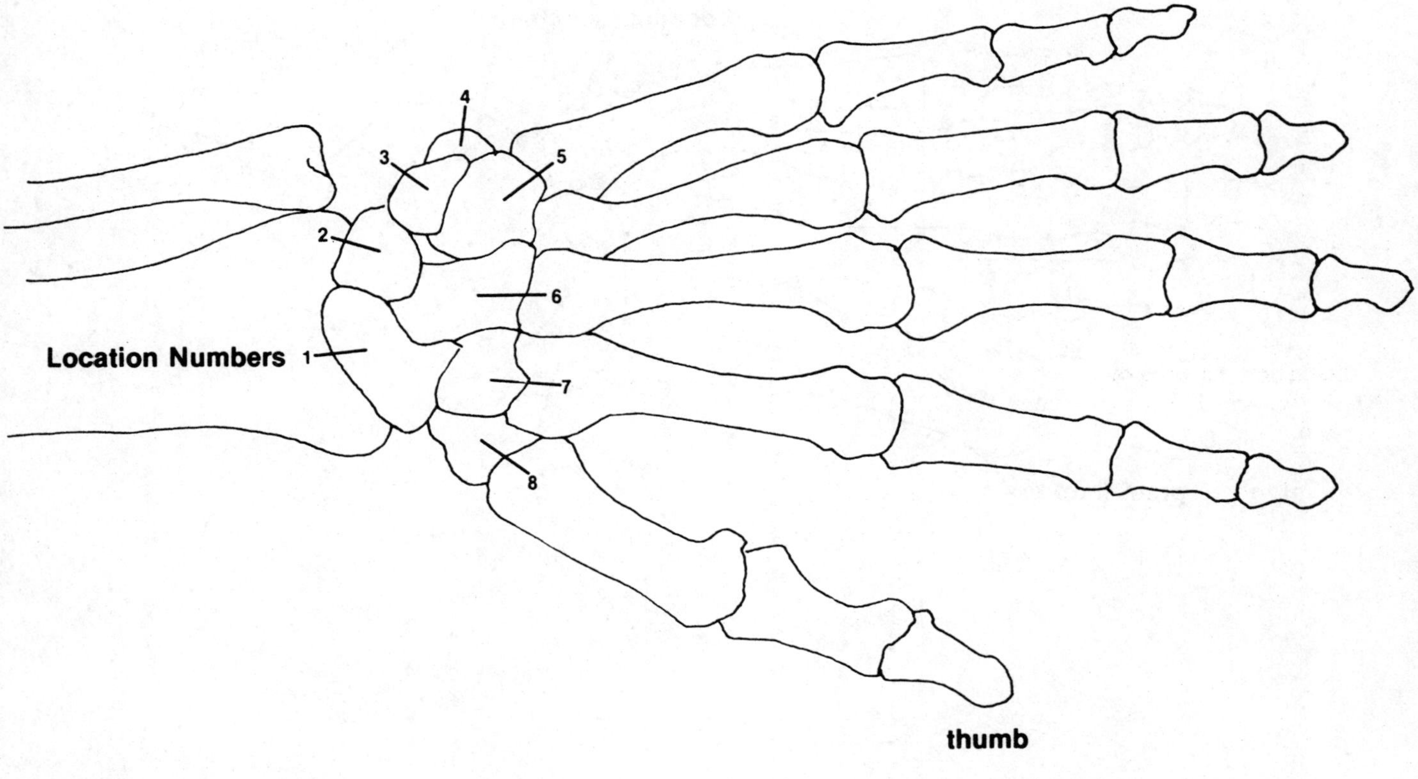

INDIVIDUAL INSTRUCTION
TARSALS
(Ankle Bones)

BONE NAME	NUMBER (left)	NUMBER (right)
TALUS*	1	1
CALCANEUS**	1	1
NAVICULAR***	1	1
CUNEIFORM	3	3
CUBOID	1	1

*alternate name: astragulus
**alternate name: os calcis
***alternate name: scaphoid

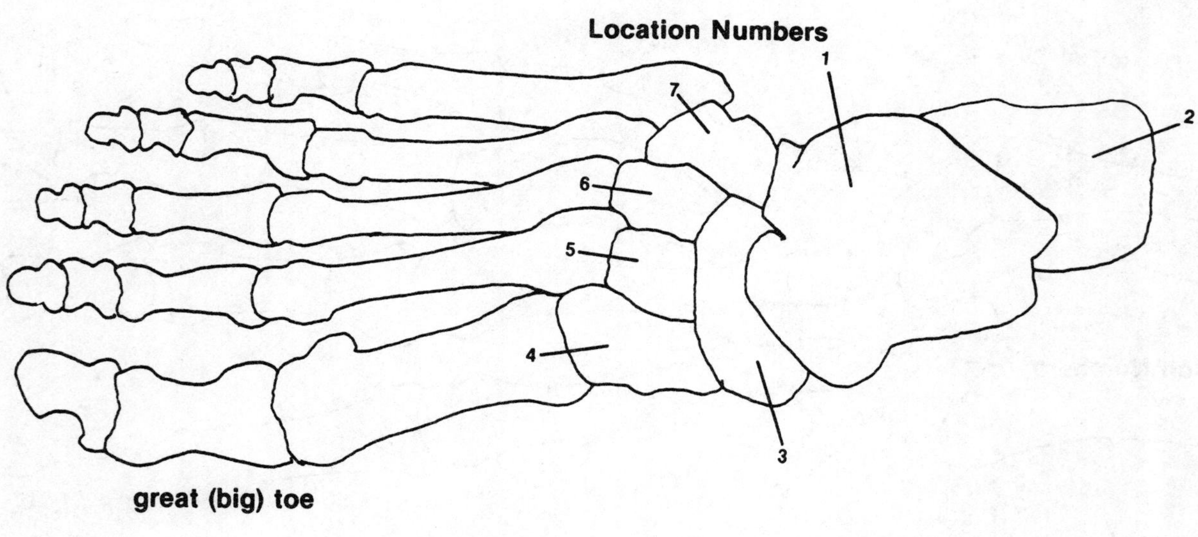

To learn the names and locations of the individual tarsal bones, use the same learning system that was used for the carpal bones.

The individual tarsal bones will be learned by studying the right foot in the following sequence: starting with (1) the talus (ankle bone), then down to (2) the calcaneus (heel bone), then forward on the inside (instep) of the foot to (3) the navicular, then forward to (4) (5) (6) the three cuneiforms, then laterally to (7) the cuboid.

top of the right foot

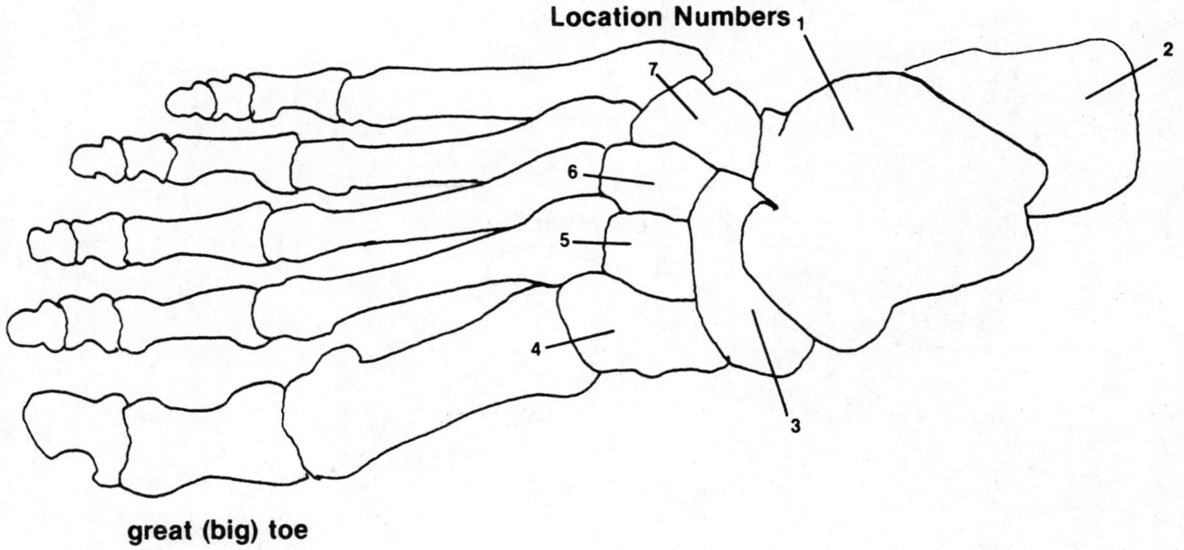

TALUS

Pronunciation: <u>tail</u> us

Talus sounds like: tail

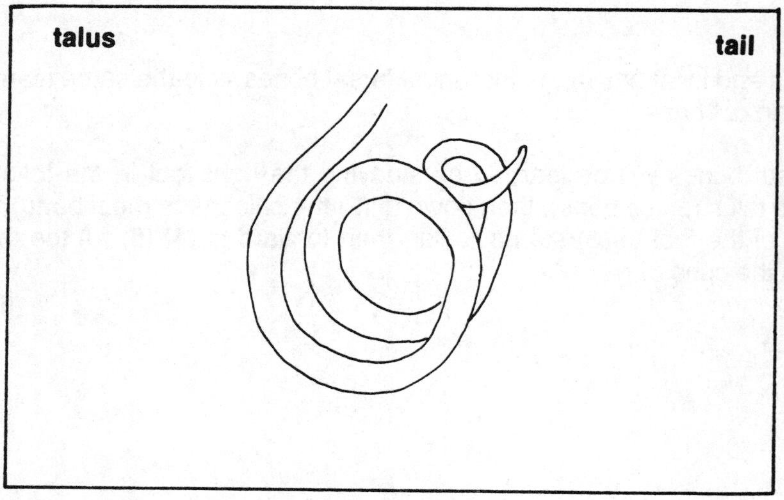

Pronounce it twice: talus — tail
talus — tail

The talus (ankle bone) rests on top of the calcaneus (heel bone). The tibia (teepee) or shin bone rests on top of the talus (tail) or ankle bone.

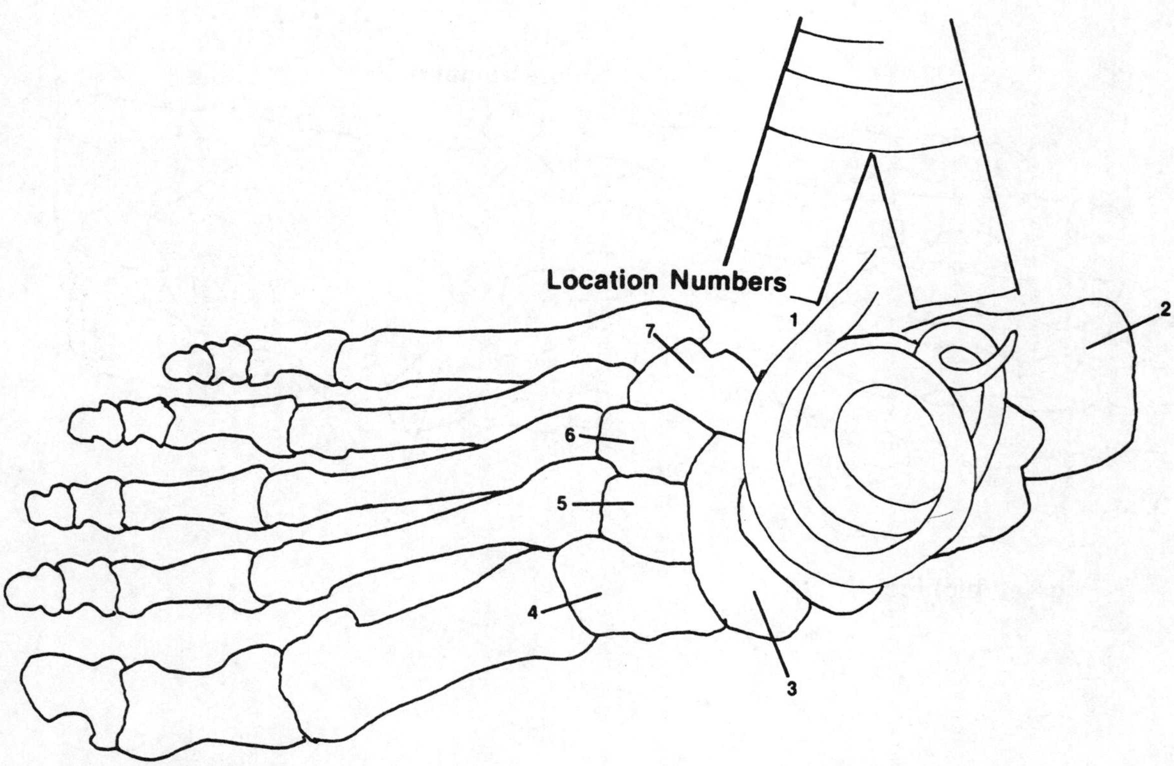

Begin to develop the sequence of the tarsal bones:

1. Out of the teepee (tibia) comes a tail (talus).

CALCANEUS

Pronunciation: cal <u>cane</u> ee us

Calcaneus sounds like: cow cane

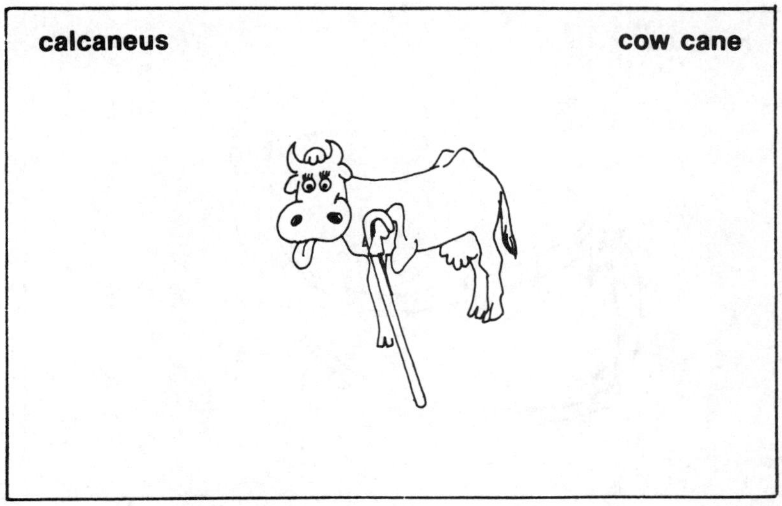

Here is a cow with a cane.

Pronounce it twice: calcaneus — cow cane
calcaneus — cow cane

The calcaneous bone (cow cane) is the heel bone.

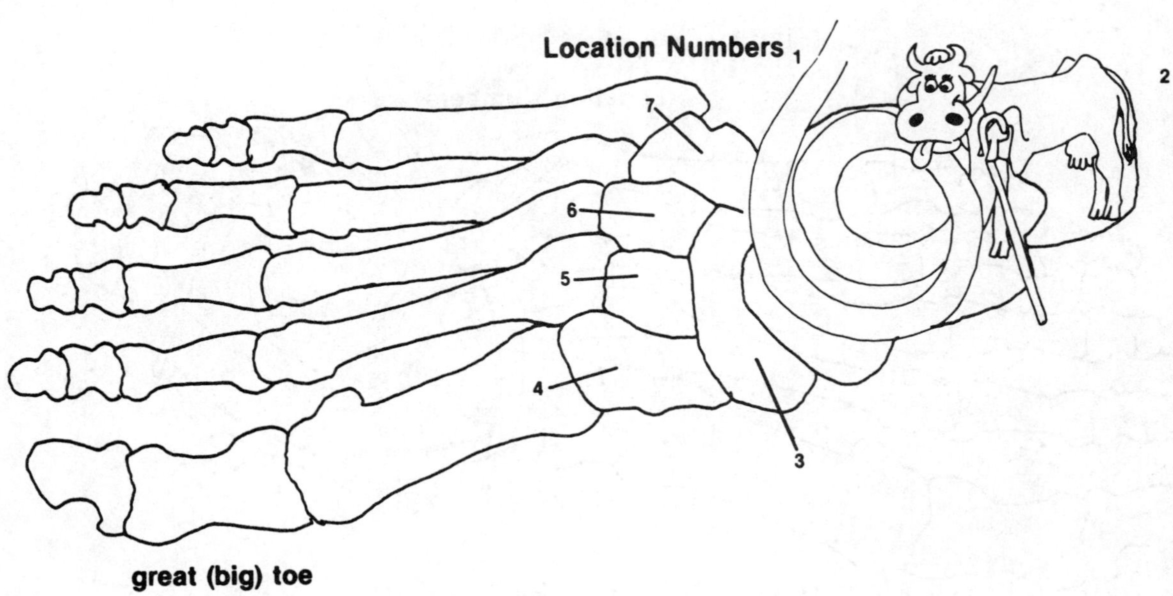

1. Out of the teepee (tibia) comes a tail (talus).
2. The tail (talus) is wrapped around the cow cane (calcaneous).

NAVICULAR

Pronunciation: nah vic you lar

Navicular sounds like: Navy collar

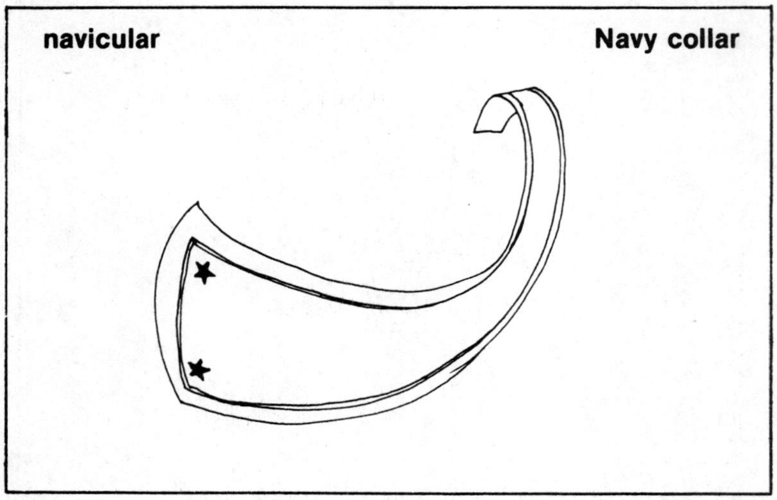

Pronounce it twice: navicular — Navy collar
navicular — Navy collar

The navicular bone (Navy collar) is located on the medial side (inside or instep) of the ankle in front of the talus (tail).

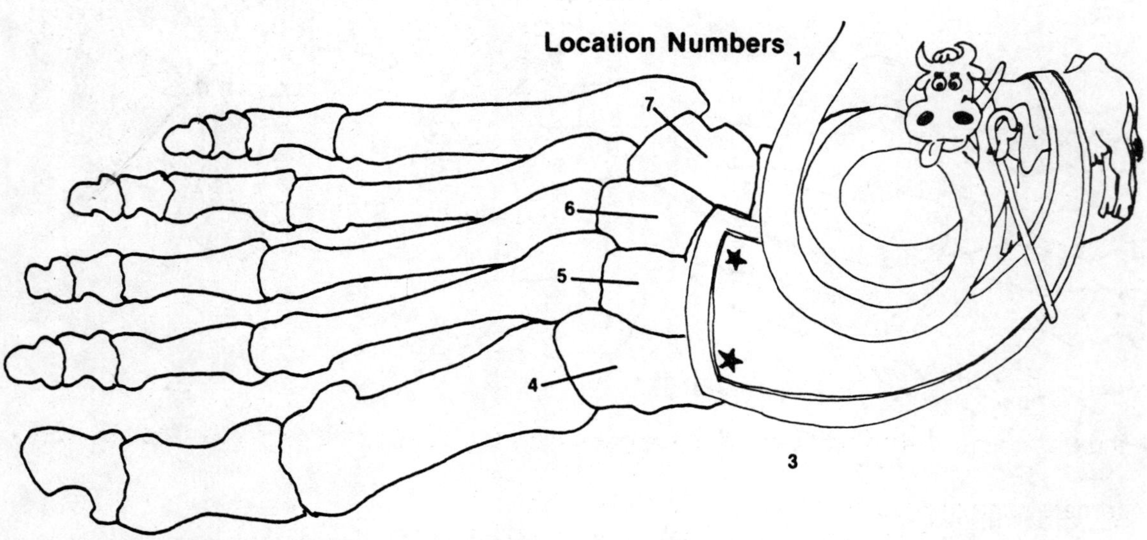

1. Out of the teepee (tibia) comes a tail (talus).
2. The tail (talus) is wrapped around the cow cane (calcaneous).
3. The cow cane (calcaneus) is wearing a Navy collar (navicular).

CUNEIFORM

Pronunciation: cue knee if orm

Cuneiform sounds like: cue knee

cuneiform **cue knee**

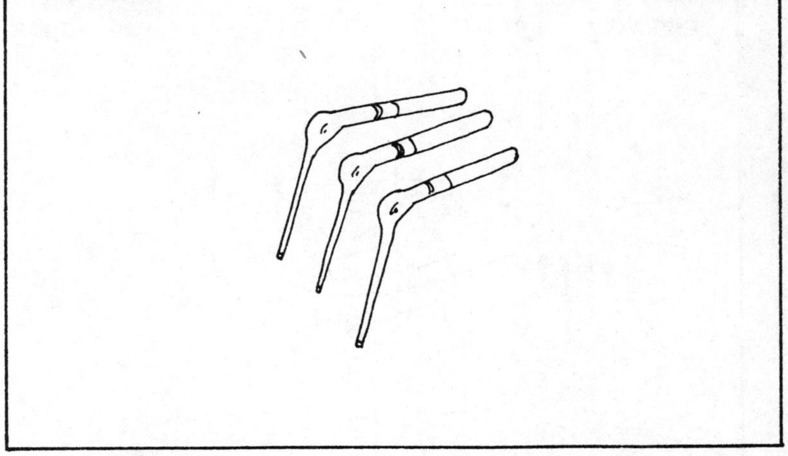

Cue sticks with real knees.

Pronounce it twice: cuneiform — cue knee
cuneiform — cue knee

Note: There are three (3) cuneiform bones.

The three cuneiform bones (cue knee) are located in front of the navicular bone (Navy collar).

Location Numbers

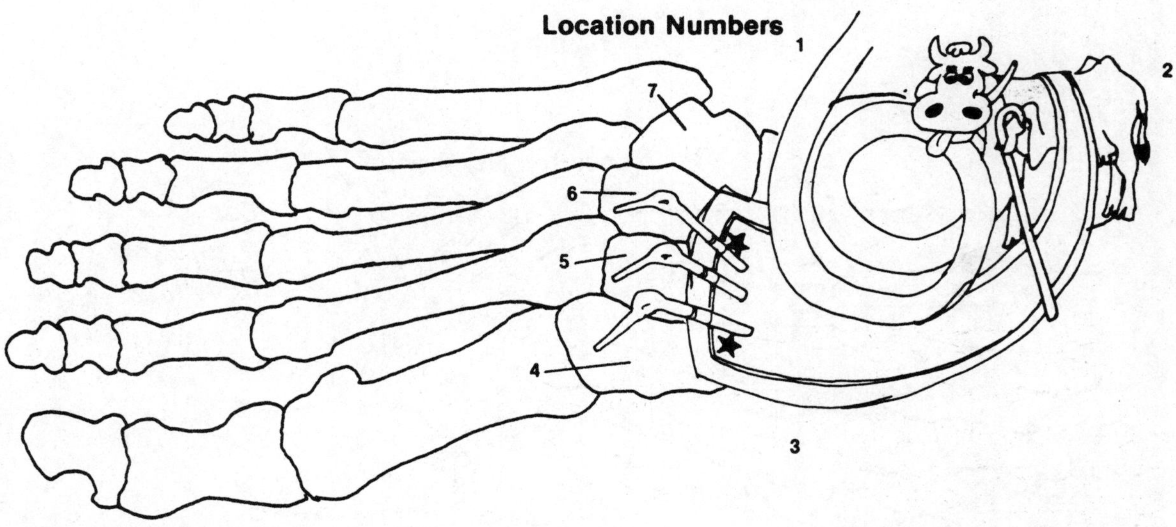

great (big) toe

The three cuneiforms are numbered from the great (big) toe side toward the side of the little toe.

Alternate names: Medial cuneiform = first cuneiform
Intermediate cuneiform = second cuneiform
Lateral cuneiform = third cuneiform

1. Out of the teepee (tibia) comes a tail (talus).
2. The tail (talus) is wrapped around the cow cane (calcaneous).
3. The cow cane (calcaneus) is wearing a Navy collar (navicular).
4. Sticking out of the Navy collar (navicular) are three cue knees (three cuneiforms).

CUBOID

Pronunciation: <u>cube</u> oid

Cuboid sounds like: cube

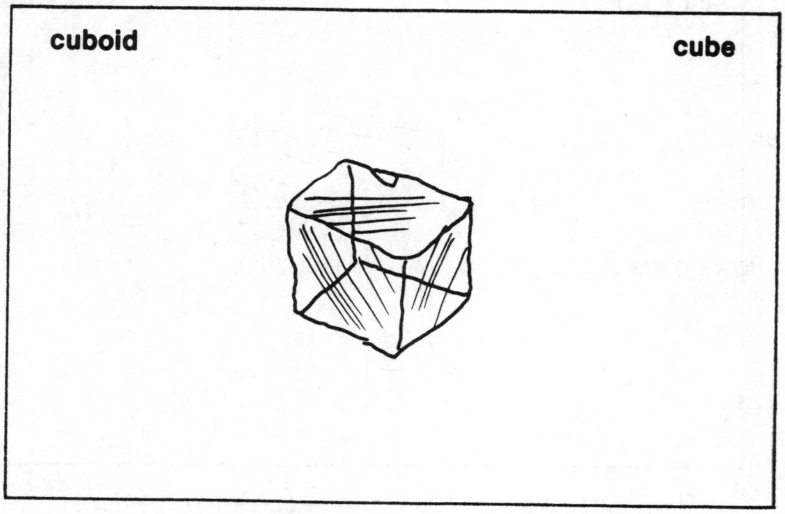

an ice cube

Pronounce it twice: cuboid — cube
cuboid — cube

The cuboid bone (cube) is located on the outside of the top of the foot beside the third cuneiform (starting on the great toe or big toe side) and in front of the calcaneus bone (cow cane).

Location Numbers

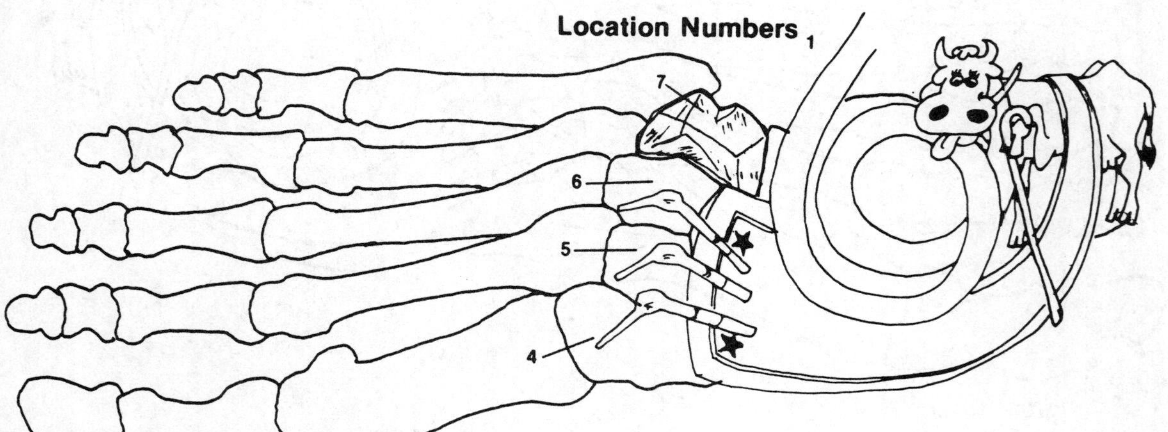

great (big) toe

1. Out of the teepee (tibia) comes a tail (talus).
2. The tail (talus) is wrapped around the cow cane (calcaneous).
3. The cow cane (calcaneus) is wearing a Navy collar (navicular).
4. Sticking out of the Navy collar (navicular) are three cue knees (three cuneiforms).
5. Beside the third cue knee (cuneiform) is a cube (cuboid).

INDIVIDUAL INSTRUCTION
REVIEW
TARSALS

Important to Remember

1. There are fourteen tarsal bones (ankle bones) — seven on each foot.
2. The tibia rests on the talus, the talus rests on the calcaneus. On top of the foot in front of the talus is the navicular (on the inside or instep). In front of the navicular are three cuneiforms. Beside the lateral cuneiform (toward the outside of the foot) is the cuboid.

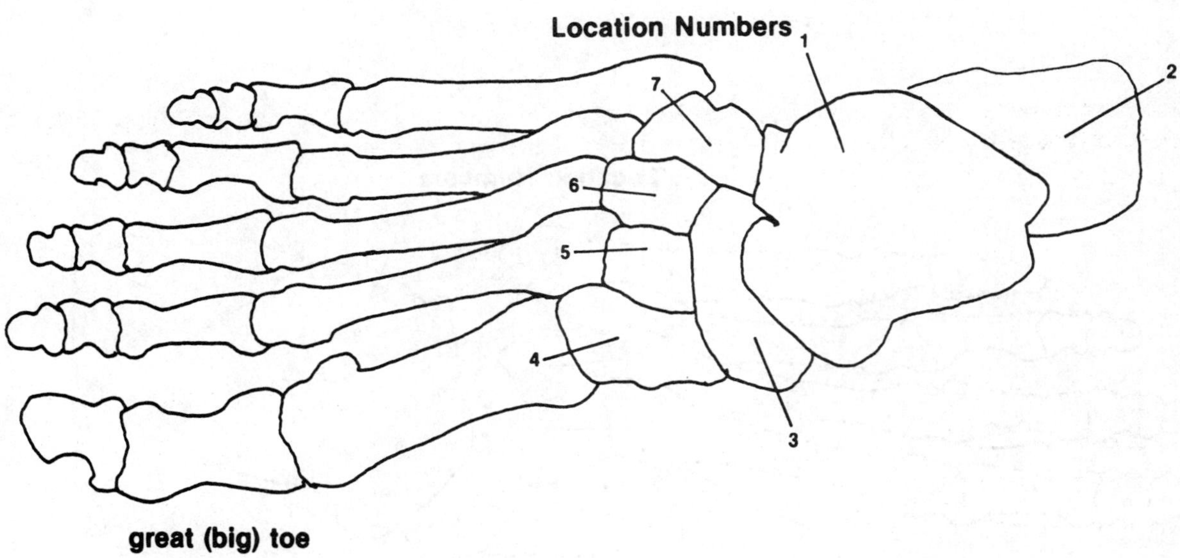

BONE NAME	**NUMBER** (left)	(right)	**AUDIONYM**
1. TALUS	1	1	TAIL
2. CALCANEUS	1	1	COW CANE
3. NAVICULAR	1	1	NAVY COLLAR
4. CUNEIFORM	3	3	CUE KNEE
5. CUBOID	1	1	CUBE

INDIVIDUAL INSTRUCTION
WORKSHEET
TARSALS

In the space provided, fill in the appropriate location number to correspond to the correct audionym.

________ CUE KNEE

________ CUBE

________ NAVY COLLAR

________ CUE KNEE

________ COW CANE

________ TAIL

________ CUE KNEE

Location Numbers

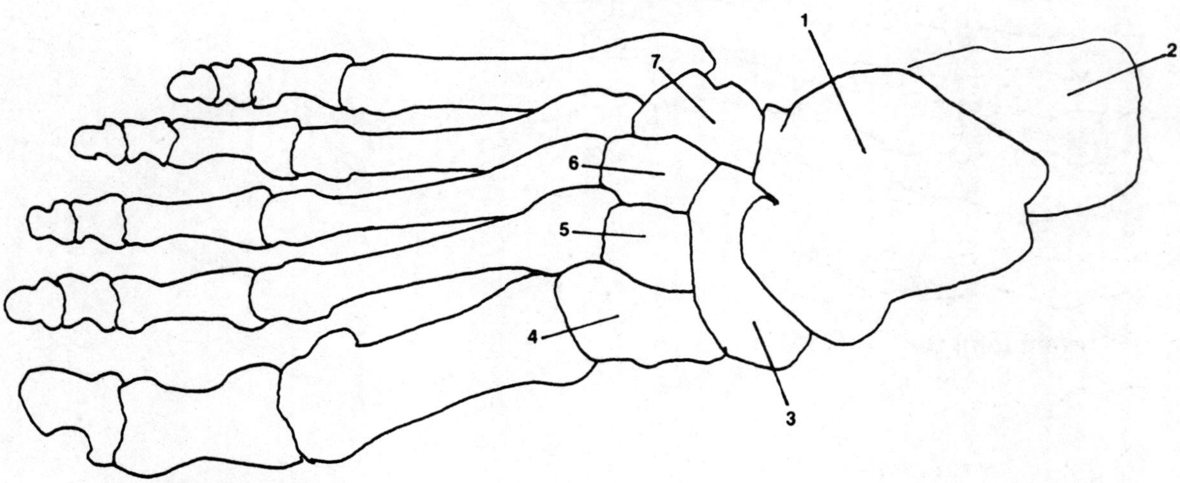

great (big) toe

INDIVIDUAL INSTRUCTION
WORKSHEET
TARSALS

In the space provided, fill in the appropriate location number to correspond to the correct bone name.

_______ CALCANEUS

_______ CUNEIFORM (Second)**

_______ TALUS

_______ CUBOID

_______ CUNEIFORM (Third)***

_______ NAVICULAR

_______ CUNEIFORM (First)*

Location Numbers

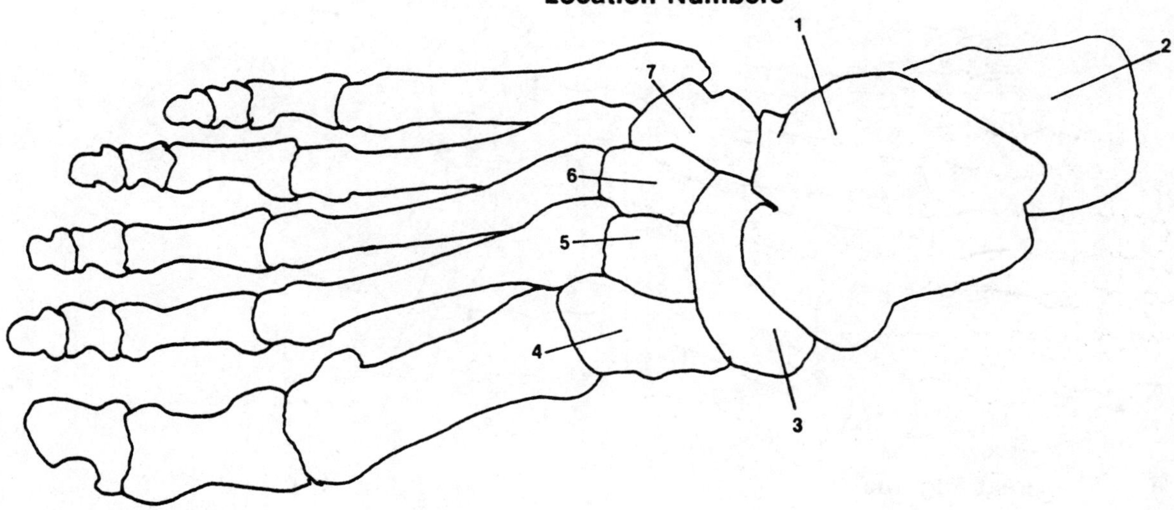

great (big) toe

*medial
**intermediate
***lateral

INDIVIDUAL INSTRUCTION
WORKSHEET
TARSALS

Fill in the appropriate audionym on the numbered line below which corresponds to the location number on the drawing.

1. ______________________
2. ______________________
3. ______________________
4. ______________________
5. ______________________
6. ______________________
7. ______________________

Location Numbers

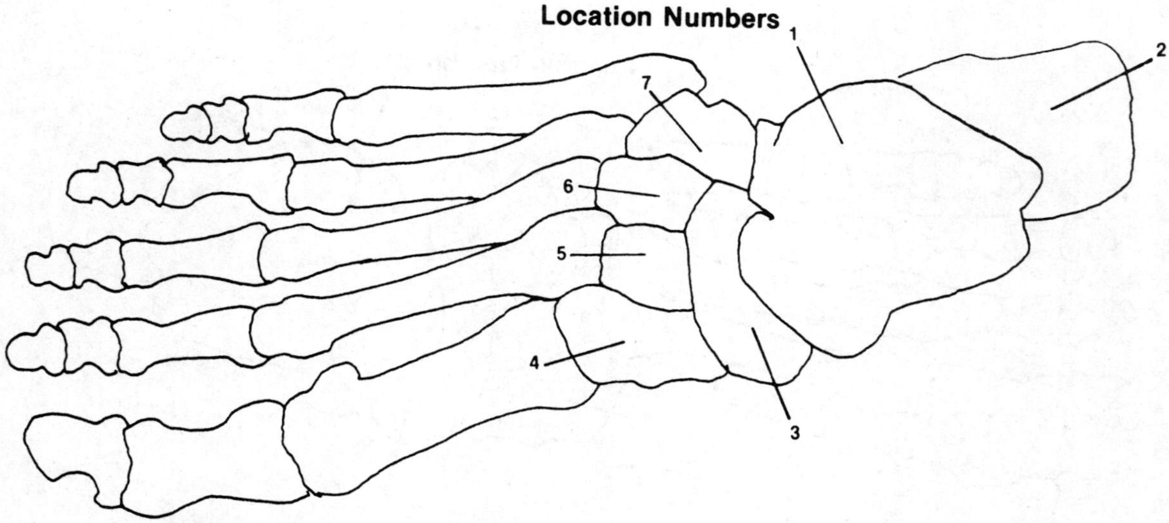

MARK AN "X" IN THE APPROPRIATE BOX

The three cuneiforms are numbered:
☐ From the little toe side toward the side of the great (big) toe
☐ From the great (big) toe side toward the side of the little toe

INDIVIDUAL INSTRUCTION
WORKSHEET
TARSALS

Fill in the appropriate bone name on the numbered line below which corresponds to the location number on the drawing.

1. ______________________________
2. ______________________________
3. ______________________________
4. ______________________________
5. ______________________________
6. ______________________________
7. ______________________________

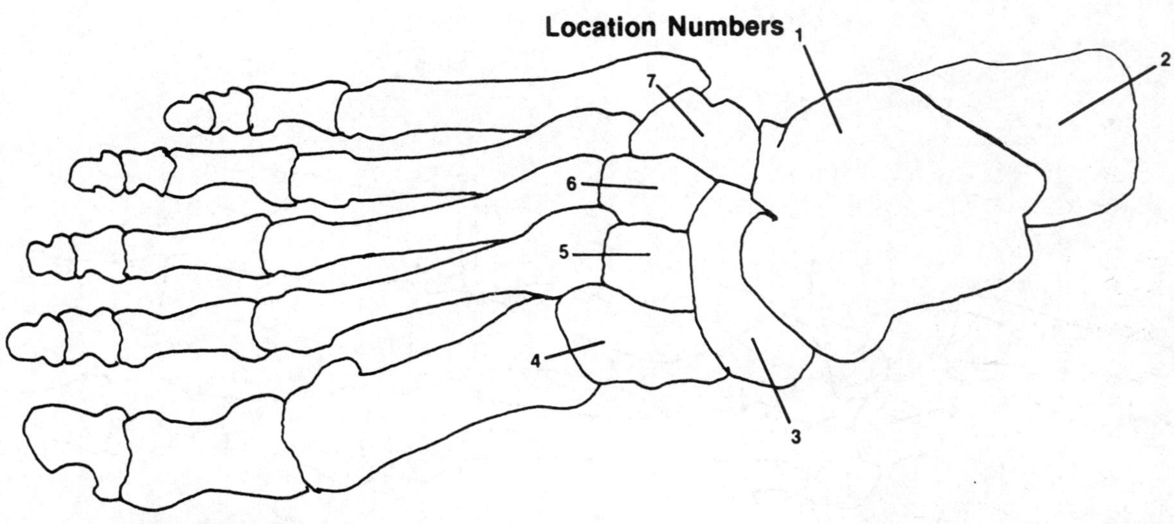

FINAL TEST
(Optional)
CARPALS

PRINT THE CORRECT NUMBER WITHIN THE PARENTHESES

( ) **TRAPEZIUM**

( ) **HAMATE**

( ) **TRAPEZOID**

( ) **CAPITATE**

( ) **SCAPHOID**

( ) **LUNATE**

( ) **TRIANGULAR**

( ) **PISIFORM**

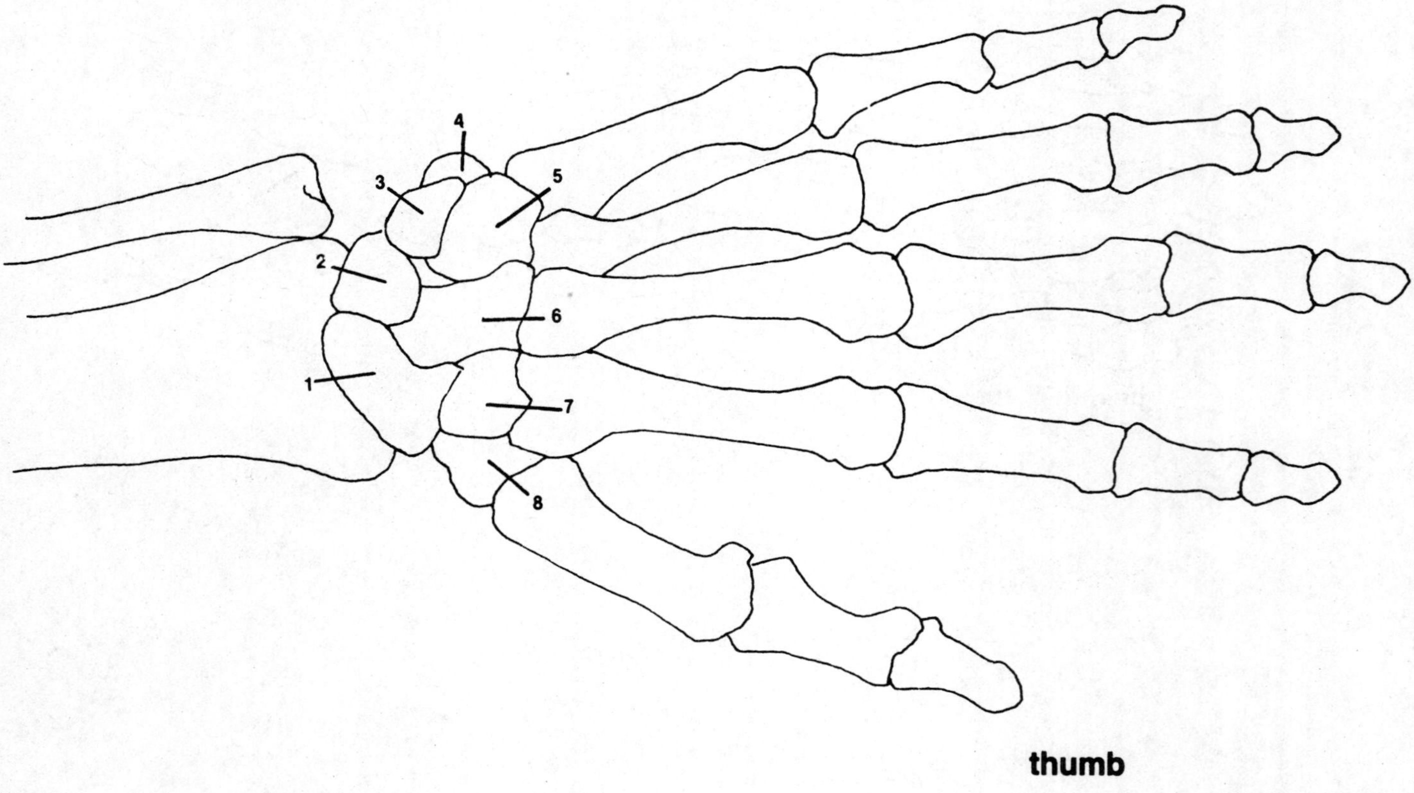

FINAL TEST
(Optional)
TARSALS

PRINT THE CORRECT NUMBER WITHIN THE PARENTHESES

( ) CUBOID

( ) INTERMEDIATE CUNEIFORM (2nd CUNEIFORM)

( ) NAVICULAR

( ) TALUS

( ) MEDIAL CUNEIFORM (1st CUNEIFORM)

( ) CALCANEUS

( ) LATERAL CUNEIFORM (3rd CUNEIFORM)

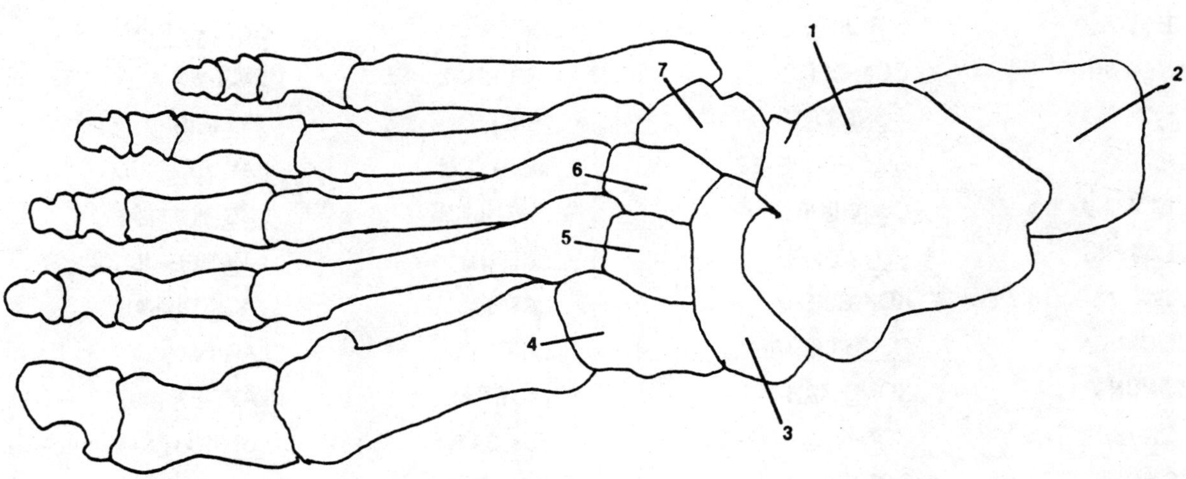

great (big) toe

PRONUNCIATION GUIDE

WORD	PHONETIC PRONUNCIATION
ABDOMINAL	AB-DOM-INN-ALL
ABDOMINOPELVIC	AB-DOM-INN-O-PELL-VIK
ABDUCENS	AB-DEW-SENS
ADRENAL	AD-REEN-AL
AFFERENT	AFF-ER-ENT
ANTERIOR	ANN-TEAR-EE-OR
AORTA	A-OR-TA
AQUEOUS	AK-WEE-US
ARTERIOLE	AR-TEA-REE-OLE
ATRIUM	A-TREE-UM
AXILLARY	AX-ILL-AIR-EE
BRACHIAL	BRAE-KEY-ALL
BRONCHUS	BRONC-US
BULBOURETHRAL	BULB-OH-YOU-REE-THRAL
CAROTID	CAR-OT-ID
CARPALS	CAR-PALLS
CAUDAL	COD-ALL
CEPHAL	SEPH-ALL
CEREBELLUM	SER-AH-BELL-UM
CEREBRUM	SER-EE-BRUM
CERVIX	SIR-VIX
CHONDR	CON-DER
CHOROID	CORE-OID
CILIARY	SILL-EE-AIR-EE
CLAVICAL	CLAV-IK-ALL
CLITORIS	KLIT-OR-IS
COCCYX	KOK-SIKS
COCHLEA	COKE-LEE-AH
CONCHA	KONG-KAH
CONJUNCTIVA	CON-JUNK-TIV-AH
CORNEA	CORN-EE-AH
CORONARY	COR-ON-AIR-EE
CRANIAL	CRANE-EE-ALL
CUBITAL	KU-BIT-ALL
CUTIS	CUE-TIS
DEFERENS	DEF-ER-ENS
DISTAL	DIS-TALL
DORSAL	DOORS-ALL
DUODENUM	DU-OH-DEE-NUM
EFFERENT	EFF-ER-ENT
EPI	EP-EE
EPIDERMIS	EPI-DER-MIS
EPIDIDYMIS	EP-I(D)-DID-I(M)-MIS
EPIGASTRIC	EP-EE-GAS-TRICK
ESOPHAGUS	EH-SOPH-AH-GUS
ETHMOID	ETH-MOID
FEMUR	FEE-MER
FIBULA	FIB-YOU-LAH
GASTR	GAS-TER
GLOSSOPHARYNGEAL	GLOSS-O-FAH-RIN-JE-AL
HUMERUS	HUME-ER-US
HYPO	HIPE-OH
HYPOCHONDRIAC	HIGH-PO-CON-DREE-AK
HYPOGASTRIC	HIGH-PO-GAS-TRICK
HYPOGLOSSAL	HIGH-PO-GLOSS-AL
ILEUM	ILL-EE-UM
ILIAC	ILL-EE-AK
INCUS	INK-US
INFERIOR	INN-FEAR-EE-OR
INGUINAL	IN-GWIN-ALL
IRIS	EYE-RIS
JEJUNUM	JAY-JUNE-UM
JUGULAR	JUG-YOU-LAR
LABIUM	LAY-BEE-UM
LACRIMAL	LACK-RIM-ALL
LARYNX	LAR-INKS
LATERAL	LATT-ER-ALL
LUMBAR	LUM-BAR
MALLEUS	MAL-EE-US
MANDIBLE	MAN-DIB-B'L
MAXILLA	MACK-SILL-AH
MEDULLA	MEH-DULL-AH
MEMBRANOUS	MEM-BRAN-US
METACARPALS	MET-AH-CAR-PALLS
METATARSALS	MET-AH-TAR-SALS
NASAL	NAZE-ALL

WORD	PHONETIC PRONUNCIATION
OCCIPITAL	OCK-SIP-IT-ALL
OCULOMOTOR	OCK-YOU-LOW-MOW-TOR
OLFACTORY	OL-FAK-TOE-REE
OPTIC	OP-TIC
PALATINE	PAL-AH-TINE
PARIETAL	PAR-EYE-IT-ALL
PAROTID	PAR-OT-ID
PATELLA	PAH-TELL-AH
PELVIC	PELL-VIK
PENIS	PEA-NIS
PHALANGES	FAH-LANGE-JEZ
PHALANX	FAY-LANKS
PHARYNX	FAR-INKS
PINEAL	PIN-EE-AL
PINNA	PIN-AH
PITUITARY	PI(T)-TO-IT-AIR-EE
PLEXUS	PLEX-US
PONS	PONZ
POPLITEAL	POP-LIT-EE-AL
POSTERIOR	POSS-TEAR-EE-OR
PROXIMAL	PROX-IM-ALL
PULMONARY	PULL-MAHN-AIR-EE
RADIUS	RAY-DEE-US
RENAL	REE-NALL
RETINA	RET-IN-AH
SACRUM	SAY-KRUM
SAGITTAL	SAJ-IT-ALL
SAPHENOUS	SAH-FEE-NUS
SCAPULA	SCAP-YOU-LAH
SCIATIC	SIGH-AT-IC
SCLERA	SCLAIR-AH
SCROTUM	SCRO-TUM
SEBACEOUS	SEA-BAY-SHUS
SEMINAL	SEM-IN-AL
SOMATIC	SOW-MAT-IC
SPHENOID	SPHEEN-OID
STAPES	STAY-PEAS
SUBCUTANEOUS	SUB-CUE-TANE-EE-US
SUBMANDIBULAR	SUB-MAN-DIB-YOU-LAR
SUDORIFEROUS	SUE-DOE-RIF-ER-US

WORD	PHONETIC PRONUNCIATION
SUPERIOR	SOUP-EAR-EE-OR
TARSALS	TAR-SALS
TEMPORAL	TEM-POR-ALL
TESTES	TES-TEEZ
THALAMUS	THAL-AH-MUS
THORACIC	THOR-AS-IK
THYMUS	THYME-US
TIBIA	TIB-EE-AH
TRACHEA	TRAY-KEE-AH
TRIGEMINAL	TRI-GEM-IN-ALL
TROCHLEAR	TRO-CLEAR
TYMPANIC	TIM-PAN-IC
ULNA	UL-NAH
UMBILICAL	UM-BILL-IK-ALL
URETER	YOU-REE-TER
URETHRA	YOU-REE-THRA
UTERUS	YOU-TER-US
VAGINA	VAH-JIE-NAH
VAGUS	VAY-GUS
VENA CAVA	VEE-NAH-CAVE-AH
VENTRAL	VEN-TRALL
VENTRICLE	VEN-TRICK-'L
VENULE	VEN-YULE
VERTEBRAE	VER-TE-BRAE
VESTIBULOCOCHLEAR	VES-TIB-YOU-LOW-COKE-LEE-AR
VISCERA	VIS-ER-AH
VITREOUS	VIT-REE-US
VOMER	VOME-ER
ZYGOMATIC	ZYE-GO-MAT-IK